WENDY COOK is a writer and speaker on nutritional issues. The first wife of satirist Peter Cook, she gained a reputation as a hostess in the 1960s and '70s. Born in 1940, she studied art at Cambridge where she met Peter Cook. Later they lived in London and New York during which time Wendy developed cooking and entertaining as her creative motif. When their daughter Daisy developed asthma and conventional medicine had little effect, Wendy began a journey of discovery of complementary treatments and alternative ideas. She studied macrobiotics as well as Rudolf Steiner's approach to nutrition and agriculture ('biodynamics'). Having discovered how life-changing nutrition can be, she devoted herself to cooking and teaching in clinics, communities and schools. More recently she was resident at Schumacher College while simultaneously studying for a degree in Waldorf Education at Plymouth University.

D1504880

HILLSBORO PUBLIC LIBRARIES
Hillsboro, OR
Member of Washington County
COOPERATIVE LIBRARY SERVICES

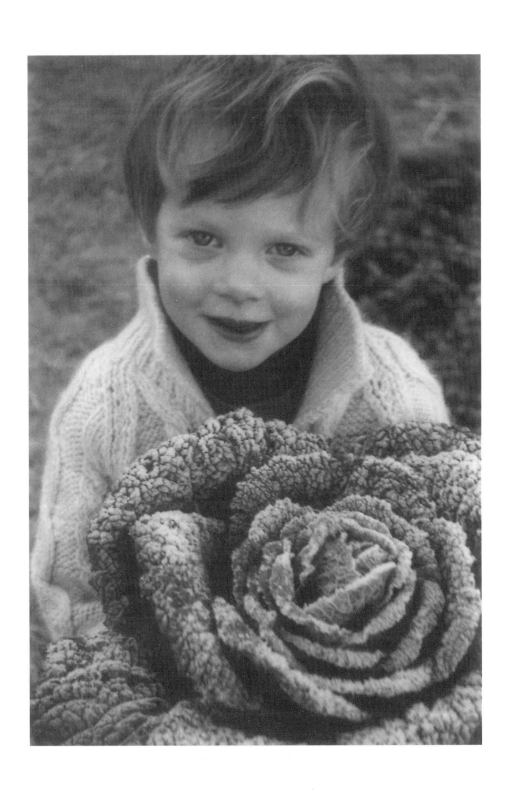

FOODWISE

UNDERSTANDING WHAT WE EAT
AND HOW IT AFFECTS US

THE STORY OF HUMAN NUTRITION

WENDY E. COOK

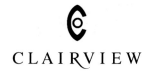

CLAIRVIEW

HILLSBORO PUBLIC LIBRARIES
Hillsboro, OR
Member of Washington County
COOPERATIVE LIBRARY SERVICES

Clairview Books
An imprint of Temple Lodge Publishing
Hillside House, The Square
Forest Row, East Sussex
RH18 5ES

www.clairviewbooks.com

Published by Clairview 2003

© Wendy E. Cook 2003

Wendy E. Cook asserts the moral right to be identified as the
author of this work

All rights reserved. No part of this publication may be reproduced,
stored in a retrieval system, or transmitted, in any form or by any means,
electronic, mechanical, photocopying or otherwise, without the prior
permission of the publishers

A catalogue record for this book is available from the British Library

ISBN 1 902636 39 2   *3072 9718 /04*

Cover by Andrew Morgan Design
Front cover photo by Daisy Cook. Back cover photo by Daniel Allan
Typeset by DP Photosetting, Aylesbury, Bucks.
Printed and bound by Cromwell Press Limited, Trowbridge, Wilts.

Dedicated to my daughters
Lucy and Daisy

CONTENTS

ILLUSTRATIONS AND CREDITS

Selby's son with cabbage, frontispiece: photo by Selby McCreery

Cross-sections of courgette and apple, p. 2: photos by Selby McCreery

Vortex ring, p. 2: from T. Schwenk's *Sensitive Chaos*, reproduced by permission of Rudolf Steiner Press

The Cook family, p. 8: reproduced by permission of *The Daily Mirror*

Early herdsmen, p. 21: Louvre, Paris

Afghan farmer with grain, p. 26: reproduced by permission of Christian Aid

Egyptian mask, p. 29: reproduced by permission of the British Museum

Nike, p. 34: Acropolis Museum, Athens

Flowing water, p. 34: from T. Schwenk's *Sensitive Chaos*, reproduced by permission of Rudolf Steiner Press

Young Roman, p. 39: Palazzo Torlonia, Rome

Old Roman citizen, p. 39: Palazzo Torlonia, Rome

Medieval monastery, p. 45: drawing by John Platt

'Self-portrait' by Louise Courtnell, p. 58: National Portrait Gallery. Reproduced by permission of Louise Courtnell

Cow, p. 61: photo by Selby McCreery

Biodynamic preparations, p. 70: photo by Selby McCreery

Biodynamic compost heap, p. 75: photo by Selby McCreery

Monoculture in the USA, p. 75: photo by John Page

Lily of the valley, p. 84: reproduced from T. Schwenk's *Sensitive Chaos*, by permission of Rudolf Steiner Press

Bread wheat, p. 93: drawing by John Platt

Rice and rice grain, p. 96: drawings by John Platt

Maize, p. 98: drawing by John Platt

Common and foxtail millet, p. 100: drawing by John Platt

Demeter/Persephone, p. 101: Scala, Antella

Two and six rowed barley, p. 102: drawing by John Platt

Oats, p. 103: drawing by John Platt

Rye, p. 104: drawing by John Platt

Correspondences in nature, p. 128: magnified human pineal reproduced by permission of Dr Jenny Luke and Professor L.J.A. Didio; cauliflower and calcium carbonate crystal photos by Selby McCreery

Derek with baskets of biodynamic produce, p. 133: photo by Selby McCreery

Experiments on the sensitive crystallization process, p. 141: photos reproduced by permission of Dr U. Balzer-Graf

Beetroot, leek and chard, p. 155: photos by Selby McCreery

Apple and briar rose, p. 159: photos by Selby McCreery

French farmer preparing bread oven, p. 173: photo by Jacquie Sarsby

Rising dough, p. 173: photo by Jacquie Sarsby

Grains, p. 177: drawing by John Platt

Electron-micrograph pictures of potato and wheat starch, p. 182: photos reproduced by permission of Mary Parker, Institute of Food Research, Norwich

Tomato plant, p. 184: photo by Selby McCreery

French bean plant, p. 189: photo by Selby McCreery

Breast feeding: p. 197: reproduced by permission of Daena Rose

Jersey cows, p. 206: photo by Selby McCreery

Olive tree and branch, p. 214: drawing by John Platt

Lime and silica, p. 233: drawings from Ernst Haeckel's book *Kunstformen*. Supplied by June Woodger

Garlic, p. 249: photo by Selby McCreery

Vegetable chopping, p. 274: drawing by John Platt

Basket of Hubbard squash, p. 280: photo by Selby McCreery

Family meal in Janet's kitchen, p. 301; photo by Daniel Allan

Paris in a Brussels sprouts patch, p. 309: photo by Selby McCreery

Lettuces, p. 310: photo by Selby McCreery

ACKNOWLEDGMENTS

Maarten Ekama was involved in an earlier version of this project and has continued to give me support and material. Louise Freisenbruch turned my copious notes into something I could present as a project to a publisher – a deed of love and patience. Dorothy Fagan gave help with editing in the early stages. Tim Dyas and Janet Allan lent their beautiful homes as setting for front and back covers. Christine Rawstorne baked the special loaves as part of the meal shown on the back cover. My daughter Daisy took the picture on the front in Majorca, and Eva Zsiray, a professional baker, personified the principle of Hestiatoria.

Daniel Allan took the pictures of the family meal. Selby McCreery took most of the other photographs and entered into the illustrating of five-pointed stars within an apple and slices of courgette with verve and enthusiasm. Jackie Sarsby provided pictures of her lovely French farmer baking his weekly supply of bread. John Platt was a delight to work with as he provided weekly harvests of drawings of grains, herbs, olive trees and monastic eco-systems.

Richard Smith, Richard Thornton-Smith, Alan Brockman and Michael Duveen, all experienced in biodynamic agriculture, have supplied me with material and checked my agricultural writings for which I am very grateful. Margaret Jonas of the Rudolf Steiner Library has been most helpful in advising me and supplying me with appropriate anthroposophical books and publications. Dr Ralph Twentyman, Dr Marthe Kiley-Worthington and Gunnel Minett have kindly given me permission to quote from their books. Dr Jenny Luke and Professor L.J.A. Didio gave permission to use images of the human pineal gland. Mary Parker of the Institute of Food Research, Norwich, was extremely patient in working with my requests for electron-microscope pictures of cereal and potato starches. Annie Wingfield and June

Woodger helped with research. Dr James Welch of Elm Farm Research Centre kindly gave information on cereal content.

Louise Courtnell gave kind permission to use her 'Self-portrait', which won the National Portrait Gallery BP prize in 1991. Thanks also for help from the Biodynamic Agricultural Association, Elm Farm Research Centre, the Soil Association and the Food Policy Department of Thames University.

I would not have been able to finish this manuscript without the dedicated editorial help of Susan Hannis who achieved surgical miracles in 'snipping and tucking' my unwieldy sentences and format. She was able to help me bring clarity into some of the more difficult concepts I have been struggling with in the book. I shall miss our Friday morning meetings which kept me focused and gave me the courage to go on with the rather ambitious spread of subject matter. Many thanks also to Eileen Lloyd for her fine copy-editing. Finally, gratitude to my publisher, Sevak Gulbekian, who saw the potential in my earlier manuscript, and has put lots of energy into achieving the final product.

Any errors left in the text I take responsibility for.

I have had a great deal of freely given time and energy, for which I am overwhelmed and full of gratitude.

*'One who understands nutrition correctly
understands the beginning of healing.'*

Rudolf Steiner

PREFACE

I have a strong memory of a May lecture given by John Davy (a former science correspondent to *The Observer* and later vice-principal of Emerson College[1]) in the mid-seventies. His talk followed an earlier presentation by Uri Geller and amongst other things he said something like this: 'It is all very well for us to be impressed by somebody who can bend spoons and stop watches and it is indeed unusual, but how many of us are aware of the daily miracles that surround us? Like the human capacity for uprightness (in defiance of gravity), and that the plant strives upwards towards the sun.' This gave me food for thought. I began acknowledging these daily miracles and looking and listening more closely to what confronts me in life and how I interact with it, for the universe is pure *revelation*.

The Western way has been involved in the exploration of physical matter, a path that could lead us back to the world of spiritual dimensions, but the connections have to be rediscovered and relationships recognized. Each phenomenon reveals something important. When we understand its essential nature and see it not as an isolated entity, we may start to recognize the role that it is playing in the world. Whether it be plant, star, animal, rock or human being, when we discover its activity (for all are constantly moving and changing), we will be changed too.

Forms display an exquisite underlying intelligence, as seen in the elegance of the snowflake, the mystery of the human eye, or the five-pointed star within the apple. What are these forms saying to us? We shall explore this question. Can we look at stellar movements, impressions of sea on sand, soup in a pot, listen to a piece of music and see them all as varied expressions of the one cosmic ordering force?

Rudolf Steiner was one of the people able to perceive such relationships, but at the same time he was a scientist who wished to present a participative

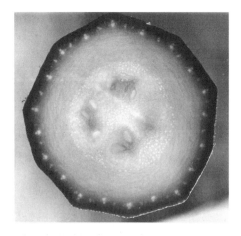

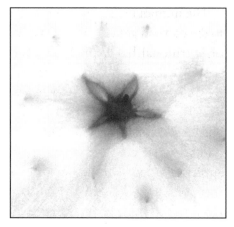

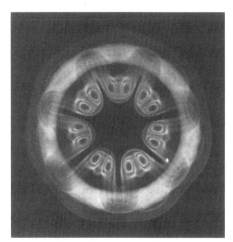

Some of the forms we find in nature: cross-section of courgette (top left), apple (top right), and a vortex ring rising upwards through water (bottom)

epistemology, leading to practical application in many spheres of life. He was not seeking for the supernatural and the sensational. His earlier translation of Goethe's scientific works, introducing the 'Ur- plant' or 'plant archetype', laid the foundations for a more artistic and inclusive approach to natural science. Steiner made many references to nutrition; he gave it a great deal of importance, both for its interface with agriculture and from the therapeutic/medical perspective. But these lectures tend to be scattered amongst educational, agricultural and medical publications, making it quite hard to see a full picture. Dr Rudolf Hauschka and Dr Gerhard Schmidt have, however, developed these ideas and their books have been of great value to me.

The human being's relation to food gives an indication of his relationship to the earth in general, and though we may hear a great deal about the effects of nutritional habits on health we seldom hear about their effects on our consciousness. I feel this to be an important consideration and in the first part of the book I have endeavoured to look at (albeit only in a thumbnail sketch) the human journey in its quest for food and some accompanying changes of consciousness. The journey sees the human 'descent' into earthly and material concerns from a previously more 'dreamy', but spiritually secure, relationship to other kingdoms. Today many people wonder whether the earth, her plants and creatures will survive the onslaught of Promethean man. Only a new kind of understanding of our own place in this complex world of interactions will bring about the necessary reordering of priorities. And this has to be a real paradigm-shift; you cannot put new wine into old bottles. We cannot go forward with insight if we have no real understanding of the past. In a very future-oriented culture, history is history and peoples of bygone ages are often considered primitive. But were they?

Next we try to orient ourselves to the current agricultural situation, and ask 'How can we heal man's relationship with the earth?' We take a look at what biodynamic agriculture offers in the way of healing for the earth, and then we focus on the constitution of the human being. How do the 'subtle bodies' experienced by the ancient Greeks and physicians such as Paracelsus fit with current concepts of the human constitution? Or do they? We ask, 'What have been the basics of human nutrition for millennia — since the early days of the inhabitants of Çatal Hüyük?' The next chapter presents the cereal grains, each with their biography and some of their mythology.

In Part Two we investigate the mystery of human digestion, where accepted theories have been based on the principles of conservation of matter, test-tube chemistry and the laws of thermodynamics, the prevailing paradigm in many people's minds and practice. Rudolf Steiner has presented us with something quite other. He describes the nutritional processes in the human being as a kind of 'anti-physics' and 'anti-chemistry' — difficult concepts, but I think worthy of real consideration.

Do we think of ideas, beautiful landscapes, music as being actual nourishment; that our breathing and absorption of sunlight are all connected to our nutritive process? We take a look at their effects on the human organism. Then follows a piece examining the various issues around vegetarianism, such as what happens to domestic animals if we stop eating them.

In Part Three we look at building blocks of nutrition. Some foods are necessities, others have the role of stimulation, some are questionably not foods at all, some provoke allergies. How can we understand these things more deeply and clearly?

Finally, in Part Four, we look at some of the practical and aesthetic aspects of cooking, planning menus, the shared meal, and children's food.

INTRODUCTION

Why would I want to write such a book? The story begins with my own childhood. I was born at the beginning of the Second World War and I spent my early years growing up in the agricultural area of Bedfordshire. Food was rationed and remained so till the early fifties. My childhood apprehensions imagined a lifetime of ration-book management, juggling those little coupons that represented tiny amounts of protein, sweets or clothing. I learnt from my father how to eke out the sweetie ration – by cutting razor-thin slices of Mars bars and jelly babies he was able to make large expanses, like colourful gardens on a plate. My mother and I would go gleaning in the pea-fields, going over the mounds of stalks looking for the peas that had been missed by the pea-pickers. This was an exciting treasure hunt. Horses were still a common sight ploughing the fields, patient, strong animals; hayricks were often still built by hand. Most of my friends were the sons and daughters of farmers, so I spent a lot of time in mud and hay, communed with the elemental beings and learnt to know the signs of seasonal passings.

My mother was a born gardener despite a childhood in the sooty streets of Manchester. Without even a window box to remind one of nature, she was the kind of person who could stick a seemingly dead-looking piece of stick into the ground and it would take root. We had about an acre of garden which seemed vast to a child, with all sorts of nooks and crannies, barns with owls and such a variety of fruit trees, vegetables and flowers. There were plums, apples, gooseberries, blackcurrants, redcurrants and a magnificent pear tree whose luscious fruits, wrapped up individually and a stored in an old chest of drawers, lasted us most of the winter. A freshly dug root of new potatoes with mint and at least three other vegetables was a satisfying meal. They were all compost-grown. Out on our bicycles as a family, if we came across horse droppings my father would ceremoniously scoop them up, put them in a container specially kept for the purpose and onto the compost they went, with grass cuttings, old woollies, tree prunings and vegetable peelings. I marvelled at how all these things rotted, changed their form and smell completely and could be reused as 'black gold' on the garden. To this day I make compost wherever I am, and am fascinated by the whole process of decay and metamorphosis.

The women ran a great deal of the agriculture during the war and all of those left at home, kids included, got involved on some level. We were exhorted to 'dig for Britain'. Parks and flower-beds were given over to vegetable growing; most people knew how to grow them. It was a matter of survival, and neighbours exchanged surpluses. Real hunger is unforgettable. My mother was also a good cook of the plain north country variety. She was keen for me to learn to share this activity and allowed me to experiment on occasions. I became fascinated by choosing, mixing and watching the miraculous transformation of the various ingredients.

My parents, whose own possibility of university education had been removed by the war, like many others, insisted that getting an education was the only way out of the arduous grind of work on the land or simply being obliged to do work that was incompatible with your nature. My father was a civil servant, previously a city dweller, and longed to be free of the smell of rotting cabbage fields and to be in some more intellectually stimulating environment. My sister and I, scholarship winners to the local grammar school, were pressed to fulfil our parents' unfulfilled ambitions. So I witnessed the trend of young people moving off the land, disdaining this work, and often severing themselves from centuries of accumulated experiences of farm and countryside management. Fertilizers were more and more used (nitrates were a by-product of the manufacture of bombs) and farming was becoming more and more mechanized, meaning fewer people were needed in agriculture.

At my grammar school I took a good spread of arts, crafts and sciences. One of my most useful courses was domestic science where we each had our own kitchens. We invited staff members to lunch. Besides the cooking and menu-planning, we learnt about flower-arranging, how to serve guests and about how to develop good conversation around the meal-table. We were taught how to market, what to look for in qualities of freshness (something that I was already quite well schooled in), how to budget, how to clean a room properly and how to iron. The boys also joined us for this, so it was not just gender based. It was good fun and was to stand me, and others, in good stead for the rest of my life.

I went to study art at Cambridge and found it intoxicating to be in such an exciting international community. My wellies were ditched and I joined in enthusiastically with the emerging exploration of new ideas, new fashions, new freedoms and the breaking of old taboos. Cooking became more and more interesting to me and though I was living on a minute budget I managed to make exotic menus for very little money. The often poorly fed undergraduates were enthusiastic guinea-pigs for my culinary experiments.

It was at Cambridge that I met my husband-to-be, the satirist Peter Cook, who was definitely intent on breaking taboos and could bewitch an audience without effort. I lived in a former pub, 'The Prince of Wales', owned by two philosophy graduates, which became a real salon – a place where good food, extraordinary witty, humorous and serious conversation flourished. Humour can be devastating, as when the jesters in Shakespeare's plays bring most incisive insights. While you laugh you create a space for new possibilities. So it was a kind of alchemy that developed around our dining table.

Later, living in London, this creative outreach continued. Like many people in the sixties I became a devotee of Elizabeth David, and dinner guests spent time in the aftermath of a evening *chez* Cooks picking out the rosemary branches from their teeth. We discovered herbs in a big way. Some of the people who shared our table were Peter Ustinov, John and Cynthia Lennon, Paul McCartney, Jane Asher, Dudley Moore, Alan Bennett, Jonathan Miller, Terry Downes (middleweight boxing champion), Joan Collins, Malcolm Muggeridge, Bernard Levin, Alan Bates and David Frost. The delight was to be able to select an interesting potion of contrasting folk who might not otherwise bump into each other and to create an appropriately magical meal to enhance a sense of well-being and stimulate conversation and new ideas.

Peter Cook and partner Nick Luard ran a satirical political nightclub called 'The Establishment' where politicians, actors, artists, jazz musicians and journalists mingled. It was the early sixties! It was the place to be! This heady and intoxicating life changed substantially when I became a mother. We had two beautiful daughters, Lucy and then Daisy. Daisy developed eczema and then severe asthma. Peter had suffered from asthma as a child and I had been bronchitic, adding to this hereditary burden. I did not breast-feed Daisy, as I had been convinced by others of the convenience of bottle-

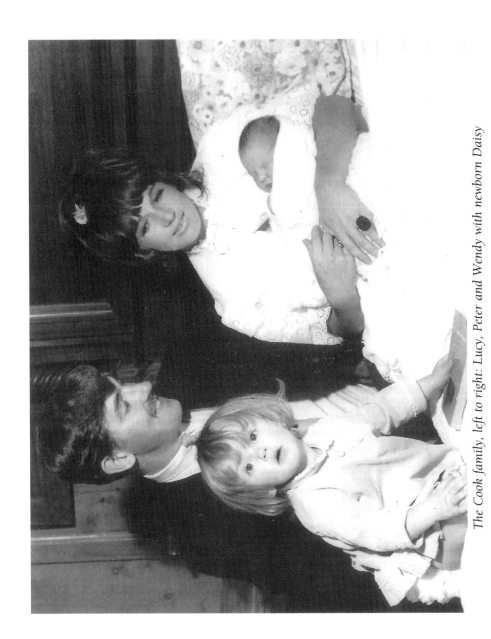

The Cook family, left to right: Lucy, Peter and Wendy with newborn Daisy

feeding. If only I had known then what I know now; alas we are not taught anything about parenting and child-care or the really important things in life. Anybody suffering from asthma or parenting an asthmatic child will know the acute anxiety that surrounds this condition and how complicated the picture can be. In those days in a severe attack adrenalin injections were given by the doctor, with violent side-effects. Daisy often needed to be taken off to hospital to be in an oxygen tent and she was given steroids which made her tremble. Her little chest was becoming the typical barrel-shape of the asthmatic. Then there was physiotherapy. I had to be very vigilant and tried to orchestrate playtime with friends as over a certain decibel pitch of excitement I knew she would start heaving. Asthmatics cannot breathe out when having an attack. I was anxious and frustrated, but despite having access to the best medical advice the condition persevered and became quite central to all our lives.

I knew that there had to be another way of healing this condition. Looking for this other way became my path, to retrieve some of my own inherent wisdom as a mother, to remember some of the home cures that my mother used to administer and to discover new ways of regarding illness and how best to treat it in its own unique context. This journey took me away from the exciting life of theatre, television and financial luxury; few people can deal well with that amount of glamour and success when in their twenties. It had been an extraordinary experience but it was not an atmosphere that I felt conducive to child-rearing.

Daisy and a young friend, now seven years old, had become determined to become vegetarians. They had seen lovely frisky lambs and calves and chickens happy in nature, but seen dead animals in butchers and made the connection with what was on their plates. They didn't want any of that, and this wasn't a three-day fad either. Although I had always provided lots of vegetables and salads at that time, my repertoire for vegetarian dishes was confined to cheese omelettes or cheese soufflés. Vegetarianism after war-time rationing was linked to poverty and considered cranky, which was I suppose why the most famous vegetarian restaurant in London in the sixties was named 'Cranks'. (In 1889 the 18-year-old Mahatma Gandhi, then a law student in London and vowed to vegetarianism, had walked the streets of the city for many hours seeking a vegetarian eating house before he found one in Farringdon Street.) Now these young folk were bringing a new kind of sensitivity.

I had been told about a community in the North of Scotland where vegetarianism was the underpinning for their spiritual and physical life together. There were stories of how they grew vast cabbages and had converse with the nature beings. I decided to go and explore Findhorn with Daisy and Lucy. Daisy flourished in the clean air, and the wonderful fresh and vital vegetarian fare made us all feel very healthy. I met environmental activist and writer Paul Hawken whilst there. He told me how he had cured his asthma by following a macrobiotic diet and put me in touch with Aveline Kushi with whom I subsequently studied for four years. I learnt a meditative approach to the preparation of food, about the seven grains and the importance of the acid/alkaline balance in a meal.

I also met an interesting family where the six children were highly individual, confident and creative. My children quickly struck up friendships. I learned that these children were at Michael Hall, a Rudolf Steiner school in Sussex. It was at this school that Lucy and Daisy were to spend the rest of their education, where therapeutic activities were subtly inherent in the whole way of teaching.

While the girls went to school I went to Emerson College, a Steiner centre for adult training in education, sculpture, biodynamic farming, music and painting. There was also a course in catering and nutrition, and after a foundation year I was drawn to the kitchen. The food supply was mainly sourced from the kitchen garden and the farm. We had local biodynamic milk and yoghourt, cheese and eggs. I introduced tamari, miso and some seaweed, which wasn't perhaps appreciated at the time (the mid-seventies), being so foreign to our Western palate, but it was a place of experiment. Now, over 25 years later, these are familiar ingredients in Emerson's kitchen as many of the students are Asian – Japanese, Korean and Chinese.

I studied nutrition from Rudolf Steiner's perspective with Dr Gerhard Schmidt, a visiting medical lecturer, and did as much as I could to learn to understand the principles of biodynamic agriculture, a lofty subject that can appear strange to the modern mind, involving as it does a study of planetary movements in relation to the growth and harvesting of plants. The best educational elements were the products themselves, even superior to those of my mother. So I have spent a lot of my life proselytizing about biodynamic food. I practised Goethean observation exercises with Hugh Ractliffe and Dr Margaret Colquhoun and gradually began to view life, education, agriculture, nutrition, the human being's relationship to nature, and indeed to the cosmos, from an increasingly enlarged perspective – but one I realized I already knew deep down, intuitively.

Through a balanced programme of philosophical-spiritual study, craft work and work in the gardens and kitchen, ideas became practice and new experiences on a physical level led to new perceptions on the level of ideation. Altogether it was a splendidly creative time and I made many interesting friends. Later I taught vegetarian cookery at Michael Hall school, and worked in clinics and with medical initiatives trying to understand more and more deeply the concepts that Rudolf Steiner was pointing to in the field of nutrition, leading of course into many other areas because all are related. I wanted to bring these concepts into line with my own experiences and developed so many questions which the answers given by current nutritional science fail to satisfy on anything more than a superficial level. I was particularly interested in the questions of quality, the more subtle effects of the kind of heat used in cooking, and the whole community-building aspect of sharing work and food.

Together with some other interested people we bought a 60-acre traditional mountain farm in north Majorca as an experiment. The setting and life-forces on this piece of land were powerful. It had been abandoned for 40 years and nature had run her course. There were terraces that had been devoted to cereal growing and threshing, terraces of olive trees, a lime-kiln and the foundations of a charcoal-burner's dwelling. There were acres of forest, providing shade, wood for charcoal and, lower down, terraces for fruit orchards and vegetable growing. Natural-rise bread baked regularly in a stone wood-fired oven was delicious and sustaining; water came from a deep spring whose emergence from the great mountain had inspired the Moors to fashion a beautiful 'temple' to house it. We cooked over wood fires and had only one solar panel to bring a little electric light into the house. We had milking goats, a sheep, ducks and chickens and a large donkey (*somera*) to plough with.

Many people came to help us and experience this paring away of technology and convenience luxuries. The food, sun-drenched and full of flavour and aroma, was unforgettable. We were properly hungry because we had laboured and sweated. The seasons were clearly marked by their contingent products, of such wonderful diversity. How many millennia had it taken of painstaking plant-breeding to produce such a variety?

Although this experiment was not very long-lived, for various reasons it left a deep impression upon me and many of our visitors. It intensified my respect for the farming fraternity — there is so much to learn about agriculture to do it well. It had been an almost biblical type of existence in its simplicity, and this is how much of our world stills lives.

However, it is possible to get on a plane to the USA and witness a vastly different scenario, one where great machines programmed by computer distribute fertilizers and pesticides in a vast landscape, a monoculture of wheat. There are no people, no weeds, no trees, no birds and no insects. And I imagine the great and sad voice of God, of a designing intelligence, saying, 'What have you done with the garden with which I entrusted you?'

And yet more questions pour forth. How come there is so much malnutrition in the world when there are grain and butter mountains, wine lakes, vegetables ploughed back into the soil, and where food policies are creating a new kind of slavery? Bio-technology professes as its motive the solving of world hunger but in fact seeks to monopolize and exploit seed culture and destroy the wonderful genetic diversity created over millennia by small farmers. Meanwhile, millions of Westerners suffer from diet-related illnesses and there is a serious crisis of meaning in our society, 'soul starvation', manifesting often as depression. Young children suffer from Attention Deficit Disorder and hyperactivity. Why are children 'yo-yo-ing' in their addiction to salt and sugar (sweets and crisps)? Why are so many children taking drugs, incidences of violence and vandalism increasing? I'm sure that we all have our own theories to why all this is happening, but how can we change these tendencies?

Steiner had some interesting insights which provoke a quite different way of seeing our world. He spoke of the evolution of food habits as giving a clue to unfolding human consciousness. He spoke about different epochs in nutrition, the current one emphasizing the mineral. It is a fairly new phenomenon that many Western people are taking mineral supplements, now a hugely lucrative industry. How can we put this strange development into context?

Do we ever ask ourselves how come we have products on our plates, many of which are mildly poisonous, consciousness-altering, addictive and deleterious to health? (Animals on the whole tend not to injure themselves by consuming inappropriate foods, if left to wisely forage.) Often these are plant-based products that have vastly changed agricultural societies, economically and socially, as they strive to provide cash crops like coffee to the detriment of their own indigenous food-growing capacity. What did Steiner mean by saying that we build ourselves primarily from the (formative) forces that have gone into growing the plants? Was it that a different chemistry and physics was at work within the human being? How could it be that extensive eating of potatoes and legumes (particularly soya and peanuts) could create an increasing tendency towards materialism? How could it be that vegetarian nutrition could support spiritual work better than a meat-eating diet, but that not everybody actually could manage to be a vegetarian even if they wanted to?

If everybody became vegetarian what would the fate of the domestic animals be? (The cow is central to the fertility of the soil in biodynamics, as well as giving valuable dairy products.) Why are there now so many people apparently not able to tolerate milk and wheat products, staples of mankind for millennia? During nine thousand years of agriculture it used to be the honoured job of the high priest to cut the first furrow, so how come that nowadays many disdain work on the land, indeed any form of manual work? In the USA there are more people in the gaols than working on the land!

Why are we so alienated from nature? Could our nutrition be exacerbating this tendency? The family mealtime is disappearing, where adults and young people learn to take care of each other, where the rudiments of conversation are cultivated, where the gifts of the earth are savoured, where we learn hospitality and gratitude.

These and many other questions have furnished my quest. As soon as one question is seemingly answered another springs in its place. I am not a doctor; my life has been spent gardening and feeding people. I've always tried to learn as much as I could about my profession, observing the phenomena. I love to share my insights and I love to teach. Cooks and gardeners are on the whole notoriously badly paid and unless they are television personalities the kudos is not great either. However, eating is probably one of the last things that any of us will willingly give up. I hope to throw some light on the importance of this great craft, art, science. All good cooks know something about alchemy, and in alchemy we learn about the deeper aspects of substances and their interactions – and the greater cosmic influences.

I believe we are here to be good materialists and that means understanding substance. When we think of a teaspoon of honey as representing approximately 2000 hours of work on the part of the bee, rather than only the sum of its constituents, we start to perceive it on an energetic level. Appreciating this may elicit quite a different response from that of the reductionist science we have been almost exclusively taught. I think we have to bring these aspects together, and in this book I have tried to do so. All I hope is that you can develop the attitude that one of my wise teachers, Dr L. Mees, recommends: 'When you meet a new and unfamiliar idea, don't say "No", just say "Oh!"' Just live with an idea and, if it has truth, it will like a plant germinate, root and transform other ideas.

PART ONE

THE HISTORY OF NUTRITION

A study of the evolution of food and human consciousness

Studying the rise and fall of civilizations can show us the story of mankind's development. From a simple childlike condition, where life went on within a timeless mythological consciousness, gradually knowledge of an earthly and practical kind increased, sometimes at the expense of wisdom. Skills developed and were often forgotten again. But the aspect that shows a continuous upward incline is the development — hand-in-hand with awakening to the physical world — of an awakening to self-awareness. We do not stop to consider how very long and intricate this development has been; it goes back over many millennia. We take for granted the degree of self-awareness we are familiar with and the outlooks that accompany it. Some consequences of our own outlook, however, are very clear — in particular the strong urge and increasing ability to control living processes.

In order to understand ourselves now, we need to appreciate where we have come from. Without that how can we orient ourselves usefully towards our future? So it is time we really tried to understand something of our human evolution in a new and different way. To look with 'new eyes' we might start by trying to appreciate what it was like to look through the eyes of the ancients. Rudolf Steiner gives interesting pictures of our earliest beginnings:

... as the human family developed, its original unity with the cosmos began to be veiled in darkness. The process involved working through three states of consciousness, which led them from spiritual heights into the depths of the earth . . . It was from these depths that the individual has the possibility to find the original forces for the unfolding of freedom. Thus the human soul went through phases that could be described as 'sleeping', 'dreaming' and beginning to 'awake'.[1]

The gradual awakening process has been accompanied, as we shall try to show, by different phases of nutrition. The variety of foods and methods of preparation have also evolved and the communication arising out of growing, cooking, preserving and trading food is one of the main stories of humanity. This chapter will highlight defining moments in the story of food, dealing primarily with the Caucasian peoples. Journeying thus we may come to see more clearly where we are today and that the historical process is neither haphazard nor arbitrary.

Our beginnings

Our journey begins in the allegorical Garden of Eden — the ultimate expression of the 'radiant energy of Creation', familiar in world mythology. Everything there was provided, but for those original occupants there had to be something more. Adam and Eve (representatives of humanity) wished to eat of the Tree of Knowledge; they wished to know what the gods knew; they wished to 'know' each other. And so it was that in eating the forbidden fruit before they were prepared for that knowledge, they were cast out naked from this beneficent garden into a world where they had to become familiar with the earth and its laws and its constraints. They were now to find their own food and to cope with pain and death, the woman to experience the pain of childbirth and the man to develop courage and strength, and to learn through physical labouring. Mankind was to become free by going into and beyond the physical, developing individuality and self-governance, but also remembering his divine origins.

The hunter-gatherers

The earliest peoples were hunter-gatherers led by shamanic priests who, according to Steiner, possessed a kind of clairvoyance, but on a low, dreamlike level. Their cave paintings, which represent the most striking and accomplished work of Palaeolithic art, are images often of animals incised or painted on the surface of the rock. An example is the powerful portrayal of the Wounded Bison from the caves at Altamira, northern Spain, so eloquently expressing the power and dignity of the creature as it gives up its life. These cave paintings are believed to be part of hunting rituals for the men of the period known as the Old Stone Age (or Magdalenian period, estimated at 18,000 years ago). By making a picture of the animal they were able to visualize the particular beast they would meet in the forthcoming hunt, and thus magically gained power over the animal's soul. The ritual helped to draw man and animal together. Animals were experienced as part of their own soul; the bull expressed elements of their own metabolism and their physical strength, whereas the deer expressed something of sun-related sensitivity. While men were engaged in hunting, the women of the tribe were responsible for the gathering of an enormous variety of wild plants – knotgrass, clubrush, berries, rhizomes of the canna lily, roots of asphodel, fungi, acorns, wild grain and snails. They may have acquired over many generations a real and diverse knowledge of the edible resources available and deliberately left tubers and seeds behind, eventually creating little patches with digging sticks for the food plants to grow.

Even today there can be found fields of wild grain (spelt) growing as thickly as cultivated grain. In the 1960s, archaeologist J.R. Harlan experimented with a flint-bladed sickle to see what a prehistoric family in Turkey might have been able to harvest. In one hour he managed to gather enough wild wheat to produce more than two pounds (1 kilo) of clean grain. What is more, this grain proved to be much more nutritious than the modern, cultivated variety.[2] It was discovered that lightly roasting wild grains would make threshing – dividing the seed from the chaff – easier. The roasting was accomplished in pits lined and covered with heated stones.

During this Cro-Magnon period the human being developed most basic skills, practical and artistic. The caves with their amazing depictions became silted up; some were discovered 11,000 years later, in 1895, in southern France by children playing.

Eventually, reliable and abundant supplies of foods and the ability to build their own homes must have been significant factors in the development of settled agrarian communities. However, the arrival of farming was certainly not sudden, nor was it simple.

After the melting of the glaciers, the Great Flood

The story of a devastating flood that almost destroyed all life in the world occurs in the legends and belief systems of all the peoples of Mesopotamia and the eastern Mediterranean, from the Sumerians to the Hebrews who wrote down the experiences of Noah. Let us try to imagine ourselves in those times.

Tribal life was strictly ruled by priests, who as initiates had direct insight into the divine ordering of the world. In the migrations which followed the melting of the ice these shamanic priests played an important role in guiding their people to new lands. Then, and for some time to come, 'the human community looked up to the starry heavens and the knowledge that man still had of the stars showed him unmistakably that their forces lived within him and that he belonged essentially to the cosmos.'[3] One of the important leaders of the time was Noah, who guided his people towards central Asia. He was known to the Indians as Manu and in the Persian epic of *Gilgamesh* as Utnapishtim, and the image of his ark is also found in many other cosmologies. Noah was also known as the father of the 'Seven Holy Rishis', the wise teachers of the ancient Indians. The nations issuing from the descendants of Noah were called Aryans, which means 'Light-bearing'. Amongst these were the ancient Indian peoples and the Persians. According to Steiner, the Indians developed first and turned their steps towards the south-east, to the river basin of the Indus known as Septa Sindhave.

The age of milk and honey
(during the Age of Cancer, 8426–6266 BC)

The tribes of the Indian Aryan stream still lived a nomadic life with their cattle, whose milk was their principal food. This milk was instrumental in building bodily substance or *kapha*, one of the basics of Ayurvedic medicine,[4] and the basis for their soul/astral body (see Chapter 3); they began to be more connected to the earth and less 'dreamy'. They also continued to gather wild food and did not eat their animals; eating meat was forbidden and the cows were revered as sacred. This is the age best described as the 'age of milk and honey'. Even today the phrase evokes images of abundance and carefree ease. However, in trying to penetrate the quality of these times we should not think of this richness solely as an outer condition, some kind of prehistoric pacific paradise, but rather as a condition of real peace and inner harmony. The human being of these times felt at one both with nature and the gods, receiving their gifts with a feeling of serenity and security. It was a state of being that can perhaps best be compared with that of a young child whose parents surround it with protection and guidance, keeping at a distance for these few precious years all the influences and difficulties destined to come later in life.

The gift of milk from cows and honey from wild bees, as two particular foods, were more than a symbol of humanity's living relationship with the gods. The Milky Way is not so named simply because it is brighter than other regions in the night sky, but because humanity perceived the region as a source of 'cosmic milk' or *prana* which gave nourishment to the whole hierarchy of gods and spiritual beings who have their home in the starry cosmos. In a similar way, any bright group of stars is called a 'galaxy', derived from the Greek word for milk (*gala*).

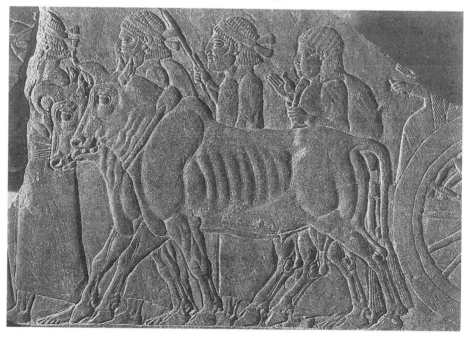

Early herdsmen, bas relief (Mesopotamia)

These early peoples relied on the Rishis for their connection with the high spiritual world in which divine beings, the devas, were beheld. It was still possible to make use of the old inherited gift of clairvoyance (through the use of the pituitary and pineal glands, according to Rudolf Steiner), and they were helped to perceive these elemental worlds by means of an inner schooling. The outer or sensorial world was regarded as *maya*, or illusion. They knew that all natural phenomena were the work of the devas, but that these beings could only be reached in an inner way; all was threaded together in a web of karma.

In the space of thousands of years the Hindus developed this path further and further. It came to expression in the Vedanta, in the systems of yoga, in the *Bhagavadgita* and in other works, and later was in a certain sense crystallized in the teachings and the revelations of Buddha. So the people were not primarily involved with the sensory earth-world but with the invisible higher spheres; it also meant that they did not come to grips with the possibilities of the earth-world, including the development of agriculture.

Much later the Hindus developed a system of categories of foods, which came from a deep insight into the different qualities of foods and their effects on the human being. The first was *Sattvic*, providing strength from within and recommended for those doing spiritual work – the Brahmins, the scholar-priest caste. Sattvic foods are considered to be pure foods which keep the mind-body-spirit balanced, clear, harmonious and strong. They include fruits, grains, vegetables, seeds, certain herbs, milk, yoghourt and honey, giving an approximate acid:alkaline balance of 70:30.

Foods from the *Rajasic* category are indicated for kings, warriors and traders. They include many more stimulating foods: fresh meats, wine, spices, garlic, sweetmeats and eggs. This combination encourages competitive, aggressive and sensual behaviour. Acid:alkaline ratio 50:50.

The *Tamasic* category includes stale, decayed, decomposed, overcooked or reheated foods. These are foods that have no spark of life left in them, and form the larger part of the diets of the lowest castes. (The acidic pole tends to dominate.)

The categories come from the Ayurvedic system and though it may seem over-simplified to us these days, it shows profound knowledge of both people and food substances.

The ancient Persians
(during the Age of Gemini, 6266–4106 BC)

We now turn to the next important Aryan tribe, the Persians, who settled in areas of southern Turkestan and who later extended towards the highlands of Iran, Persia and Medea. At an early stage they developed an outer perception and the kind of thinking that connects with observation. They were still conscious of the existence of a spiritual world active behind the normally visible world, and they still possessed great power over the forces of nature, which were subsequently to withdraw from the control of humanity. Their teachers were the initiates who were the guardians of the oracles and had command of inner forces, particularly of fire and the other elements. Their leader was Zarathustra (considered by some to indicate a certain initiatory level, not an individual, so there was more than one Zarathustra, causing confusion amongst historians rather like the ubiquitous King Arthur).

Zarathustra brought the prophecy of the great 'Sun Spirit of Light' known as Ahura Mazda, creator of heaven and earth and source of light and dark. The conspicuous monotheism of Zarathustra's teaching had an inbuilt dualism: the Wise Lord (God) has an opponent, Ahriman, who embodies the principle of darkness. However, both mankind and spiritual beings are free to choose whom they want to follow. Thus the world is divided into two hostile blocks, whose members represent two warring factions. On the side of the Wise Lord are the settled herdsmen or farmers caring for their cattle and living in a definite social order. On the other side are the followers of the Lie (Druj), who are thieving nomads, enemies of orderly agriculture and animal husbandry. So Zarathustra encouraged his people to be the first agriculturists.

Here I would like to retell part of a Persian legend, where Yima is guided by Ahura Mazda to become the first tiller of the land.

Now Ahura Mazda gave Yima a gold sword and a gold decorated whip for the purpose of cultivating the soil, and he consecrated him first king of the kingdom of Iran. The earth was filled with men and cattle, dogs and birds and blazing red fires, but soon it became too small to contain all. When the afternoon came, Yima went up to the stars; he touched the earth with his gold sword and pierced it and spoke: 'Enlarge, O holy earth, augment and split open, O yielder of cattle and men.' In this way he made the earth larger than it was by a third, so that all its inhabitants could walk upon it with pleasure.

After many years, Ahura Mazda called Yima to make it known that humanity, now become wicked and materialistic, would be overtaken by severe winters during which huge masses of snow were to come down from the highest mountains. This and the floods, which would inundate the lands after the snows had melted, would cause a third part of men and cattle to perish. For the protection of his people, Yima was charged to prepare a 'var', that is a fenced place or a kind of stronghold, 'a day's journey long and wide'. There he was to take men and cattle, dogs and birds and the blazing red fires. On arrival he was first to drain off the water, put up boundary posts, then houses made from posts, clay walls, matting and fences were to be built. There was to be neither suppression nor baseness, neither dullness nor violence, neither poverty nor defeat, no dwarves, no cripples, no long teeth, no giants, nor any characteristic of the evil spirits.

'Thou blessed Yima, child of the sun, expand the earth, split it apart like wise men, expand the earth by tilling it ...'

From this ancient legend we learn how the Persians, through Zarathustra, now took in hand the cultivation of the soil. The 'gold sword' forms the archetype of the plough, received from the Sun God himself. Through the use of the plough they became amongst the earliest growers of corn, and indeed many of the food plants we use today originated from that time. The Zend Avesta, or Holy Book of the Persians, can be regarded as the first agricultural handbook.

Excavations in 1960[5] led by Russian archaeologists in Turkmenistan (the country of origin of the Iranians) uncovered one of the oldest known agricultural settlements, consisting of small rectangular, one-roomed houses, loosely grouped together with small courtyards in which it seems that cattle were kept. These settlements lay on arable land, so that each farmer had immediate access to his own field from the home. Impressions of wheat and barley grains were found in the walls together with agricultural tools with bone handles.

Other legends go on to tell us how Yima, seduced by Ahriman, left the way of God and fell to lying. He also induced the people to eat meat, which had not been the practice of these people, to whom milk was the most revered of drinks. Indeed, a sacred drink was made from milk mixed with the juice of a certain plant. This drink was called *soma* by the Indians and *haoma* or *hom* by the Persians. It was first put through a fermentation process and sacrificed to the gods by means of the 'blazing fires', then it was drunk during the ritual – it induced a kind of holy enthusiasm.[6] This cult, and its various rites, was later extended and ordered by the priestly class of the Magi. At its centre the eternal flame in the Temple of Fire was constantly tended by priestly service and the *haoma* sacrifice.

The early Persians were surrounded by nomadic tribes who had little understanding of private property and would take the cattle of the settled farmers. We can see how, by erecting fences to keep in the cattle and creating boundaries between the 'wild' and the cultivated, tensions were created between those who still led a nomadic, almost childlike life and those who wanted to cultivate and develop their land and culture. For it was out of these settled agricultural communities that the great civilizations arose.

So the change-over from hunting to husbandry was accompanied by profound changes in the human's perception, not only of himself, but of his relationship with his world, where he became custodian of a piece of land. The story of Cain and Abel is an archetypal image of these two streams – the nomads and the new farming fraternity. (We should not attempt to rigidify the story within the flow of time. Real myths and legends have their being 'out of time' and are therefore true for all time.) Cain is described as an agriculturist and as such was able to develop a kind of independence. He was beginning to understand the laws of nature and gain some control over them. He was able to store grain – a tremendous advantage. Abel was a shepherd who moved about with his flocks, gathering food and using animals' milk. Cain 'slew' Abel, actually meaning that the new way of life, anchored as it was in the soil, provided a surplus that could enable other activities to develop, superseding the nomadic way of life in many places.

Early settlements

One of the earliest settled human communities to be found is Çatal Hüyük in Anatolia, in modern-day Turkey. It existed around 7000 BC and its popula-

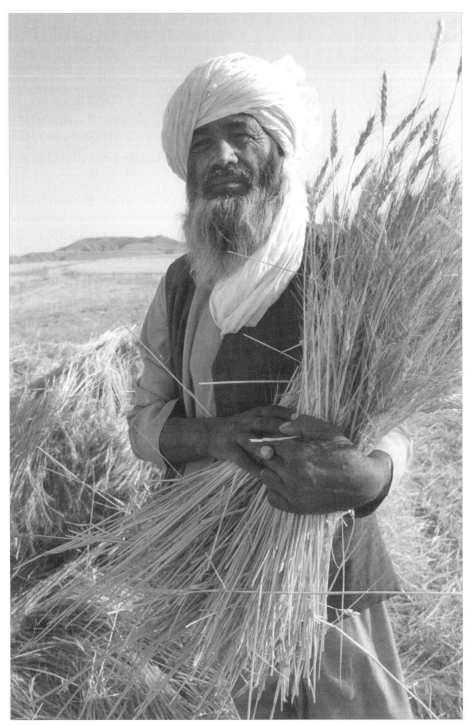

Afghan farmer with grain

tion grew to an estimated 5000, 'a community with extensive economic development, specialized crafts, a rich religious life with ritual ancestral burials, a surprising attainment in art and an impressive social organization'.[7] In this great city the houses did not give out onto the streets but were accessed by ladders through the roofs (somewhat reminiscent of a honeycomb!). There have been found remains of oak, juniper, pistachio, apple and pomegranate trees, as well as barley, wheat, onions, lentils and shepherd's purse. The inhabitants developed superior sharp tools from obsidian, a volcanic glass, and they were known to have traded with this. Jericho, another famous city of the time, was a shrine to the Mother Goddess situated by an oasis in the Jordan Valley.

The hearth was central in the living space and cereals were ground on a back-breaking saddle quern; the bread must have been somewhat gritty and full of bristles and chaff with this technique. Nevertheless the diet was an improvement on the earthy roots, tubers and snails of the hunter-gatherer period. Much of the cooking would be done in pebble-lined pits, using heated stones which enabled a combination of roasting, steaming and smoking. The foods were wrapped in leaves or seaweed. Now we have the prerequisites for the development of cooking – a hearth and an open fire. As this was still a pre-ceramic age there were no pots, only wooden vessels.

In Mesopotamia a culture thrived on the flood plains between the rivers Tigris and Euphrates which reflected developments occurring throughout the Near East, and here the creation of pottery undoubtedly had a significant impact on how people prepared, stored and cooked their food. There were also dome-shaped ovens known as *tannurs*, which are still in use today. Irrigation systems were developed and now two forms of plough were in use, one with a seed hopper allowing fields to be sown and tilled simultaneously. With the invention of the wheel and cuneiform writing came huge changes of life-style, and with clay tokens developed to represent surpluses of food came the beginning of a money currency and the problems that might follow.

The epic of *Gilgamesh* from Babylonia is the first story to be written down. It shows how humanity begins to realize the separation that death brings. Gilgamesh is devastated by the death of his close friend Enkidu; thereafter his journey becomes a search for immortality, and for a lost plant that bestows immortal life.

The Egypto-Chaldean epoch: cereals and the vine (during the Age of Taurus, 4106–1946 BC)

The Egyptians were still under the guidance of priestly initiates or Pharoahs and selected people were trained for initiation into the temple mysteries. The chief gods were Osiris, god of the sun, and Isis, goddess of the moon, from whom we are all supposed to be descended. The great Egyptian teacher Hermes saw to it that these chosen people prepared themselves during earthly life for communion with the 'Spirit of Light'.

Egypt grew out of a narrow green trench cut by the Nile, extended from two to twenty miles wide by the efforts of the population. In this unique location with its special climate, flora and fauna, a new urban culture arose. Their treasure was the silt brought down every year from the melting of the snows on the mountains of Abyssinia, worth more than any gold. It is estimated that in 7000 years of cultivation the Nile has received the equivalent of three hundred times the total area of topsoil that would cover the whole of Europe.[8] The Nile would begin its yearly rise in late July and crested in October. To time their agricultural activities the Egyptians carefully noted the beginnings of each annual rise, and over half a century of observation led them to create the first solar calendar of 365 days (then divided into three four-month seasons of 120 days each, plus five extra days).

Nourishment by now is no longer experienced as a direct gift from the gods. What the gods gave were skills and insights into the construction and use of implements to till the soil, and insight into the development of food crops. It became necessary to labour for one's daily food and all levels of society were involved in this work, either directly by putting their hands to the soil or indirectly by carrying responsibility for the fertility of the soil, the supply of seeds, times of sowing and harvest, as well as distribution. Everything was geometrically balanced according to cosmological principles, following the heavenly bodies. In particular, kitchens were placed towards the east.

In Egypt, as well as spirituality we meet sensuality – the beguilements of food perfumed with spices, beautiful dancing girls, music, gold ornamentation, scents of incense, immense temples and tombs. The food offered would be grilled fowl, dishes of wheat and barley, pulses flavoured with onions, leeks and garlic (they were particularly fond of garlic and onions, as an inscription on one of the pyramids testifies). Children would wear

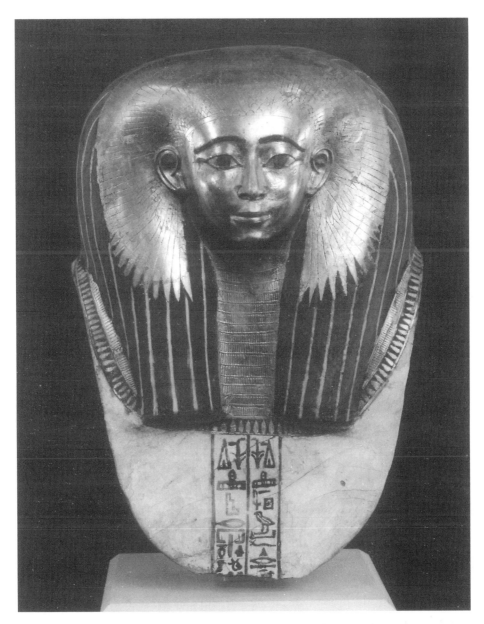

Egyptian mask. The Egyptian Pharaoh presents a remote figure with an almost trance-like expression. Is he listening to 'the music of the spheres'?

necklaces of garlic for protection. Dates and figs were cultivated, as well as melons, cucumbers and pomegranates.

The crops of wheat and barley flourished, as did the population, which seems to have multiplied more than a hundredfold in a few centuries. Fermentation processes were developed; 40 per cent of the grain was used in beer-making, the brewing done by the womenfolk using the red barley of the Nile. The knowledge of fermentation must have led to the making of leavened bread (see p. 169).

Only the Pharoahs were allowed to use spices as they were held especially sacred. We shall see how in time the demand for these aromatics were to bring about great changes. Trading practices began and Egypt traded with Eritrea and Somalia, which produced the honoured incense used in temple ritual. Looking at the image of an Egyptian Pharaoh we can observe a tremendous stillness, attentiveness and remoteness. The expression in the eyes is somewhat trancelike, the ears listening (listening to the cosmos, to the music of the spheres?). The ornate headdresses seem to extend the whole majesty of the head, whereas the rest of the garments are by contrast quite simple. The leaders of the Egypto-Chaldean people were developing this powerful kind of observational intelligence. Their study of astronomy led them to geometry and star-based architecture. The building of the largest pyramids could only have been done with esoteric knowledge. (The pyramids were used for initiation rites, where the acolyte was taken to the threshold of death.)

Hermes derived their writing system from his capacity to read 'stellar script'. The worship of cats was part of their cosmology and the presence of the cat family in the mysterious Sphinx confirms this understanding. Anyone who killed or caused harm to a cat would be severely punished.

Might the Egyptians be seen in one sense as the first real materialists? The practice of mummification and the burial of dead royalty in tombs surrounded by household items and sacrificed servants suggests a real attachment to the physical world and an intention to return to their own familiar bodies, possessions and retinues when they were resurrected at a future time. Drought, famine and invasions brought about the decline of this great empire.

Although beer had been the favoured drink of the Egyptians, wine began to become popular in the New Kingdom (1400 BC). And now with the appearance of bread a great advance was accomplished, a portable food made of flour. Pounding grains has had really far-reaching effects on human nutrition; reducing grains and seeds to smaller particles can facilitate a more complete digestion.

Around 1250 BC emerged Moses, the foundling from the Egyptian bulrushes. He became the leader of the Twelve Tribes of Israel, distinguished by their faith in the one God, Yahveh. (Perhaps Moses had been influenced by the monotheistic Pharoah Amen-Hotep, married to the beautiful Queen Nefertiti.) The enduring faith of the Hebrew people despite manifold obstacles has enabled their powerful contribution to survive through the streams of world civilizations.

Some other cultures

Let us briefly look at some of the foods being used by other cultures at about the same time. In Thailand dietary remains have been found from those early times consisting of peas, beans, cucumbers and water chestnuts, and there is evidence of rice cultivation. The people of the Indus Valley had a varied diet which, as well as rice or wheat, included dates, coconut, bananas, pomegranates and a type of melon. Grain dishes were cooked in sesame oil; spices used were turmeric and ginger. In Mesopotamia the dates of the date palm were used as a fruit and also to make a thick syrup to sweeten puddings. Indeed the date palm was said to have 360 uses — even the pits could be transformed into charcoal.

In China south of the Yangtse rice was cultivated and foxtail millet was widely grown, spreading from village to village across central Asia. Millet was also grown in the Sahara area (the wheat and barley of the Nile not being suitable), red rice in the area of the River Niger, and Kenyans grew finger millet. Cave dwellers in the Tamaulipas Mountains of Mexico had begun to domesticate types of squash, chilli peppers and beans; further south in the Tehuacan Valley we find the development of the most important staple food plant of the Mayan and Inca civilizations — maize or Indian corn. The people of this area also began to cultivate the potato and tomato, both members of the poisonous nightshade family.

The olive tree began to change the landscape in the Mediterranean. Its oil was in great demand and its geometrically linear terraces appeared along the hillsides, giving the setting for our next culture — the Minoan civilization. This rose to its fullest expression by the third millennium BC on the Mediterranean island of Crete. It was an intriguing culture with the Minotaur (the bull) and the journey to the centre of the labyrinth as main features of its central cult. It was both spectacular and long-lasting. The Mother Goddess, femininity and fecundity were worshipped. It was a joyful, creative, energetic culture. Here pottery came to an unsurpassed expression. Delicate vessels and figurines were decorated with lively depictions of bare-breasted python goddesses, bees, dolphins and octopus. Great earthenware amphoras were made to store their wonderful wines and oil. The trading of their famous herb-perfumed olive oil and wines with the tang of resin (retsina), as well as the sale of their Mediterranean oak for boat-building made them wealthy and influential. The great palace of Knossos is a testimony to their special achievements.

The role of wine

Dusky are the avenues of wine,
And we must cross the frontiers, though we will not,
Of the lost fern-scented world:
Take the fern-seed on our lips,
Close the eyes, and go
Down the tendrilled avenues of wine and the Otherworld.

From D.H. Lawrence's *Grapes*

According to Rudolf Steiner it was important for evolving humanity to become thoroughly awake to the importance of concrete existence, so that they could learn from it all that could be learned. As long as the human being felt that he was still a citizen of the spiritual world and considered physical life only a small part of existence, he would not take the possibilities offered by earthly life seriously enough. He would not apply himself to the opportunities for growth found only in earthly existence and might well have dallied his time away, never developing its potentials. The only way an appreciation of concrete physical existence could be aroused in man was to deprive him of the memory of his higher existence for some time. Then he would come to know only his present physical state and would consequently be impelled to apply himself seriously to it.

One of the substances that contributed to this forgetfulness was wine. Instead of feeling harmony with the gods as previously, wine allowed the human being to feel in harmony with himself and his friends. The soul adjusts, shrinking in order to fit more comfortably in the body, but it also brings with it forgetfulness. The active principle of alcohol is as a counterforce to the upwardly striving nature of the human spirit, temporarily paralysing it.[9] This concept of Steiner's that wine was needed for its shrinking effect upon the spiritual part of the human being is a hard one, but we can possibly understand that without it we would never have engaged fully into the implications of physical embodiment.

The Graeco-Roman epoch
(during the Age of Aries, 1946 BC–AD 215)

We now come to the time of the Greek civilization. The oracle sanctuaries were still operating and a few individuals such as the sibyls retained vestiges of the old clairvoyance, while others could attain it by training. The Orphic and Eleusinian mystery schools were centred in Greece. In Pythagoras' school at Crotona, Italy (established in 525 BC) the old wisdom teachings worked on. He had obtained knowledge of geometry from the Egyptians, arithmetic from the Phoenicians, astronomy from the Chaldeans, and from the Zarathustrans the secret teachings about man's relationship to the spiritual worlds.[10]

One of the lasting monuments to Greek civilization is the Greek temple. The proportions of Greek architecture, using the Golden Mean, expressed a perfect balance between heavenly and earthly principles, gravity and lightness, known now as 'architectural order', and uniquely demonstrated in the temples. There is an internal consistency, a mutual adjustment of parts that gives these structures a quality of wholeness and organic unity. Within such a structure the human could have an experience of his own uprightness, being made aware at the same time of the meeting within his own physical and spiritual natures of the dynamic tensions of creation – how he was in himself a 'hieroglyph of nature'.

Greek society was an outdoor society and the first Pan-Hellenic Games were held at Olympia in 776 BC. There was still enormous plasticity in the human form; the fluid form of the etheric presence can be sensed in the fine flowing drapery of garments shown in the friezes on public and private buildings. The Greek needed beauty and proportion in everything; anything that was ugly or disproportionate would make him feel physically ill.

Everything flourished. The Muses inspired great poets and writers. Philosophy, logical thinking, new concepts were emerging in the various schools and disciplines. The art of disputation and debate grew through the

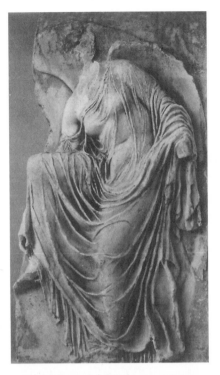

Nike, from the balustrade of the Temple of Athena Nike. The Ancient Greek period represents a high point in spiritual and physical integrity. Rhythm flowed through life as manifest in architecture and sculpture

The vital presence of the etheric, which is seen in the fluidic drapery of Nike, is echoed in this picture of flowing water (bottom)

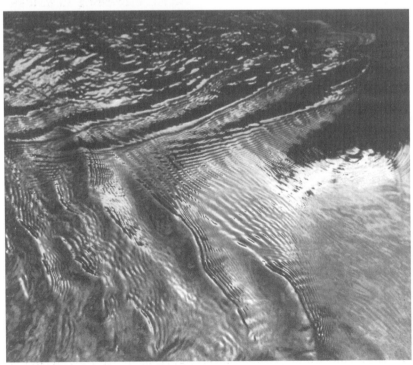

influence of the great minds of Athens. They sought to find rational order and ideal balance in every aspect of nature and human activity. In Plato and his disciple Aristotle we see two complementary philosophies which have greatly influenced our own thinking today. Aristotle, the son of a doctor and therefore exposed to medical and scientific thinking, formed the Lyceum school of philosophy in 367 BC. His view of the cosmos incorporated learning from previous schools, including the Ionian, and provided a comprehensive and empirical system based on logic and natural science. The human body was placed in high esteem and an emphasis was placed on the value of observation and classification. Plato had espoused a more mystical and transcendent system. His was a spiritual path which led, through a search for divine law and personal spiritual exercises, to union with the divine origin. The emphasis in his school was always on the beyond, the invisible eternal hidden within the visible.

When we look at what the Greeks were growing and using for nutrition we find, certainly amongst the masses, a certain purity and simplicity of diet. Food was seen as a sun-product, of which the cereals wheat and barley were the sacred life-giving staples. Vegetarianism played an important role in Greek philosophy, which considered the ethical aspect of eating. In addition to cereals, the Greeks used figs, grapes, pomegranates, spinach, beets, mallow, hyacinth bulbs, nettles, marrows, celery, olives, the original carrot (which was white), artichokes, asparagus and honey. The milk of goats and sheep was made into curd cheese and flavoured with poppy seeds; green herbs were used for culinary and medical purposes, and occasionally fish was eaten. Meat was not part of everyday fare, usually only appearing at times of religious sacrifice, when a sheep or goat was offered.

The Demeter myth
The fruitfulness of the earth was attributed to the divine earth mother, Demeter. Her activity, her force could be experienced instinctively. In the Eleusinian Mysteries the neophyte received, after being prepared by a long fast, the draught of barley, consisting of a mixture of roasted barley, water and mint. It was an 'initiation drink' through which he perceived the goddess Demeter.[11]

The use of salt
It was at this time that salt began to be used as a seasoning. It was considered

holy and used with great care. This denotes a new step: the human being now takes in an element of the mineral kingdom as a separate item in his nutrition. Eating salt like this had a relationship to the developing powers of thought and logic in particular. (See Chapter 14, on salt, p. 218.)

> Here is a Greek dish as described by the Roman writer Pliny:
>
> 'Soak some barley in water for three days and then leave it for a night to dry. Next it is dried by the fire and then ground in a mill. It is mixed with three pounds of flaxseed, half a pound of coriander seed and an eighth of a pint of salt, previously roasting them all. This mixture would then be shaped into loaves and baked.'
>
> A remarkable understanding of the processing of grain in order to make it more flavourful and digestible.

Homer speaks of the 'dark sea-red wine' from Lesbos, doctored with barley meal and curd cheese, and taken as a restorative. Fish baked in fig leaves, and Cappadocian loaves made with milk, oil and salt were dishes for the more sophisticated. The sacredness to the Greeks of the domestic hearth expressed *hestiatoria* – the principle that all hearths are shared with the gods.

> 'The genuine master chefs of the time were expected to have a sound knowledge of astrological cosmology, architecture, geometry, natural history, military strategy and of course medicine.'
>
> 'Not merely politics, but all religious experience found expression in the ritualized consumption of food and drink'[12]

The decline of Classical Greece

We are now at one of the critical points in the human story. Up till now these great cities, palaces, temples, pyramids and irrigation systems had all been achieved through group co-operation. It is thought that the pyramids were most probably built not by slaves but by farmers and their families while their land was flooded by the Nile. They all worked together to do whatever was needed in order to help integrate the Pharoah into the solar cycle, so he could bring forth the necessary wisdom to guide their daily lives – rather as the whole bee-hive works tirelessly to give the queen bee the necessary conditions to lay her eggs. Although there is a hierarchy, everyone honours it – true even in the democracies of the Greeks. But all this was to change, and as all cultures have a flowering, they also have a decline.

One of the factors in the decline of Classical Greece was Dionysus, god of wine, inspiration of the great Dionysian revels. There are vivid descriptions of processions with giant wine presses filled with grapes being trodden by 60 satyrs, all singing a vintage song while the wine gushed everywhere. One can imagine that this revelry led to excesses and it is well known that the Bacchanalian rites became decadent and orgiastic. The gateway between the spiritual and the physical world was steadily receding.

Meanwhile, Aristotle had a special pupil, the young man destined to become Alexander the Great of Macedonia (356–323 BC). While Greece had become myopic, arrogant and weakened by her self-preoccupation, Alexander amassed huge armies. He swept through Greece, Egypt, Babylon, Persia and northern India, taking the Greek language and customs into the vast empire that he conquered, fired by a vision of a united mankind. However Alexander died young (also affected by Dionysus) and his great empire did not have enough stability to hold together. Later, out of this dissolution Rome arose as the focus of a new empire. The Greeks also absorbed a great deal from the conquered peoples and brought back new ideas, knowledge and skills from the East to the West. However brutal the conquest, the suppression is always accompanied by some degree of assimilation; even when partially absorbed the vanquished still react on the victor, so as to transform him – a process the academics call endomorphosis or interfecundity.

The Romans

By 146 BC Greece had been conquered by Rome, and by 100 BC the Romans began to play a dominating role in the Mediterranean and beyond. The mission of the Romans was to spread out and colonize, implanting their culture into 'barbarian lands'. Their ability with counting, organizing and directing is legendary. Linear thought patterns seem to crystallize into straight roads to move their legions rapidly from one place to another. Architecture and sculpture become more gravity-laden. No longer do we see the flowing lines of drapery as on Greek sculptures; instead a serious kind of rigidity begins to appear. Julius Caesar decided to reform the calendar –

time itself is something to be controlled. Discipline and order were enforced upon people, often by violence, and gladiatorial displays and cruel spectacles such as bear-baiting led to a fear-based society, with excesses of all kinds. Amongst the manifestations of these extremes were the notorious orgies of gluttony and feasting where diners after eating hugely would be given a feather to tickle their throats to make themselves vomit, so they could start feasting all over again.

> Trimalchio, a character of the author Petronius, was always throwing banquets:
>
> 'The guests were offered a hare, tricked out with wings to look like Pegasus, a wild sow with its belly full of thrushes, quinces stuck with thorns to look like sea-urchins, roast pork carved into models of songbirds, fish, geese...'[13]

Here I want to describe a Roman sauce called liquamen that found its way into practically every dish. It was made from a mixture of fish (anchovies or mackerel) fermented for six months with salt in a ratio of 5:1 (giving what is now called enzymic proteolysis). Then old wine, shellfish or other things were added, creating a cheesy, salty flavour. (Perhaps our Lea and Perrins sauce has something of the same quality, but certainly more refined!) Apicius has a recipe for patina of pears to make your hair stand on end. He speaks of pears pounded with pepper, honey, cumin, oil, eggs and liquamen, baked together into a kind of custard.[14]

Although many fresh foods are eaten – asparagus, artichokes, cabbage, kale, broccoli – in general the diet is now departing from the pure, vital sun-quality so cherished by the Greeks. People are eating rotted, fermented foods, meats, animal fats, vinegar, salt and spices which have a hardening, 'mineralizing' effect. They are all Tamasic foods.

From being farmers the Romans turned to being warriors, and for many war was their *raison d'être*. They drew up many laws to do with land and property ownership, citizenship and trading. Society was subject to form and order imposed upon it (our own judicial system has its roots in these times). In their efficient way they were also responsible for many inventions, such as in the area of milling. After thousands of years of grinding grain laboriously in a backward/forward motion, it was discovered that with

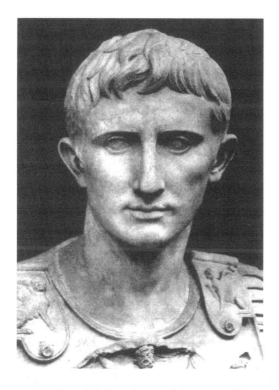

Might the face of this young Roman express the beginnings of a new kind of self-consciousness?

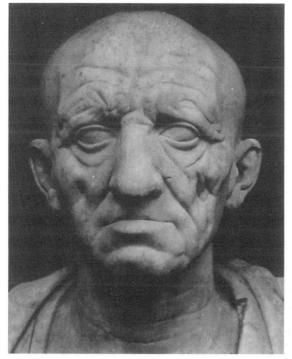

This old Roman citizen appears to be permeated with gravity and weight of responsibility

circular millstones and a donkey walking in a circle the whole process of milling became significantly more efficient. So the Roman miller-baker became one of the first to produce flour in bulk and to mass-produce loaves of bread.

Roman cooks employed large quantities of spices bought from Arab traders. Pepper was valued like gold, and appears in almost every one of Apicius's recipes. Now pepper is a stimulant, but it also acts as an irritant. The role that spices played was somewhere between culinary and medicinal; they activated both the senses and the digestion. Hippocrates used peppercorns medicinally in combination with honey and vinegar for feminine disorders. Salt increased in use as a condiment. Soldiers in the imperial army were paid a *salarium*, their wages, partly in coin and partly in salt (hence our word 'salary').

During its later days the glittering displays of Rome masked a moral and spiritual bankruptcy: 'Indeed, the whole development of reason now seemed to have undercut its own basis, with the human mind denying itself the capacity for genuine knowledge of the world, while reason and verbal skills were coming to have a less than impeccable reputation.'[15]

The Beginning of Christianity
(during the Age of Pisces, AD 215–2375)

The teachings of Jesus of Nazareth drew from the many mystery schools around the eastern Mediterranean and the rich traditions of the Israelites, encompassing resurrection and reunion with God. They also owed much to the context of the Graeco-Roman period.

> The old idea of the initiate-king has been raised to a new and more inward level, that of the individual spiritual Self, and no longer looks back to an atavistic loss of identity. The 'Kingdom of Heaven' is to be achieved, not through outward action, but by a breakthrough in consciousness.[16]

The emphasis was on reconnecting with the soul and spirit through a process involving scrupulous self-examination. Many of his parables are to do with a person's relationship with himself in his social and natural environment. They are stories of relatedness, bringing a new kind of morality into a divided world. The people he chose to surround himself with were simple, heart-filled people, and women had a special place in this group. What emerged from these teachings was a call to break the binding and often suffocating blood-ties of tribe or civilization, to find one's own spiritually nourishing family and personal freedom. After centuries of bondage to duty and obligation, the human being could *begin slowly to make his own choices.*

Before Jesus' great sacrifice on the cross he initiated a new cultus in the form of a shared meal. Here earth elements, bread and wine, are sacralized to act as a leaven, Christ's body and blood, working in the human body, soul and spirit.

I am the Bread of Life,
I am the Fine Vine.

Placed into the Passover setting this community-forming, symbolic meal[17] became the centre of a new religion, Christianity. Jesus as Christ reminded us that death was but a transition.

By the close of the fourth century Christianity had become the official religion of the Roman Empire and began to take on the warlike, patriarchal and legalistic images of Roman society.

The early Christian centuries and the meeting of cultures

In the Greek world emphasis was given to the human psyche with its ability to interact with the physical world and the development of logic. Rome took this logic and used it to explore the material world. Christianity bought a new moral-ethical dimension. When the Muslim religion arrived in the Mediterranean world all of these influences were fused within it, especially strongly in Spain. The synthesis of these diverse cultural impulses brought tremendous intellectual insight and artistic creativity.

The Arabs had dominated the spice trade, by which they gained great wealth and knowledge of many nations and cultures. They set up great centres of learning and new traditions of investigation, including medicine, mathematics and astronomy, strongly centred on spiritual values.

The Christian empire of Byzantium, which had inherited much of Greek learning, was now divided by controversies over dogma and saw the exodus of many learned 'heretics' to the more tolerant Zoroastrian Persia. There at Jundishapur they met Syrian, Hindu and Persian scholars and amongst their studies of science, art and religion they developed a particular interest in dietetic medicine. Their cooking, which had been raised to a high art, was a fusion of influences from Persia, sweetmeats from Egypt, black truffles from the Arabian desert, and dishes such as cous-cous and moussaka.

> A dish of the nomads called *hais* sounds both nutritious and medicinal:
>
> '1 lb of breadcrumbs to be kneaded with $\frac{3}{4}$ lb of stoned dates, the same of almonds and pistachio nuts ... some honey and coriander kneaded together with some sesame oil ... this made into balls and sprinkled with powdered sugar'[18]

As the Arab cuisine brought together recipes and ingredients from many sources, so the Arab mind was also receptive to all the intellectual influences of the known world. Works they studied included the writings of the Greek physician Galen; these were transported to a medical school in Salerno, Italy, flourishing under the care of the Benedictine monks of Monte Cassino. This school was noted for its eclecticism and freedom from dogma. The Muslim influence contributed an important emphasis on hygiene and dietary practices. The Arabs also had a profound understanding of agriculture, building extraordinarily strong and beautiful irrigation systems; water was particularly esteemed and precious in their culture.

> There is an old Cordoba agricultural calendar dated AD 961 which shows they were still working with the wisdom of the stars. It is based on the solar year and gives the position of the stars each month. How closely their lives were woven into the seasons and how they loved all the signs and activities of the times of year —
>
> *For the month of January:* 'at this time the water in the rivers feels tepid ... The sap rises in the wood of the trees, birds mate. The falcons of Valencia build their nests and begin to mate. Horses feed on young shoots. Cows calve and the milk yield increases. Now is the time to plant grain, to put in stakes for the olive and pomegranate trees. The early narcissi bloom. Trellises are put up for early vines. Purslane should be planted and sugar cane harvested, beet preserved and syrup prepared from bitter lemons.'

In February: 'the young birds hatch. The bees propagate. The sea creatures stir. The women begin to tend the silkworm eggs and wait for them to burst. The cranes make for the river islands. Saffron bulbs should be planted and spring cabbage sown. Truffles can be found now and the wild asparagus grows. Mace begins to send out shoots. This is the month to send out letters to recruit summer labourers. Storks and swallows return to their homes . . .'[19]

As the strength of the Roman Empire declined, life returned to basics in many areas. Indeed, these early years of Christianity were beleaguered by severe famines, plagues and attacks on crops. One such attack was the first outbreak of ergotism in AD 857 in the Rhine Valley, from which thousands of people died, poisoned by their daily bread. Ergot is a strange fungus that grows on rye crops (see p. 104), but is not now common in Britain.

So the centuries after the fall of the Roman Empire were times of con-solidation. The diet of the rich and poor was not too dissimilar. Most people were obliged to live upon bread, water and ale and a *companaticum* (i.e. that which goes with bread), usually vegetables and pulses, simmered together in a cauldron that was seldom emptied, with the addition of whatever else might be available – if you were lucky a hen or a rabbit or some dumplings. As the traditional rhyme goes, 'Pease pudding hot, pease pudding cold, pease pudding in the pot, nine days old.' Not a pleasant prospect!

Frumenty was a nutritious grain dish, either sweet or savoury, made by soaking hulled wheat in hot water for 24 hours in an earthenware crock and placing it in the hearth; this was then eaten flavoured with milk and honey or some of the remains from the companaticum. It would be eaten for a great deal of the time.

The Middle Ages

It was to be in the monasteries that culture flourished in Europe in the Middle Ages. Here was the seat of learning where also arts and crafts were studied and taught. The arts of gardening, cooking, baking and brewing, calligraphy and illuminating manuscripts thrived in these stable communi-ties. Prayer, meditation and chanting also helped to focus their efforts on a higher reality. Though the royal courts might show a fashion in imported delicacies, the monastic communities demonstrated sound ecological practice usually leading to a high degree of self-sufficiency.

Such a community would be centred on the church as the place for worship, the living quarters of the monks for sleep and study. Beyond this stretched the medicinal garden, planted with many varieties of herbs, the vegetable garden, the fruit orchards, the coniger for rabbits, the pond for carp, beehives for honey (also used in the making of mead), fields for grain and surrounding woods for the acorn-grubbing pigs. Not only was this very practical, it also had a wonderful aesthetic that harmonized with the landscape.

The great Gothic cathedrals such as Chartres were built on ancient sites, on a place where telluric currents worked through outcrops of granite and lime. They were prehistoric places of pilgrimage. All the Gothic cathedrals sprang up within a space of two hundred years.

We might see in the figure of Francis of Assisi (d. 1226) the converging of the teachings of both Christ and Buddha. The example of this man's life, his relationship to sun, moon, brother, sister, beast, bird and flower, shone as a beacon in the darker ages to follow.

By 1095 the Crusades had begun and in AD 1115 the compass was invented. These events and more were preparations leading up to the flowering of Medieval Europe.

The growth of the medieval towns in Europe, the formation of the craftsmen's guilds, and surplus time and money all contributed to a degree of individual freedom hitherto unknown. Greek and Roman cities and towns had been based on slave labour, but the medieval town was founded on the work of free people, for whom the motivation of money began to play an ever-increasing role.

Questions were beginning to be asked, and one of these questions was to do with the reality of the substances consecrated for the Christian sacrament. The awe of the mystical was fading. People began to look beyond the boundaries of Europe and the Mediterranean. The account of Marco Polo's journey to the fabulous East was published around 1300. Desire for spices intensified, causing chaos in the spice trade; so many middlemen were taking their percentage that many countries decided to trade directly with the Spice Islands. This, of course, in turn stimulated the shipping trade; new, stronger ships, now with three masts instead of one, were built, making them faster and no longer dependent on oar-power.

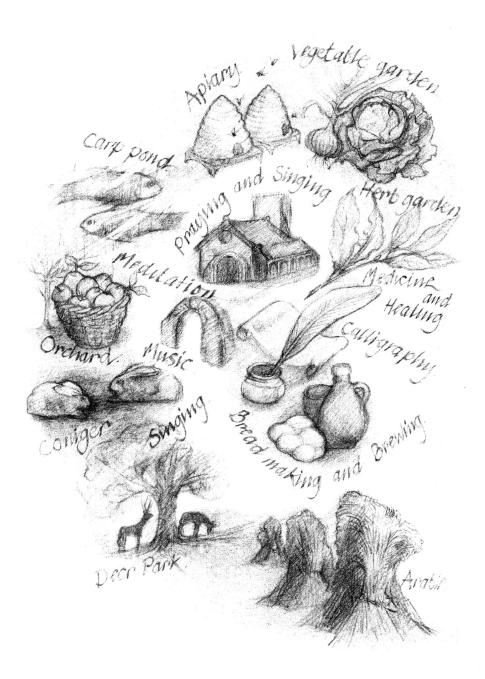

The medieval monastery was often a fine example of good ecological principle

Venice alone was estimated to be bringing 2500 tons a year of pepper-corns and ginger to Europe; pepper was still as precious as gold. Then there were cinnamon, nutmeg, cloves, coriander, turmeric, cardamom, saffron, vanilla and many other spices.

The value of spices

What was it they were seeking at this particular time that spices offered – those minute gifts of nature, seeds, roots, bark, so laden with aroma and flavour?

Spices have the capacity of stimulating and awakening the senses. They make possible the realization of many potentials in nature and the human being by virtue of broadening the palate and creating an interface with far-off exotic places. Eventually everyone would want to go there. If we can imagine being fed for a lifetime on a diet of turnips, swedes, barley and wheat (as opposed to a subtly spiced curry or some of the other culinary delights we have described), I think you may agree one would perhaps remain a little dull in consciousness.

The age of exploration

Spices generally have an expansive effect and, for the human being at this point of his development, they encouraged his need to know, to explore and to colonize the world. In the figures of Christopher Columbus and Vasco da Gama we meet two men whose destiny was to discover new lands and cultures and new foodstuffs; their journeys were to change the known world very significantly.

The existence of the Americas was already known in certain circles;[20] it was also known that the development of these countries would speed up the increasing materialistic tendency in the West. Columbus had access to certain maps and began his journey without the blessing of the Church. In 1492 he set off, sponsored by Queen Isabella of Spain, ostensibly in search of 'spices and Christians'. As a result of his discoveries in the New World many new foodstuffs, and with them new impulses, were brought to Europe and spread around the world. Maize, or 'Indian corne', was introduced to Europe to become a staple in Northern Spain, Portugal and Italy, and later the Balkans. Potatoes, tomatoes, red and green peppers, peanuts, vanilla, tapioca and the turkey were all discovered and brought back. All of them have made an increasing impact on the diet of the West.

To Asia from the Americas went pineapple, papaya and sweet potatoes. Chilli peppers and potatoes became the staple food of the Sherpas in Nepal by the nineteenth century. Maize, manioc, sweet potatoes, groundnuts, beans and later pineapples served to augment the narrow variety of food plants in Africa. Christopher Columbus carried vegetable seeds, wheat, chickpeas and sugar cane with him when he returned to the Caribbean on subsequent voyages. He was an extraordinary man – voyager, botanist and horticulturalist. Columbus had found the New World and by his fourth voyage in 1504 he had discovered the West Indies and settled at least 20 islands, but now he was a dying man, returning to Spain with tobacco but also with syphilis. Much blood was spilt in all these adventures.

To Colombia in 1543 went wheat, barley, chickpeas, broad beans and vegetables as well as the first cattle. Bananas, rice and citrus fruits (natives of Asia) were in turn transplanted to the New World. It was as if the whole world was one big garden; the soil must have been still fertile and receptive.

The Renaissance produced wonderful works of art dedicated to reproducing nature as exactly as possible. In Leonardo da Vinci we meet an artist not only striving for beauty but also for accuracy in scientific research. He dissected the human corpse, hitherto a complete taboo, to record what was working physically beneath the human skin, taking the analytical approach a step further.

Coffee and other stimulants

Coffee now began to make an appearance (see also pp. 251–2). Originating in Kenya or Ethiopia, it spread to Arabia where many of the new ideas in science, medicine and mathematics were thriving. Quickness of thought and an ability to work well in the world of numbers was characteristic of the Arabs. Coffee contains the stimulant caffeine; its flavour and aroma and stimulating propensities are only produced when the bean is roasted and ground, which could be seen as a further intensification of the ripening process. (Even to the point of being rather 'mineralized'. The seed is the most mineralized, dense part of the plant and its inherent flavours become intensified and released through grinding.)

In 1637 an Englishman, John Evelyn, wrote of meeting the first person he had ever seen to drink coffee, 'a Greek who was studying at Oxford'. The practice became very popular and many coffee-houses appeared, becoming centres for the discussion of ideas. Journals were read and intellectual pursuits generally followed, being quite distinct from the atmosphere in alehouses. Samuel Pepys gives a good impression of London coffee-houses in his diaries.

The delights of tea-drinking were also being discovered. In1657 the first public tea sale in England took place, but tea carried with it a different mood from coffee and found itself more at home in salons where diplomatic 'chit-chat' was cultivated. Chocolate also started to become popular, especially with the Spanish (see pp. 255–6).

These three new substances taken in the form of drinks, which have a quicker effect on the blood-stream than foods that have to be chewed, were taken up cautiously at first and then with great fervour in Europe and America. They work on the nervous system as stimulants and cannot really be classified as truly nutritional substances, but they too have played their part in man's awakening, mainly by stimulating intellectual processes. Unfortunately, they do tend to develop addictions and over-use of coffee particularly can lead to serious health problems.

The other seemingly incongruous food plant which was introduced into the Western diet was the nightshade or *Solanaceae* family, all members of which have a lesser or greater degree of poison in them. They are the potato, the tomato, the capsicum or bell pepper, chillies, the aubergine or eggplant, and the tobacco plant. The potato, at first treated with great suspicion, was later embraced enthusiastically as a staple. Previously humanity had been nourished by the starchy cereals but now we see the beginning of a wide-spread consumption of new foods that stimulate the head processes, unlike the cereals which nourish the totality. To this last group of foodstuffs we can also add cane sugar, which came to be demanded in increasingly greater quantities.

Such trends brought about significant changes in agricultural practices and the beginnings of a globalization of food, along with *changing chemistry both in the earth and the human being*. In addition, plantations of tea, coffee, cocoa and sugar all used slaves who suffered great hardship, poverty and social ills.

Towards rationalism

In the seventeenth century scepticism and dissatisfaction over the understanding of man's relationship to the earth and the heavens brought forth a particular constellation of men whose ideas appeared in the short period of 1596–1666. These philosophical and scientific ideas gave a new interpretation of man's place: he was seen as created by God purposely to have dominion over nature, in a world observed to operate in a mechanical, measurable way. The initial wonder and interest with which people of the Middle Ages such as Paracelsus viewed the world of nature was to give way to a ruthless pursuit of methods to harness nature in a purely utilitarian fashion, motivated by desire for control, power and wealth. In the early sixteenth century, Copernicus in effect deposed the earth from its central position as hub of the universe, and the human being was thereby also dethroned, his values apparently of no real importance in the vast impersonal universe. Some of the key thinkers who followed were Bacon, Kepler, Galileo, Newton and Descartes – all men of religion. When taken out of context, their work led to a duality which was a simplistic interpretation of their philosophies. Science, art and religion became separated and the basis was laid for Darwin's theory of evolution – 'the survival of the fittest'.

Bacon studied the measurable, calculable world and thought he was freeing matter from contamination by theological superstition. He proclaimed, 'Let us unlock all of nature's secrets.' Descartes discovered analytical geometry and divided the physical world from the mind; soul was equated with mind, and all possibility of an inner vitalizing principle was dismissed. With Descartes came doubt. Newton formulated a way of understanding why all the planets remained in orbit around the sun and why heavy objects fell back to the earth – the concept of gravity – but he was in fact looking at the whole creation and its God-given laws.

Christianity and the Church gradually lost power, particularly over the minds of the intelligentsia. As the background to these battles for the minds of men, I would like to remind us of the new foods that have been available – potatoes, sugar and chocolate – and the increasing consumption of salt, coffee, tea, along with tobacco and opium.

The growth of city life

The seventeenth and eighteenth centuries saw the growth of city life. New professions were created, merchants' associations were established and universities expanded to include sciences as well as classics and the arts. The world population had grown to over 500 million. Foods had to be transported in from the countryside and each city had its own great market. Rotting produce, blood and offal thrown into the cities' rivers created terribly unhygienic conditions, often resulting in plagues of disease. Fraudulent practices arose amongst tradespeople, who saw their customers as merely a means of monetary gain. Wooden nutmegs, junipers sold as peppercorns, flour adulterated with alum (a whitening agent), brick dust in cocoa, tea adulterated with used dried tea leaves stiffened with gum, pepper contaminated with floor-sweepings and other trickery were commonplace. These frauds could be detected by increasingly strong microscopic lenses, and they gave rise to the first indications of loss of trust in the foods people were buying and eating. The city dweller thus soon began to lose contact with nature and the community of agricultural life, and the bonds that had always held people together by mutual respect were quickly eroded. Strong and punitive laws had to be introduced to deal with such swindling.

The French Revolution of 1789, with its high principles of equality, liberty and brotherhood, sought to throw off the stranglehold of the aristocracy (at this time the cost of a loaf of bread was equivalent to a working man's daily earnings). New ways of baking bread with special yeasts were introduced as the old, naturally leavened bread was considered unhealthy by the scientific fraternity. New specialized yeasts were introduced (see p. 171).

The Napoleonic wars resulted in the blockading of British ports; Napoleon had identified England as a 'nation of shopkeepers' and knew what would hurt. Coffee and sugar were scarce but soon chicory root was used as a coffee substitute and sugar beet developed as an alternative source of sugar. Food science and chemistry were well on their way.

The age of ore and oil

We now come to the Industrial Revolution in the nineteenth century which brought further radical changes. Iron and steel made it possible to build huge, intricate and powerful machines. The population of England is esti-mated to have more than doubled during the hundred years between 1800 and 1900 and could no longer be properly fed. Grain was therefore imported from America, and tea from India and China in greater and greater quantities. Railways proliferated, enabling all classes to travel and made possible the rapid transport of goods.

British factory workers lived on a diet of tea, bread and potatoes, with perhaps a little bacon at the weekends. Bread was already being made from sifted flour. Fresh fruit and vegetables were seldom eaten and, predictably, the health of the working people declined. Little fresh air or sunlight com-bined with appalling pollution and long hours in gruelling factory condi-tions led to many diseases, tuberculosis being the most common. Children were sent to work in the factories often by the age of seven. The Romantic poets and artists, Keats, Coleridge, Wordsworth, Ruskin, Goethe and Schiller, protested at what they saw as a terrible dragon unleashed in Eur-ope, but particularly in England in the Industrial Age. However, nothing was to stand in the way of this dragon; even larger gaps widened between the rich and the poor, now without the benign patronage of the feudal system. A burgeoning and increasingly prosperous middle class set the pace for a new consumerism and French-style ten-course dinners became the rage.

Darwin's contribution to the story of life widened the split of the human being from any heavenly connection. The popular perception of Darwin's work reduces man to a 'sophisticated ape'. The universe was irreversibly moving, in Darwin's scheme, towards dissipation and 'heat death'. After the Civil War (1865) America quickly started to change from an agricultural nation to a manufacturing one. Agricultural products were processed into transportable commodities. Breweries, flour mills, tanneries all grew like mushrooms. Canning, freezing and chilling enabled meat and other foods to be transported long distances, and this encouraged the proliferation of cattle farming. Canned meat from Australia was half the price of fresh meat from England. Texas ranchers were to clear the Great Plains of both bison and Indians (who had relied on them for meat and skins). Freezing processes began, using volatile chemicals such as liquefied ammonia; ice became increasingly in demand and was used extensively in the fishing industry.

Scientific knowledge continued to be applied to questions of food pre-servation. The French microbiologist Louis Pasteur in 1895 identified cer-tain micro-organisms as responsible for the spoilage of food. The discovery of this new world of microbiology set up a terrible aversion to germs and a subsequent combative approach to their elimination. Pasteurization was developed to sterilize food products selectively by heating them to 72°C.

These hygiene requirements led eventually to standardization and pre-packaging, with brand names. City life for the wealthy began to focus on new fashions in clothes, food delicacies and novelty. The expansion of the population, of trade, of scientific discoveries and inventions was to bring such great and rapid change as had never been possible before, when horseback, boat or foot had been the only means of transport.

The England of Queen Victoria conjures up an image of colonial self-satisfaction. Countries had been conquered and divided up with little thought for natural boundaries, ethnicity or language, a lack of sensitivity that led to centuries of conflict. England presided over a vast colony that gave rise to the feeling that she had a right to transport her way of life anywhere else in the world. This kind of life appeared to have an outer stability, the strength of iron, but society was utterly repressed on many levels (reflected in the corsetted bodies of womenfolk, not an inch of whose body should be exposed). Table manners were carried to a farcical level where the butler was obliged to measure a two-foot space between diners in case there was any bodily contact between men and women! It is small wonder that there has been a strong reaction to such prudishness.

Everything had to be standardized, from bicycles to sewing machines, even time – Greenwich Mean Time was created. Business required that the trains run on time! All measurements were standardized, to enable the precision needed for mass-production. Of course there is a practicality in all of this; the problem was that in such a drive for rationalized efficiency there was little room for the eccentric, the magical or the mystical, even heaven with its chubby cherubs seemed to be utterly gravity-laden.

By the end of the nineteenth century the sign of the age had become clear. The first wave of the Industrial Revolution was over, the grossest injustices had been apparently corrected, and a sense of material complacency seemed to settle over the civilized world. The main purpose in life now was the production of material goods. The supply and distribution of agricultural products no longer dominated life. Thanks to the railways, the effects of crop failure in one region could be minimized by transporting from another. Scientific and technological progress dominated many aspects of life and within a generation would start to control the life of the farmer as well.

Initially the raw materials that fuelled the industrial age were iron ore and coal, but with increasing diversification a variety of metallic ores were exploited and the most important energy source became oil. Ore and oil are the materials upon which our modern life is founded. They do not bring harmony or a sense of health, instead they hold out a promise: *a seductive promise of a life of comfort and luxury*. Human ingenuity has achieved tremendous control over ore and oil. However, it does not enquire into their origins, nor has it had much concern over the consequences its products have on creation. These substances are put to work for man, carrying out his most egotistical and most selfless desires with equal efficiency. There seems to have been little place for questions of ethics or morality in the world of technology; the position taken is often, 'If we *can* then do!' But oil and ore are substances with no spark of life in them.

The petrochemical era

The petrochemical industry became firmly established after the Second World War and began to produce many products hitherto not present on the earth, such as artificial fertilizers, pesticides, fungicides, plastics, then food additives, colourants, preservatives, stabilizers, pharmacological drugs, and many others, all having particular brand names. The spread of their popularity was achieved by abundant advertising.

Psychiatrists Freud and Jung had made their mark in many ways, mostly upon the educated classes. The work they had begun on the hidden, suppressed desire-life was taken up by many advertising companies and politicians, who studied how to manipulate people's desires. The emerging individual found himself offered an endless stream of things to crave for. Freud built upon Darwin's perspective, but now brought convincing evidence for the existence of a submerged and unconscious life in the human being that directed feeling and behaviour. Jung focused on the dream-life and its ability to access a pool of 'collective unconscious', a world of archetypes and symbols. Contemporary with Jung was Rudolf Steiner, who founded the Anthroposophical Society in 1913.

It was soon realized that desires could be continuously stimulated by new products, as long as there was money to buy them. So began the necessity to work for more money, and to have credit facilities. The banks and governments would then have a large source of credit as well as taxes to finance their projects. Money has become a new god. Here was the beginning of a very cynical development – seeing people as consumers to be exploited by the manufacturing and advertising conglomerates.

The fascination with science as a panacea to end all ills took hold of the consumer's imagination. In relation to food, new processed convenience foods appear to have been met with enthusiasm by a population tired of post-war austerity and having to do everything 'the hard way'. Because these new foods had to be transported and stored for periods of time, food chemists were inventing diverse ways of making this possible. Drying, freezing or canning all change the taste, texture and colour of foods (not to mention their nutritional quality), but apparently this was not a matter for concern, to begin with at least.

Colourants were added for a good appearance; for taste, various powders such as monosodium glutamate or cyclamates (artificial sweeteners). Anti-caking agents were added to prevent the lumping of substances such as salt, sugar and powdered milk; emulsifying agents to help homogenization of substances that would normally separate (such as fats and milk), and sequestrants to stop trace minerals causing fats and oils to go rancid or to prevent cloudiness in soft drinks. The use of chemical preservatives was seen as the cheapest method of preserving food and the number of artificial substances permitted for use in the food industry now runs into huge catalogues. Many health problems have been traced to the ingestion of these substances, children often being the most vulnerable. If the cost of consequent medical treatment were included in the cost of manufacture we would have very different statistics. Luckily the public is becoming sensitized to this problem. Pressure groups have been formed which have had some effect in, for instance, the labelling of foods, though there are still loopholes as we shall see.

In the realm of agriculture, science has also held sway over the past 50 years (see pp. 64–7). Experimentation in plant breeding, as with cereals, has resulted in all kinds of distortions with the use of mineral fertilizers. Lady Eve Balfour, founder member of the Soil Association, once remarked that the use of such fertilizers merely amounted to the 'art of making water stand upright'. Lodging (being easily blown down) of cereals and distortion of gluten content were amongst some of the results. Further experimentation showed that new, so-called improved cultivars, unless they receive sufficient water, strict pest and disease control, together with abundant fertilizer, do less well in poor soil than the lower-yielding traditional varieties. Some countries end up with 'grain mountains', where others starve. Now we have biotechnology and genetic modifications, whose advocates insist their motives in pressing forward with this technology are to solve world hunger.

Meanwhile there is an increasing incidence of gluten intolerance, the reasons for which are not completely understood (see Chapter 4). But it is in the hybridizing of wheat, forcing it to contain more and more gluten, that part of the problem lies, making it totally unbalanced. Therefore it is not the wheat, that 'sun-related' grain that has fed humanity faithfully for thousands of years, that is at fault but its qualitative manipulation.

To find real answers to these growing problems we need to remind ourselves of the larger picture. Pest control has its definite limitations, since most of the chemicals used tend to destroy not only the pests themselves but their predators (e.g. ladybirds, which eat aphids), not to mention the bees and butterflies, which are needed for the pollination process. Despite chemical treatments the pests and fungal diseases become stronger and more tenacious. Fifty years of what amounts to chemical warfare in agriculture have shown only too poignantly a lack of insight into the finely balanced, integrative forces at work in nature, and this at great cost to the environment and human health, both psychologically and physically.

Diseases of our time reveal increases in conditions linked to diet and the environment, such as heart disease, asthma (one in five children in Britain is a sufferer) and respiratory diseases, diabetes, cirrhosis of the liver, cancers, coeliac disease, candida, ADD, so the list goes on. The government gave the largest percentage of a recent budget to the National Health Service for more hospitals, doctors, nurses and technology. Many people expect to have a heart by-pass or a hip replacement or some kind of serious medical intervention in their lives. Our lack of health costs billions of pounds annually, but where is the budget for health education, nutrition and cooking classes and gardening in our schools? Where is the emphasis on good organic agriculture and husbandry without resorting to poisons, leading to mass illness?

Another recent phenomenon is the extraordinary proliferation of fast food chains, serving cheap take-away food, often eaten whilst walking in the street. The British, eager to take on an American life-style, are the highest consumers of fast foods in Europe. But we should surely take heed that 'every day, in the USA, roughly 200,000 people are taken sick by a food-borne disease, 900 are hospitalized and 14 die. One quarter of the USA's population suffers a bout of food poisoning each year, as a result of the nation's industrialized and centralized food system'.[21]

Here in Britain there are those who are proud that our agriculture involves less than 2 per cent of the population, and this figure is dwindling rapidly. After the foot-and-mouth crisis more farmers have left the land and their children are leaving too. For many men and women release from the arduous yoke of agricultural work, which never really ends, may be a relief, but for many it is a sadness, a tragedy. As for the rest of us, we have not yet felt the true impact of this revolution. One day perhaps not too far in the future we will realize that we cannot eat money. None of us would advocate returning to medieval times and I personally am grateful for much that science has brought us, but some of these possibilities have been gained at the expense of the rest of humanity. Science and technology can only be truly helpful when integrated with a truly moral/ethical understanding of life.

There is an apparently huge range of choices for the privileged minority in this world. Certainly we are given that impression when we walk into supermarkets with their vast areas of products, but one only has to observe the contents of another shopper's trolley to have a pretty good idea what kind of household they run and what the family mealtimes are like. Many people are buying 'photographs of meals', for the gaily coloured, appetizing meals pictured on the packaging seldom measure up to the frozen factory meals inside – they are 'virtual meals'. Britain buys over 80 per cent of her food from supermarkets (Soil Association figures). In having so many choices, are we awake to what we are choosing? What are we supporting with those choices? How much support do we give to our local farms?

Our journey has taken us from the beginnings of settled communities where the tension arose between the 'childlike nomad' and the bounded territory of the first settled farmer, past the first priestly directors of cultivation to the star wisdom of the Egyptians and Chaldeans, the exuberant Minoans, the Greeks with their nature oracles – all these peoples had the Mother principle of fertility and fecundity at their core, their lives had lightness, creativity and abundance.

From the Roman Empire onwards there emerges the hero-warrior, the patriarch, the rise of the nation state with its boundaries and flag, and participative, intuitive and inclusive feminine qualities were subsumed in what was to become the scientific-technological age. Humanity certainly lost its original connection to the spiritual worlds and to food as sacred substance; now we in the West live in a largely secular society. In the blinking of an eye we have dismantled so much of what formerly nourished humanity, gave it hope and vision.

How is it — presuming all events to be random or chance — one event bears fruit and another does not? What would have happened if Goethe's theory of colour had prevailed over Newton's? How would it have been if Al Gore had become President of the United States rather than George Bush in these particularly daunting times? What soil had been prepared for Darwin's ideas to take such firm root? Goethe once said, 'There is nothing so powerful as an idea whose time has come.'

We can see how clever the human being has become, but specialization has brought fragmentation and our relationship with our planet needs to be reconstituted — a matter of great urgency if we are to survive. Surely no other creature would foul its nest the way the Western impulse has pillaged the planet and scattered its detritus. We need now to create a different set of imaginations from which to work, a new loom upon which to weave our notion of creation, if we are to heal the wounded Anfortas, reconnect with our story, and heal Mother Earth.

Our food will play a vital part in any kind of spiritual renewal; it is one of our most important interfaces with the planet and the human family. If food is not vital — fully alive — then we will find it difficult to have inspiring ideas. What we grow and what we import has an enormous impact on the earth, and when we look at the journey of origins we can see that most of the foods and drinks since the discovery of the Americas have an acidic and mineralizing effect on both the human constitution and soil chemistry (see Chapters 14 and 15). To remind you, some of the main food items that have spread around the world during the last four hundred years are: potatoes, tomatoes, soya, grapes for wine, rapeseed, coffee, tea, cocoa, sugar, peanuts, the use of extra salt and mineral supplements. Many of these 'foods' have a one-sided effect upon the brain and nervous system.

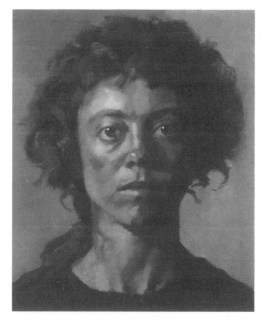

A young twenty-first century woman: independent, conscious and alert

Look at the faces of the Egyptian and the Romans (pp. 29, 39). Can you detect a densifying process, something descending and solidifying? What meets you in their expression? In the face of the twenty-first-century woman can we detect a new impulse?

Rudolf Steiner spoke of three different developments in the human journey. The first was the 'time of the sentient soul', when early childlike people lived in their vivid pictorial imaginations in a dreamlike consciousness. Next came the 'intellectual soul development', a waking-up stage in which the Western stream particularly has been immersed; and then (through the individuation process and capacity for independent choice) 'the consciousness soul' development, where the human being will have the opportunity for ethical individualism and a growing world awareness, but *through a heightened ability for self-consciousness and self-regulation.*

Upon this gifted stage, in its dark hour,
Rains from the sky, a meteoric shower
Of facts ... They lie unquestioned and uncombined.
Wisdom enough to leech us of our ill
Is daily spun, but there exists no loom
To weave it into fabric.

From Huntsman, What Quarry?
by Edna St Vincent Millay

Our task now will be to see if we can discover the 'loom'.

AGRICULTURAL METHODS

As I mentioned in the Introduction, my childhood was spent in the agricultural area of Bedfordshire. Despite the background of war and ration books I nevertheless experienced life and nature as abundant. From a tiny packet of seeds we would have a garden full of lettuces, cornflowers, radishes. How could this tiny seed grow into something as big as our cabbages? It was a miracle, no less.

Since we had no television at that time (the late forties) the outdoor world was our playground, and living with the seasons gave great comfort and safety. I watched the hedgerows and knew the nests and the birds that laid their eggs in them. To this day the rare sight of the heavenly blue of a clutch of blackbird eggs still brings a tremble of awe in my heart, for that vulnerable preciousness of bird life. The hedgerows represented a slice of condensed history – some of them went back to good Queen Bess's time. They were full of hips and haws, sloes, blackberries and hazelnuts in autumn and in spring perfumed blossoms and garlands of honeysuckle. They were as beautiful as they were useful, to birds, insects, field mice, beetles, grazing cows and to humans. Harvesting wild food was part of our seasonal rhythm.

Blackberry jam on a slice of newly baked bread was a treat, as were the first strawberries of the season with top of the milk. I loved getting up early in the autumn to search for field mushrooms which were plentiful in those days, dew-covered white domes with tender pink gills, nestling secretly in lush grassy knolls. The field had to be impregnated with cow pats for the mushroom spores to flourish; nothing cultivated approaches their flavour. These fields were usually full of wonderful wild flowers and herbs, buttercups, milkmaids, clovers, ragged robin, plantain and wild sorrel, to name but a few. The cows seemed to love this variety of plants and, need I say, the milk was incomparable in its creaminess and flavour with what is sold now.

Of course, you can still find fields with wild flowers and ancient hedgerows, but they tend to be in places where agribusiness has not prevailed, such as South Devon where I live now. Here is one of the attractions that drew me – the splendid hedgerows with high banks, studded with a procession of wild flowers from February onwards – snowdrops, primroses, violets and miniature daffodils, which give way to bluebells, red campion, stitchwort and marguerites, in turn eclipsed by waves of magenta foxgloves ('like Red Indian braves' said D.H. Lawrence), all in a landscape of small farms flanked by the moors and their granite outcrops.

My friend's father had cows and was somewhat entrepreneurial. He decided to try his hand at making ice-cream. This was cause for great excitement in the village. We had to take bowls from home to receive luscious scoops of creamy stuff; it couldn't be hoarded because most of us didn't have fridges, so it was a treat, and a rare one, too. Here was the beginning of what became a thriving business, a farmer diversifying from one of his basic products and realizing a lot of 'value added'. Another neighbour started with yoghourt, which took longer to catch on, the sourness being quite foreign to the British who by now had developed a very sweet tooth.

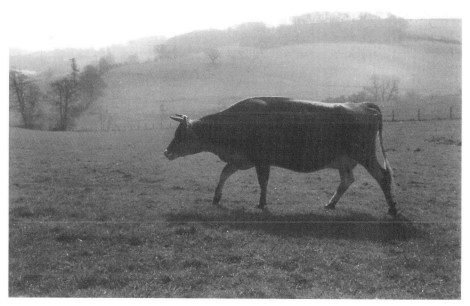

The cow with her marvellous digestive capacities and fertility is prominent in biodynamic agriculture

The present crisis and its history

Now our farming industry is in crisis. The year 2001 saw the slaughter of 10 million cattle in the foot-and-mouth epidemic, over half of them healthy. (I have found a figure of 95% in an article. We hear that 50% of all farmers harmed by the foot-and-mouth epidemic are determined to leave agriculture, their average age being 50. In June 2002 the *Western Morning News* gave the weekly suicides of farmers as more than one a week.) The sight of those vast pyrrhic heaps is etched indelibly in our memories. Before that it was BSE.

> BSE – bovine spongiform encephalopathy – 'In England the disease became widespread in beef cattle as a result of the unnatural practice of feeding them parts of carcases of sheep infected with scrapie (the ovine form of BSE). Human cases of this fatal brain disease that result from eating the meat of infected cows are well documented.'
> Dr Andrew Weil, *Eating Well for Optimum Health*.

What will future generations excavating these burial pits make of our culture? Many farmers left their farms or tragically took their lives, unable to face the future, and the knowledge of farming practices accumulated over generations went with them. Even in conventional farming a vast amount of agricultural knowledge is incontestably being lost at a terrifying speed. The broadcaster John Humphrys has commented, 'If we compressed our time on earth into one 24-hour period the past 50 years would register as a microsecond. We have done more to disrupt the cycle in that micro-second, that blink of an eye, than in our entire history.'[1]

How did this come about? In Chapter 1 we looked at some of the defining moments of millennia of patient cultivation and plant breeding. Thousands of years have passed in this unhurried process of observing soil, skies, plants and cosmic rhythms, of experimenting, taking risks, experiencing crop failure, famine and abundance. Much had happened to drive people off the land in the intervening years, beginning in Britain with the Enclosure Acts. By the seventeenth century over six million acres of common land had been annexed and enclosed.[2] British agriculture virtually collapsed after the repeal of the Corn Laws in 1846. Later, in the Depression of the 1930s, there was a further dramatic fall in agricultural prices, bringing more resentment against the ruling classes.

The folly of this lack of insight was realized when war was declared and Britain, whose lifeline depended on imported food and other goods shipped from her colonies, was found to have only three weeks' supply of wheat and one month's supply of sugar. We had been importing more than 22 million tons of food and animal feed, requiring a fleet of 3000 merchant ships to criss-cross the Atlantic. When German U-boats put an end to that, food rationing was quickly introduced.

> *Wartime Rations* —
> An adult's weekly allowance at one point in 1942 was: 2 oz butter, 4 oz margarine, 8 oz sugar, 2 oz oatmeal, 4 oz cheese, 2 half pints of milk, and 1 oz of tea. 1 lb of preserves (jam, marmalade, honey etc.) had to last four weeks. Fresh eggs and oranges all but disappeared. You had to register with a particular grocer and butcher. It is said people were healthier on this. Rationing ended in 1954, meat being last to be derationed.

During the war food policies were directed at maximizing agricultural production; everybody was exhorted to 'dig for Britain'. Ornamental and park gardens were dug up to grow food crops and many women took to the land with the Land Army. Those of us in Britain who had survived the food shortages continued to suffer rationing of some items including bread (not rationed during the war). It was said by many that people were healthier during these years, but it must have depended on whether there was access to fresh vegetables (not rationed if you grew them). There was as well a large psychological factor, because people became united and purposeful, prepared to make sacrifices, all of which contributes to a nation's health. In response to the shortages much food was brought in from North America under the aid programmes.

Conditions were therefore set for the state to intervene to ensure an increase in food supplies and to guarantee incomes for farmers. (In England in1950 there were more than a million families earning their livings from 450,000 mixed farms of varying acreage, but farm wages failed to compare with wages in industry.)

Government aid to the farming population took the shape of protection of domestic markets, support of prices, official purchasing at set prices, and subsidies to producers. The policies varied slightly from one country to another. Support of prices meant that the price of any given crop could be raised to 40 per cent above its world market price. Of course the consumers paid for this. In Paris between 1952 and 1954 there were the Green Pool Talks, where 15 countries including Britain tried to set up a Common Market, but the many disagreements and complications meant that little was achieved. The next stage of decision making was in July 1958 when Sicco Mansholt, vice president of the commission with responsibility for agriculture, convened a conference with the following objectives: a single market, community preference and financial solidarity plus an unstated principle that farmers should receive an income equivalent to that received by other sectors. By January 1962 the Common Agricultural Policy had set common policies in cereals, eggs, fruit, vegetables, wine and pig meat. Sugar was omitted.

> It was easy to see the direction in which the community was moving: it was insulating itself from the world market and setting in motion a complex system of intervention managed from the centre.[3]

With the incentives of subsidies, new forms of agricultural mechanization and artificial fertilizers, the traditional ways of farming – natural fertilization with manures, crop rotation, diversity of crops – quickly changed, for now the emphasis was on efficiency.

It is possible to see how many farmers' confidence had been eroded over the centuries and here was an opportunity to give a new impulse to the land. The new system must have appeared attractive and, with the terrible suffering of the war behind them, many people were ready for a new beginning. But how many really understood what kind of Pandora's box was being opened with the new technology, or what the eventual outcomes might be?

Agrochemicals and health

Instead of enriching the land with animal dung, sackfuls of nitrates (a by-product from bomb-making) were spread upon it. These were followed by herbicides to kill the weeds, and pesticides to kill the pests, and fungicides to kill the fungi. Many of these poisons had their beginnings in chemical warfare laboratories and were used in nerve gases, for example DDT. In 1939 Swiss scientist Paul Muller discovered the use of DDT to kill insects (he was awarded the Nobel Prize in 1948). It became one of the world's most notorious pesticides and was used extensively with disastrous results. A new chemical weapon had been secretly developed in Britain during the war and instead of against Hitler's armies was to be used against armies of weeds. MCPA weedkiller was marketed as Methoxone, which made plants contort and die.[4] Previously pesticides had been made from naturally occurring plant and mineral substances, but these new products were manufactured synthetically, cheaply, and appeared on the surface to be effective. Residues inevitably found their way into the water table.

Wetlands were drained, moors and pastureland were ploughed up for cultivation of more food – no matter that it wasn't being used, that it was piling up in vast quantities in grain silos. Hedgerows disappeared at the rate of more than 10,000 miles a year. Apple orchards were grubbed out; our native apples with their abundant varieties couldn't compete with the prices of unblemished Granny Smith's or Golden Delicious from South Africa and New Zealand (of course the transport involved was not reckoned into the cost and still isn't). How could our farmers reconcile themselves to this?

Bigger and more efficient machinery meant that fewer hands were needed on the land. Supermarkets proliferated and with them food technology to 'take the drudgery out of cooking'. Special relationships between politicians and businessmen began to take hold, with sometimes the appointment of people wearing both hats at once (such as the chief agricultural adviser to the Ministry of Agriculture, Sir William Gavin, who also happened to work for ICI).

Elements of a chemistry of what amounts to death, which had been used in warfare, was now being applied to farming. There was a war on pests and weeds and on anything out of place. With the extermination of the so-called unwanted elements on and in the land went untold damage to micro-organisms in the soil, which for a million years had toiled away recycling nutrients. However, it was felt by the chief movers in this scenario that we were embarking on an exciting agricultural adventure. It all changed our way of life and our landscape.

Writer and environmentalist Stefania Vignotto has said:

A landscape is the result of people living and working on it. It used to reflect the history of the place and has its own unique atmosphere. Thus the history of landscape gives rise to 'landscape art' which is a product of the creative interweaving of the human being and the creativity of nature.

The gradual dismembering of familiar landscapes had started a downward spiral of disconnection: living in degraded landscapes has increased the insecurity and disorientation of modern people. This lack of connection has wider consequences, which make themselves felt in the physical, emotional and social spheres.[5]

So began a degradation on many levels, but it was masked by exciting innovations: more choice in foods, more punchy advertising, labour-saving this and that. At the same time there was television, Hollywood movies, jazz, travel, exciting new fashions, more sexual freedom; much of the new life-style was generated in the USA. After the experience of food and clothes rationing and the horrors of war most people wanted never to see the bad old days again. Science and technology were going to solve all our problems.

Now, 50 years on, we are experiencing some of the consequences of what we have done to the earth. That 'exciting agricultural adventure' was born out of fear – fear that we could again be vulnerable by relying so heavily on imported food – and born out of a marriage of war technology with political ambition. It was hasty and went in defiance of traditional wisdom. Some smaller farmers became mere pawns. As George Monbiot has pointed out, it has meant that we are currently paying for our food three times over – first with our cash, second through our taxes to pay for subsidies to the farmers, and third through what we have to pay in clean-up, e.g. the high cost of household water.[6]

Many of the chemicals that have been used in agriculture have been implicated in human illnesses. Organo-phosphates used in sheep-dips can produce subtle changes in the human brain and nervous system, lindane – a hormone-disrupting chemical used extensively in growing potatoes – has been linked with breast cancer. And many varieties of pyrethroids, which attack the nervous system, and the organo-chlorines, which get into the food chain, have proved to be almost indestructible. Altogether there can amount to a cocktail of 500 artificial chemicals in our bodies, and residues were found in 43 per cent of all fruit and vegetables tested in 1999.

It was this poisoning of the earth and her wildlife that prompted Rachel Carson to write *Silent Spring* in 1962, and although her book caused a great stir and was an awakening call, more sophisticated chemicals continued to be developed. To this story has now been added the genetic modification of foods, introducing yet another hitherto unknown variation into nature.

In the UK cancers have increased by 60 per cent since 1950, obesity has trebled since 1960, and there are 1.4 million people with diabetes. (It has been predicted that there will be about 3 million people with diabetes by the year 2010.) Coronary heart disease accounts for 27 per cent of all deaths, and strokes, due to cerebrovascular disease, account for a further 12 per cent. One child in five has some kind of respiratory disease. Our hospitals are overloaded. (A sign of a country's health status would surely be fewer hospitals rather than more.) The argument that we are living longer must be qualified by the fact that longer lives are accompanied by debilitating and long-standing illnesses such as Parkinson's disease, Alzheimer's disease, arthritis and diabetes.

Tim Lang, Professor of Food Policy at City University, has been concentrating his recent research on the link between agriculture and health. In his 2002 Schumacher Lecture he said:

Here is a culture where young women are bombarded by images of their bodies which encourage anorexia and a self-denying approach to food, yet which encourage them to binge, to dislike themselves, to feel perpetually dissatisfied. At the same time figures on obesity are rising rapidly. Here is a culture where food is a major factor in the nation's top two causes of premature death: coronary heart disease and cancers of the breast and colon. On these, medical evidence is consensual, that excess consumption of fat and under-consumption of fruit and vegetables are the key. Yet the food industry spends an annual £600 million on advertisements which are overwhelmingly extolling the joys of sweet, fatty foods. The budget for advice on health education by the Health Education Authority, by contrast, is about £2 million a year. It is this mixture of contradictory trends and countervailing forces that leads me to pronounce that British food culture is slightly, if not significantly, mad. The challenge is to heal that madness.

Economics – the real cost

If we were to put the economics of farming and public health together, we would have a very different set of statistics. The word economics comes from the Greek *oikos* meaning 'house' + *nomia* meaning management. To manage nature's household properly we will need to develop a new way of accounting and economics. The profit motive, when applied to nature, has led to chronic depletion of the soil and a dangerous exploitation of animal and plant materials. We need an economics that takes fully into consideration the intrinsic interrelatedness and value of all aspects of our environment. For instance, it should acknowledge that our forests are vital for providing habitat for birds and animals, for their intrinsic beauty, for food, and for wood products but are also vital as air-conditioners. I would not be so churlish as to deny that some scientific advances are valuable, *but we cannot also deny that we are profoundly changing the earth and its biosphere's chemistry and inevitably our own.*

The supremely delicate balance we have on this planet came about through complex and symbiotic relationships over millions of years; the dimensions could not have been even marginally smaller or larger or this diversity of form and function could not have happened. James Lovelock, an influential scientist-philosopher, whose Gaia hypothesis sees the planet as an intelligent, self-regulating organism, speaks of a kind of Damascus experience he had:

> It was at the moment that I glimpsed Gaia, an awesome thought came to me. The earth's atmosphere was an extraordinary and unstable mixture of gases, yet I knew that it was constant in composition over quite long periods of time. Could it be that life on earth not only made the atmosphere but also regulated it, keeping it at a constant composition and at a level favourable for organisms?[7]

The popularity of the Gaia hypothesis has grown, bringing with it many positive initiatives. In *Gaia: the Practical Science of Planetary Medicine*, Lovelock calls out for healing for the earth:

> The limitation of a scientific reductionist point of view is now becoming more and more apparent, but proper measures cannot be taken until scientists acknowledge the extent of their ignorance about the earth.[8]

Traditionally it was farmers who held deep knowledge and intuition about the earth's symbiotic systems. In Babylonian times they used astronomy in their planting cycles and that custom is still kept alive by tribal people and peasant farmers around the world. But a new development started to be investigated in 1924 that can only properly be described as 'planetary medicine' and has become known as the biodynamic method of agriculture.

Origins of biodynamic farming

The initiative was taken by a group of farmers in eastern Germany who had noticed an increasing degeneration in seed strains and in many cultivated plants to ask Dr Rudolf Steiner's advice. In response he gave an agricultural course in June 1924 on the estate of the Count and Countess Keyserlinck at Koberwitz near Breslau. These lectures are the source of biodynamic methods of agriculture.

As a new impulse in farming, biodynamics arose independently of, and slightly before, other European organic movements. Although in terms of acreage it still only represents a small proportion of today's farming, it is nonetheless a worldwide movement with representation in both tropical and temperate regions. The biodynamic ideal is founded on good organic farming practice. Its relationship to the organic movement as a whole is that of providing a wider, cosmic dimension and through addressing the unseen forces behind nature it helps us understand why organic farming in general is so necessary for us at the present time.

When Rudolf Steiner was persuaded to offer his insights into agriculture, his aim was to try and correct a largely one-sided, mechanistic view of nature, which even by the 1920s had become entrenched. Steiner's approach, by contrast, offered a view of life that connected earth and cosmos, physical life with its spiritual origins and with forces that pour down to work within soil and plant to stimulate the processes vital to agriculture. But in order for these beneficent influences to be fully active the soil needs to be sufficiently sensitive, and for this to occur natural organic fertilizing materials have to be used, so keeping substances in the realm of the living. In this respect manure from the cow is accorded a special fertility status, as it is in Asia.

So by various means, organic and biodynamic farming aim to maintain a living soil, replete with organisms and actively promoting humus-formation. Organic materials, including composts derived from plant residues and animal dung, are most beneficial if they derive from life on the same farm, having first absorbed the farm's own interchange of earthly and cosmic activity. In biodynamics even more than other organic practices the farm is viewed as a living organism having its own unique individuality – in fact it is a microcosm of the living earth. Thus we see that the by-products of farming activities pass through the process of transformation and chaos to emerge as substance and vitality for the new season's production.

It is also recognized that healthy and productive farming depends on maintaining a diverse natural environment. So, rather than sweep all aside in order to maximize space for production, if we allow nature her place all our best interests will be served. This can be achieved on several levels: by the way crops are grown in sequence, by the way they can be (but all too often are not) grown close together with companion plants, and by judicious creation and management of habitats for wildlife. While birds and insects can often be viewed as enemies by farmers, the insights of biodynamics point to essential though unseen processes that these creatures bring. When

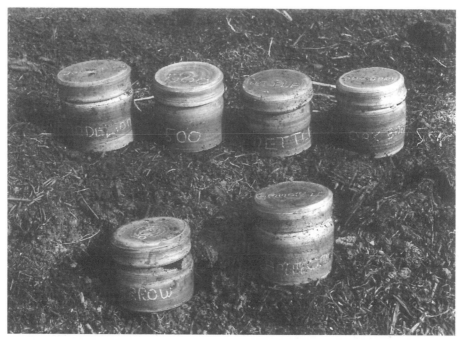

Biodynamic preparation are stored in earthenware pots in peat

these processes are missing, our plant life would be and is already becoming, weakened.

In order to work constructively with cosmic forces and to enhance their operation, special preparations[9] are used which vitalize soils and composts and which support crops in various stages of their growth. These 'vitalizers' or preparations are designed to ensure that plants grow in a balanced and healthy way. Not only does this relate to an important polarity between the roles of lime and silica (see pp. 232–5) but our food must contain an appropriate balance of planetary forces. Otherwise, according to Steiner, our body's protein (built up mainly *by the body*, rather than as currently assumed) will not be balanced either. Fertility, an indication of living, vital forces, is also becoming an increasing problem in plant, animal and human, often as a result of these dynamics not being understood clearly enough. Biodynamic preparations will become increasingly important as the earth's vitality continues to decline and we can only wonder at how much further damage has been done since Steiner's agriculture course of 1924.

All cosmic influences are of course subject to rhythmic variations: the interplay of sun, moon and planets with each other and the background of the zodiacal constellations. Alan Brockman, a biodynamic farmer in Canterbury, explains:

> Each planet has its own force field; thus each planet can, at some time or other, be seen in every part of the zodiac. The earth can be pictured as being surrounded by seven spheres of force, of which each physically visible planet is marking out its own particular boundary. These spheres were known as 'crystal spheres' (a description attributed to Ptolemy). Steiner indicated that the various leaf spirals and their positioning around the stem, or 'phyllotaxis', indicates which particular force field the plant is reacting to. So clearly plants and planets have correspondences, as healers such as Paracelsus and Culpeper well knew.[10]

Here we are not simply dealing with prosaic timings, but with specific formative influences that have created and sustained us throughout our existence. Biodynamic practice allows the timing of agricultural activities to take place in the most beneficial way for each type of crop. Using the timings of a biodynamic calendar in conjunction with other biodynamic practices will also reinforce important aspects of quality in our food products (one aspect being the trace mineral content).

Of course, these biodynamic practices raise the wider question of the conscious working of people with nature's less visible aspects. As we have seen, in bygone times they were perceived to be teeming with elemental nature beings who mediate between spiritual force and material growth. Steiner has made it clear that though in times past we have been supported by spiritual powers, increasingly it will be up to us how our future will work out. A close partnership with and understanding of the world of the stars and elemental beings appears to be of the greatest importance. Biodynamics is uniquely placed to both raise our awareness of hidden nature and play an important role in furthering human, animal and plant development in a healthy way.

A new relationship to farming and produce

If we follow the spirit in nature we put into our service both the rationale and the economy of nature, who wastes nothing. This ultimately is the basis of the life of humanity.[11]

In the biodynamic movement one of the aims is to try to take land out of private ownership. Land trusts make land available for those who have a vocation in farming but cannot afford to buy their own land. There is also a great deal of land under cultivation biodynamically under the stewardship of the Camphill movement.

Community Supported Agriculture, pioneered in the USA by Trauger Groh and Hugh Ractlliffe, is a movement that is growing steadily. The basic principle is that a group of prospective consumers gather around a farm and pledge together to provide and divide amongst themselves the costs of the products that they will receive, plus the salaries of the farmer and any helpers. This pledge also ideally includes the agreement that if a crop fails they are willing to share such a loss too. Of course this calls for trust and possible sacrifice on the part of the group, which can be up to a hundred people. One also needs capable and experienced farmers. But there is room for much creativity and diversity in such a scheme. Consumers really start to connect with a particular piece of land, usually helping with harvesting, and, if they wish, with the stirring of preparations. This is wonderfully educative experience for the children too.

Veggie-box schemes, which began in the 1980s, are an example of another development that has become tremendously popular within both the organic and biodynamic movements. Such a scheme cuts out the middleman. Customers can choose the size of box they would like to receive and for a few pounds a week receive a box of seasonal vegetables delivered to their home, usually with many optional extras as well.

Biodynamics, like organic farming, can be more labour-intensive, but mechanization is not shunned. It is a question of using appropriate technology. In this country the largest biodynamic farms are to be found within the Camphill village communities[12] where residents are involved in farming and gardening as well as food preserving and cheese-making as part of their education, so supporting the seasonal work of the farmer. At Emerson College, when I was there, the body of some 200 students could be called upon to help with the potato harvest and other labour-intensive tasks like the making of the preparations. I found it fun and interesting, and good to take exercise with a useful end-product (better than going to the gym!).

Farmers' markets are greatly on the increase all over Britain, bringing in useful additional income, and through forming co-operatives farmers have found they can resource each other and help to break the stranglehold that supermarkets have exerted on them. Other agricultural projects need the support of a school or other institution, bringing customers and making the farm part of the education.

Can organic or biodynamic farming feed the world?

(I have based this section on a paper presented by Lawrence Woodward of Elm Farm Research Centre[13] at the AGM of the Farm and Food Society, October 1995.)

The answer to this question will depend on what is meant by the word 'feed'. If it means *either* a varied diet of fresh grains, vegetables, pulses and grains, low in saturated fats, *or* a diet that is rich in higher proteins – a 'convenient' diet for a developed world life-style and high in short-term gratification – then the answer would be 'Yes' to the first option.

Several studies have put the question: 'What if the whole country went organic?' A study at Iowa State University did a projection on this involving the whole USA. They concluded that all domestic needs would be met, only export supplies would vary from year to year. As a result of this and other empirical studies, the US Department of Agriculture concluded that organic farming employed best land management as well as water conservation. But will they ever act on this? Not when faced with the conservative views of men like Dennis T. Avery, Director of the Centre for Global Food Studies: 'High yield farming is the only way to save most of our wildlife, unless we are willing to destroy three billion living human beings and abort most of the babies being born in the world today.' It is surely this kind of thinking that has paved the way for GMO propaganda.

In the UK a study undertaken by the University of Aberystwyth and EFRC reached a similar conclusion as the Iowa studies, that we could feed ourselves using organic methods. There would need to be a large reduction in pig and poultry products because of changes in feed and welfare requirements, and therefore a change in our diets to include more vegetable protein and less meat – bringing us more in line with dietary recommendations. Another study in Germany showed that the country could indeed cover her domestic food requirements in spite of lower outputs, on the basis of vegetable production.

In countries who are poor in resources, organic and biodynamic farming with their emphasis on *biological* nitrogen supply, on maintenance and enhancement of organic matter, and on soil and water protection are arguably the most appropriate farming systems and the most sensible approach to feeding people. So if this makes practical sense, what is stopping us wholeheartedly going in that direction? Presently Western Europe consumes nutrients from almost five times its agricultural area. How can this be sustainable? Imagine if in China (a country fast moving into industrialization, with a population of 1.2 billion) everyone wanted two extra beers each. The demand would be enough to use the entire annual Norwegian grain harvest. Is this sustainable?

The fact that, despite the data, not much is being done to give organic or biodynamic farming urgent priority on political agendas has little to do with their ability to provide adequate nutrition, but rather more to do with systems of distribution, subsidies, markets, finance and political structures. Control of commodity trading is critical in the world food system. Some 15 trans-national companies account for the bulk of this activity. One of the most powerful in the group is Cargill, which has been able to position itself

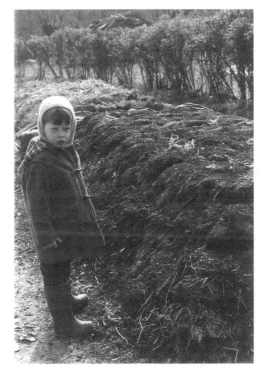

A biodynamic compost heap

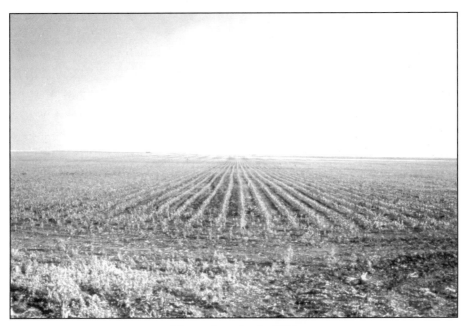

Monoculture in the USA

as feed supplier, banker, buyer of finished cattle, butcher and wholesaler — indeed, everything except the farmer, who does the real work. With such strategies the question of feeding people really seems not to feature.

Some of the changes proposed by Al Gore when running for President of the United States were quite radical, which of course is what we need:

- Write off the Third World debt
- Stop subsidizing crops like tobacco and create a favourable fiscal environment for the production of food security, not agro-industry commodities for trade
- Face up to the need for land reform in order to provide access to land so that people, especially those facing insecure food supplies, have the opportunity to grow food for themselves
- Develop a global strategy for soil and water conservation, in which organic farming would have a major role to play

But fundamentally we have to change the growth/consumption imperative that drives the global economy (i.e. our life of desires!).

THE FOURFOLD HUMAN BEING

It is indeed the physical body that is the deepest mystery, for it has to be created through a meeting with spirit and matter. Anatomy and physiology can understand a great deal about the body in its outer aspects. What it is in itself is very far away from our comprehension for we are deeply unconscious of this aspect of our life on earth, even though it is that same aspect to which we are most intimately bound. It is in this sense that we can say that the body is the ultimate mystery, involving the whole cosmos, heaven and earth, in the process of its creation.
Dr Pearl Goodwin, priest in the Christian Community[1] and embryologist[2]

The thrust of popular mainstream thinking still seems to be lodged in the Descartes/Newton/Darwin mode, which has come to omit the question of man's body/soul/spirit. The result is a crisis of meaning in our society. Our concepts of the human being, our relationship with nature, have a bearing on how we live our lives, our purpose and direction. But we have become a culture without mythology, we have lost our connection to our collective journey. Never has the need been more urgent to restore the bridge between spirit and matter. Teilhard de Chardin said in *The Phenomenon of Man*, 'To connect spirit, body and soul is important – science has provisionally decided to ignore the matter!' That thought is echoed beautifully in the following poem by Ursula Vaughan Williams:

Man without Myth
He did not know his father was a tree
Nor that his mother was a river's child,
That the sea rocked his cradle long ago
Or that the birds came crowding in from the wild
To tell him stories of their hierarchy
And teach him all the things a man should know.

He did not know his dog had ranged with stars
Nor that his horse had wings he could not see,
His cat had been known in Temples of the Sun,
All doors stand open upon infinity.
He only saw a window dark with bars
And many matters to be done.

He never saw his wife was made from flowers,
Ephemeral beauty and enduring roots,
A forest murmur and a summer scent,
He only cared for the thirst-quenching fruits
And cursed her withering and Autumn hours
And did not follow Winter ways she went.

Nor did he know history as a road
On which he too made footsteps every day,
He never used his head or heart or hand,
When comets blazed he looked the other way.
Small jealousies were something of a goad
But more than that he could not understand.

He never knew and never cared to know more than
Bare necessity could show.
Once Man and Wonder walked life side by side
He lost his Kingdom once his magic died.[3]

How does it affect us if we only see ourselves as a 'ghost within a machine', 'behind a window, dark with bars', the human body and consciousness as a prison? Where is the place for imagination, for love and compassion, for intuition and tenderness, for an ethical/moral basis to life? How is it that the divine origins of the human being have been so quickly forgotten? It is as though a veil has been drawn between us and the intangible, leaving us confused and isolated.

Where spirit was lost

A new stage of natural science began in the sixteenth century. Vesalius published a medical work on the accurate dissection of the human corpse and at the same time Copernicus published his treatise on the anatomy of the solar system. Galileo established a methodology for pursuing this new vision of things and later Descartes provided the philosophy to go with it (famously reduced to his epithet 'I think, therefore I am'). Descartes tried to relate the utterly insubstantial soul to the utterly substantial body by suggesting a link in the pineal gland, which has only served to deepen the confusion. For him soul was mind.

Newtonian science had described the motion of the planets by a mechanical paradigm. The laws he observed appeared to demonstrate that time and place and physical phenomena were the causal aspects of nature. All physical reactions were seen to have a physical cause that could be explored and analysed, like the movements of balls colliding on a billiard table. Only that which could be weighed and measured was allowed in this scheme, with the human senses limited to five: touch, taste, sight, smell and hearing (by contrast Rudolf Steiner spoke of twelve senses, see Note 17 to Chapter 5).

The limitations of that outlook continue to our time. Many people experience their bodies in a mechanical way, defining their lives in terms of three-dimensional space and linear time. Our children are taught this natural-scientific conception of the human being: that we are limited to the matter and its movements of which our bodies are composed; that there is nothing particularly special about living, as distinct from dead or mineral things, other than complexity; that feelings are simply the life of nervous tissue; that a human being is only another animal whose larger and more complex brain allows him to think.

To Darwin and his successors, evolution is the result of blind forces acting without intention or aim; the human being is the product of these forces, a process characterized as 'the survival of the fittest'. In the early nineteenth century the researches of Michael Faraday and James Clerk-Maxwell led them to a theory of electromagnetic fields. So was born the concept of a universe filled with fields interacting with each other. When Albert Einstein published his Special Theory of Relativity, it shattered most of the bases of the Newtonian world-view. According to relativity theory, space is not three-dimensional and time is not a separate entity. They are intimately connected and form a four-dimensional continuum of space-time.

More recently Rupert Sheldrake proposed in *A New Science of Life*[4] that systems are regulated, not only by known energy and material factors but also by an organizing field – a 'morphogenetic' field – forming an invisible matrix (morph = form and genesis = coming into being). These morphic fields can propagate across space and time, meaning that past events could influence other events everywhere else.

Dr David Bohm in the journal *Revisions* said the same is true for quantum physics.[5] Something happening to distant particles can affect the formative field of other particles and 'the notion of timeless laws that govern the universe doesn't seem to hold up, because time itself is part of the necessity that developed'. He wrote of an 'implicate order' existing in an unmanifested state, providing the foundation upon which all manifest order exists — the 'explicate unfolded order'. Despite such important developments in quantum physics and chaos theory, people like Rupert Sheldrake (currently investigating telepathy) are still marginalized by mainstream science. He is, however, greatly appreciated by those of us totally unconvinced by the materialistic paradigm and who seek more meaningful cosmologies. But let us now look back to find other great minds who perpetuated a more spiritual science.

Paracelsus

Paracelsus (born *c.* 1490) was known at the 'Swiss Hermes' because he was a pivotal figure, representing a fusion of the old alchemical wisdom and the new objective science. An instinctive student of the essential Pythagorean ideal, he was physician, herbalist (using the doctrine of 'similars'), astrologer, alchemist and rugged non-conformist. Among many achievements he discovered hydrogen and nitrogen and pioneered the use of mineral baths.

Although the Renaissance was founded upon a collaboration of science and esoteric tradition, Paracelsus was aware of the impending struggle between medicine and magic. He warned his contemporaries against dividing therapy from the religious life. For him the development of practical therapy depended upon an unceasing exploration of the invisible side of nature — the search for causes — and the realization that the human being was not simply a physical creature but a living soul whose inner orientation and spiritual life could profoundly affect his health.

He discovered that the most satisfactory way to learn was to observe, so he worked with herbalists, gypsies, witches, faith healers and people from the land. He burned before his own students the medical works of Galen saying,

'He who would understand the book of nature must walk its pages with his feet.'[6] Many of his writings were devoted to the subject of light. He considered it to be concerned in the nature of Being, the total existence from which all separate existences arise. Light not only contains the energy needed to support visible creatures and the whole broad expanse of creation, but the invisible aspect of light supports the secret powers and functions of the human being, particularly intuition.

Intuition therefore relates to the capacity of the individual to become attuned to the hidden side of life. As the light of the body gives strength and energy, sustaining growth and development, so the light of the soul bestows understanding; the light of the mind makes wisdom possible and the light of the spirit confers truth. Therefore truth, wisdom, understanding and health are all manifestations of one virtue or power – light. This 'light-life' corresponds to the *chi* of Eastern systems, the *mana* of the natives of the Polynesian islands and the *orenda* of the Iroquois Indians. The Greeks knew of this light, the 'ocular fire' placed in the human eye by Aphrodite as an emanation of love and life.

Paracelsus spoke of the human being as the microcosm reflecting the greater macrocosm:

> In him are contained all the powers and all the substances that exist in the world, and yet he constitutes a world of his own. In him wisdom may become manifest and the powers of his soul – good as well as evil – may be developed to an extent little dreamt of by our speculative philosophers. In him are contained all the forces and beings and forms that may be found in the four elements out of which the universe is constructed. Man is the microcosm, containing in himself the types of all the creatures that exist in the world, and it is a great truth which you should seriously consider that there is nothing in heaven or upon the earth which does not also exist in man, and God who is in heaven exists also in man and the two are but One. Each man in his capacity as a member of the great organism of the world can be truly known only if looked upon in his connection with universal nature, and not as a separate being isolated from nature. Man is dependent for his existence on nature, and the state of nature depends on the condition of mankind as a whole.[7]

So to Paracelsus the human being is woven out of the cosmos, 'containing all substances that exist therein'. This is rather like looking into the heart of a

lettuce and discovering an emerald-green caterpillar almost indistinguish-
able from its environment. The caterpillar is, on a certain level, metamor-
phosed lettuce; indeed it is woven out of the lettuce! Along with all other
living things the human being is bound to the whole universe by energy
correspondences. Everything that lives is a focus of universal life-energy; for
every star in the sky there is a flower in the meadow and heaven seems to
have inverted itself upon the earth. However, Paracelsus – this 'Luther of
physicians' – died early and it was suspected he was killed by assassins
hired by the medical fraternity.

The Copernican revolution, giving rise to the mathematization of the
world and the resulting science and technology, was an uneasy bedfellow of
the esoteric, the hidden and indeed of religion. Later this led to the perse-
cution of wise women, herbalists and midwives. The essential link between
spiritual heaven and corporeal earth had been broken.

Figures of our own time

In the last century C.G. Jung commented towards the end of his life:

> This peculiarity of our time, which is certainly not of our conscious
> choosing, is the expression of the unconscious man within us who is
> changing. Coming generations will have to take account of this momen-
> tous transformation if humanity is not to destroy itself through the
> might of its own technology and science ... So much is at stake and so
> much depends on the psychological constitution of modern man ...
> Does the individual know that *he* is the makeweight that tips the
> scales?[8]

Contemporary with Jung was Rudolf Steiner who sought to restore a unified
picture of the human being and his relationship with nature, with the divine
principle and with his own inner and outer dissonances. Steiner was a scientist, but wished his contribution to be known as 'spiritual science',
involving a deep order of contemplative enquiry.

If we want answers in life we have to define our questions and Steiner's
own work was stimulated by people approaching him with their deepest life
questions. His contributions (in education, agriculture, philosophy, re-
medial work and Christianity) usually had very practical applications. He

spoke often about the nature of the human being, the subtle bodies and the relationship to the kingdoms of nature.

Steiner's fourfold human being

(For the following I am indebted to Dr Ralph Twentyman for liberal use of passages from his *The Science and Art of Healing.*[9])

Steiner called the four kingdoms of nature the mineral kingdom, the plant kingdom, the animal kingdom and the soul/spiritual kingdom.

Beginning with the mineral kingdom, if we take a crystal of salt we will see that no matter how small or large it will present a uniformity throughout; it is so constituted that it is held together permanently by its own forces. The molecules of a mineral are unfit for growth, by their very structure. A mineral does not initiate movement and it tends towards the timeless.

A living organism, plant, animal or human, carves out for itself a characteristic space. The organism also has a time framework within which movement and metamorphosis take place. This time element unites all living things and Steiner called it the 'etheric body' or 'the body of formative forces'. During the entire time between birth and death the etheric or 'life body' combats disintegration of the physical body.

This etheric body does not belong in Euclidean space – the normal space we are familiar with in which physical bodies and forces such as gravity and electromagnetism are studied. Such forces operate between one point and another. For instance, gravity acts from the centre, so the forces of gravity diminish with distance according to strict mathematical law. Etheric forces, on the other hand, act from the periphery and work outwards. They were said by George Adams to act in 'negative Euclidean space'.[10] Such space arises from the interweaving of *planes* as distinct from the *points* of normal Euclidean space. The space we are familiar with, in which matter has its existence, 'is in reality the result of the polar interplay of centric and peripheral components'.[11] In the plant kingdom we see the play of planar forces working from the periphery, together with physical forces related to the earth centre. The plant tends to be all spread out as it grows into spatial manifestation.

The etheric works through fluid elements. Paracelsus said the vital essence of life moves through the body not only by way of its physical

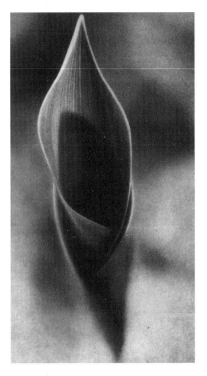

In this shoot of a lily of the valley we see how the rolled up form opens out into the flat area of the leaves

structure, but by means of a vital etheric counterpart which he called 'the vital vehicle', through which flow countless tiny streams of semi-fluid energy. The common experience of an arm or a leg 'going to sleep' is because the normal circulation is temporarily impaired, resulting from the obstruction of the vital body. As it returns to its normal relationship with the physical member there is a pricking sensation, giving an indication of the network of meshing and criss-crossing of the etheric. The glandular system is seen as a physical expression of the etheric.

In animals the developing organism at a certain stage turns in upon itself and makes a cuplike form, whereas plants grow only outwards. More and more infoldings occur, gradually creating the wonderful inner organs of the higher animals. Steiner calls this 'interiorization' – a process which gives rise to inner sensations such as pleasure, desire, pain and movement. Hence comes our ability to 'interiorize'. The new aspect that comes to expression in the animal kingdom Steiner calls the soul or the sentient element, or the astral (starry) body. The soul or astral aspect works through the principle of air and is responsible for the catabolic – breaking down – activity within metabolism. The astral body also mediates between the nervous system and the blood system with its principal gestures of sympathy and antipathy, rising and falling.

In animals, and particularly in mammals, we often observe soul qualities that relate to the human, e.g. the courage of a lion, the cunning of a fox, the benevolence of a cow. The whole world of emotions can be found collectively in the realm of the animals, embedded in a specialized form, as birds can be seen to embody an airy world of weaving thoughts. The human being shares this astral body with the animal kingdom. However, the difference between animals and humans is great, despite the commonly held belief that a human is just a highly developed primate. The basic building plan may be similar but the way in which it is carried out reveals different principles at work.

A human being is unfinished at birth, helpless and incapable of maintaining life, or of moving from place to place. Most animals are virtually complete at birth and usually only grow in size and strength until they are able to reproduce. Each fully represents their own specialization, excepting animals who live with or are trained by humans (they are altered by such contact). Only the human being keeps *omnipotentiality* – the freedom to develop or specialize in many ways.

Additionally, our orientation in space shows radical differences from that of animals. In them the spinal column is usually horizontal with the head as a continuation of the vertebrae. In the human the vertical ascent of the spine gives freedom to the head which is balanced and poised, and only the legs touch the earth. (Humans alone have a straight knee.) If we look at hands, only the human has the unique opposing thumb, allowing for versatility, creativity and delicate handling skills.

It is possible that without uprightness we could not have developed speech, which relies on the air flow through a unique vertical arrangement of the human vocal organs. We are the only creatures who say 'yes' or 'no' (familiar at the stage of around three years old when independence starts to show itself). A human being has the potential for morality, ethical individualism and freedom, and indeed their opposites.

The spiritual core in the human being – the true individuality – is referred to as the ego by Steiner (this is distinct from the everyday, selfish ego). It works through the element of warmth, coursing through the blood circulation.

The various bodies (physical, etheric, astral and soul/spiritual) work together, informing and vitalizing each other. They are all there from birth but each tends to dominate at certain times in the life of a human being.

In the first seven years of life the main activity is the building of the physical body in which the etheric is implicit. Between the ages of 7 and 14 the etheric body is given its unique stamp through rhythm and the formation of good habits. Bad habits formed during these years will be difficult to change. The years 14–21 are the period in which the astral body, through the agency of hormonal activity, brings about the start of the procreative stage with all the turbulence that accompanies these changes. From 21 to 28 the ego principle starts to make itself felt. This was the time when young people were thought to be responsible enough to have a key to the family home.

We find now that these periods are in some disarray due to the arrhythmic society we in the West have created. Nevertheless, beneath the deceptive appearance of precociously advanced young people one can still see the seven-year milestones by careful observation. Many tribal societies know and understand these thresholds in the unfolding human being and wisely create rites-of-passage that are age-appropriate to the young people, making them aware of advancing maturity and its related responsibilities.

To sum up, we have:

The mineral kingdom	relating to	the physical body	(earth)
The plant kingdom		the etheric body, working through fluids	(water)
The animal kingdom		the astral/soul/starry body, working through the nervous system	(air)
The soul/spiritual kingdom		the human ego	(warmth, fire)

The basic outlines can be traced back to Plato and neo-Platonism and to the great systems of the East. As I have pointed out, what was significant in Steiner's work was that he accepted the scientific revolution as a basis. In this way he intended to free the later movement (the Anthroposophical Movement) from contamination by psychic and occult associations and to build a clear spiritual-scientific methodology. The foundation of his methodology is rigorous natural observation.

Additional note

Steiner spoke of the chakra system, calling the points the 'lotus flowers'. Anthroposophy also recognizes the four temperaments, familiar to the Greeks and Paracelsus and recognized up to the medieval world. These were:

the *choleric*, whose fiery nature works primarily through the heat of the blood;
the *sanguine*, the 'airy' person interested in everything, whose temperament works through the nervous system in conjunction with the blood;
the *phlegmatic*, whose being is mainly embedded in the fluidic juices, slow to anger or energize;
and the *melancholic*, whose heavy earthiness makes it hard for him to see the joys of life.

We all usually have a mix of several of these temperaments, but one tends to dominate — an understanding that is found useful in the many Steiner schools around the world.

4

GRASSES AND GRAINS

The origins and mythology of the cereals

The grass family enjoys a unique position amongst the botanical families. Not only is it specifically mentioned in the biblical creation story, but three of its members – wheat, rice and maize – are the world's three most important food crops.

The family has some 4000 members (some sources say 6000) not one of which is poisonous. All over the world grass provides food for many kinds of herbivorous animals and until recently vast areas of each continent had a unique kind of grassland, each supporting a particular animal or group of animals. Best known are the prairies of North America on which vast herds of buffalo peacefully roamed for centuries and which today make up the bread basket of the world. Other examples include the veld of southern and central Africa with its many different kinds of antelope, the Russian steppes on which grazed large herds of horses, and the foothills and mountain slopes of the South American Andes with its llamas and goats. Grasses are the mainstay of animal husbandry and more than 60 species are cultivated worldwide as food plants.

What gives grass this tremendous ability to provide nourishment? Part of the answer lies in the roots. Grass forms a thick, matted growth of roots which penetrate the soil and together with it make up a separate layer. This is turf, described as a living geological stratum. A single seed can produce numerous shoots through the process of tillering: from the bottom node new shoots appear which immediately begin to grow their own roots. Some species have rhizomes, stems creeping under the earth, which send out new shoots and roots at every node. A single rye plant, grown without interference from other plants, has been found to have more than 50 miles of root hairs.

All green plant life is dependent upon the process of photosynthesis whereby carbon dioxide and water are transformed into carbohydrates in the presence of sunlight. Grass has a particularly strong affinity to light and the strong vegetative growth of grass is due to its ability to use light more efficiently than any other green plant – up to 24 per cent of the incoming light is utilized for photosynthesis, against 5–10 per cent for other plants. (As we shall see later, this is a very significant aspect of cereal nutritional quality compared with other food sources.) With grass anchored into the earth as no other plants are, the blades strive upward like spears of light that have taken root on earth.

Another reason why grasses provide so much nourishment may lie in the lack of significant flowers. There are no beautifully coloured petals, little scent; these qualities are transferred to more hidden attributes. Yet who has not experienced the wonderful fragrance of newly mown grass or of freshly dried hay? Here the chlorophyll processes are found deeply invigorating and refreshing to the lungs. Grass does not offer its vitality in colourful revelations but as nourishment to the human being and the grazing animal. This ability to hold back on natural development, and to transform it, is best shown by the cereals, which all but bypass the flowering stage and at the end of the ripening process provide a different kind of flower – flour.

From about 7000 BC onwards in the Middle East, in Asia and in parts of the Americas, small groups of people began the task of transforming the unique vitality of the roots of selected grass species into seed vitality. Through many centuries of careful, concentrated work the tiny insignificant seeds of these selected species began to swell and the seed coat became thinner – the key morphological markers of domestication. The roots became weaker and what may have been perennial species became annuals.

Even today this process of root energy turning into seed energy may be observed. Carefully dissect a young cereal plant about six inches tall. At ground level a miniature ear, tiny but complete, is visible. The grains really do grow out of the roots! Return to the field just before harvest, pull out a clump and notice how much more easily the roots part with the soil. Now the inherent qualities of light are enhanced and become visible, just before harvest as the golden wheat fields ripen in the sun.

Maarten Ekama[1]

How this task was carried out by ancient peoples remains in part an agricultural mystery and is still being fathomed. Scientific explanations are constantly being re-evaluated with new discoveries and new dating methods, but what is understood is that a new co-dependency started to arrive with the development of settled agrarian communities.

> Human beings have similarly intervened in the life cycles of many plants and animals, so that after thousands of years of selection and sheltered existence these organisms have been transformed into a rich variety of domesticated species that are highly successful in agricultural landscapes and at the same time incapable of surviving without human help. In the same way, the survival of human societies has come to depend on domesticated food sources.[2]

It is known that all the cereals were in cultivation early in the first millennium BC. Archaeological evidence indicates that oats and rye 'appeared' about 2800 years ago in different areas north of the Alps, where no wild ancestors of either are known. But in Afghanistan several varieties of wild rye are common in crops of winter wheat to this day. Millet and its southern sister sorghum were known north and south of the Alps by 3000 BC. In northern China, however, excavated village settlements have revealed that millet was domesticated already 7500 years ago.

In tropical South America, in the Amazon, Orinoco, Paraguay and Parana river basins, several species of wild rice flourish, but no attempt seems ever to have been made to take these into cultivation. The cereal of the Americas is maize, known in Mexico at least 7000 years ago, and introduced to Europe at the end of the fifteenth century and into Africa 50 years later. Long before that red rice played an important role in the diet of the West African people and even today it is preferred to the Asiatic varieties. In the Far East rice was domesticated by about 6500 BC, both long and short grain varieties were in cultivation. Short grain rice is grown in sub-tropical areas, whereas long grain rice is generally more suitable for cultivation in tropical areas as it is a so-called 'short-day' plant. Tillering in this variety is particularly marked.

Wheat and barley have been cultivated in Europe and the Middle East from *c.* 7000 BC. Domesticated einkorn wheat is one of the oldest known cultivated plants and according to recent scientific research was taken into cultivation independently in different areas of the Balkans, Turkey, Armenia and Iran. Finds of einkorn on archaeological sites date from 7500 BC. (It was still grown in Swabia in 1936, not for the grain but for use as binding straw in the local vineyards.)

Wild emmer wheat apparently arose from a cross between wild einkorn and a second wild grass called *Aegilops*. It was widespread in the Middle East, though not actually cultivated. The grains were collected by hand and probably roasted whole, as the very tough awns (see drawing, p. 93) prevented it from being ground. At some point in time, emmer with a loose-lying awn arose spontaneously and began to be taken into cultivation. Gradually different varieties evolved and the ease with which awn and grain could be separated by threshing increased. The gluten content was also increased. By 4000 BC emmer was widely distributed and in time became the wheat of the Egyptians, the Phoenicians, the Greeks and the Romans.

The bread wheat known today is now assumed to have been derived from a further chance crossing of wild emmer wheat and another *Aegilops* grass species, resulting in a wheat of the greatest environmental adaptability. Until recently every smallest geographical area would have had its own variety of wheat, and in 1976 the genealogy of 14,000 different varieties was listed.

Two of the major wheat species known to have been cultivated in antiquity have been mentioned, but today only two species are in common use: bread wheat and durum wheat. Emmer and so-called English or rivet wheat are still grown but usually only as food for livestock. Only one species of oats is grown commercially, but in hilly parts of Wales the more robust black or 'bristle oat' may still be found. Barley has two commercial species, six-rowed and two-rowed barley. There are several species of rice, including North American wild rice, classed in a different genus from the common Asiatic rice, which because of difficulties with harvesting is not cultivated on a commercial scale. Millet shows a large variety of forms. There are at least seven major species belonging to six different genera ranging from bulrush millet, which grows on a cob, foxtail millet through to sorghum and common millet with a panicle (see drawing, p. 93) rather like an old-fashioned broom.

In spite of the many species and varieties, the ancestors of these seven groups of cereals – rice, oats, rye, millet and sorghum, wheat, barley and maize – were selected for the qualities latent in each one. In those cases where the wild ancestor is known and still exists, modern science has been unable to discover them. However, what was significant to the peoples engaged in these early agricultural experiments was the interaction between the spiritual worlds, the gods and the cosmos. This has been preserved in wonderfully rich legends and myths, which still have tremendous symbolic power if we choose to work with them.

The peoples of ancient civilizations regarded the planets and stars as visible abodes of the gods and goddesses who had power over all aspects of daily life. In Mesopotamia each city state and all its inhabitants belonged to the city's particular god. Not all deities were connected to the planets or stars; for the Hittites the most important god was the god of storms, Teshub.

We can experience the importance of the sun to all plant life at any time of the year, but especially in the spring. As the sun rises higher and the days grow longer, the earth responds with a quickening, budding and sprouting activity. If this was to be the only influence, all plant life would be like a sublime rainbow of tender colours, growing continuously upwards towards the sun, ever volatile, never a truly connected element of the earth.

> There is a famous legend about Demeter, goddess of fertile culti-vated soil, who presided over the harvest:
>
> Persephone, the daughter of Zeus and Demeter, was abducted by Hades, God of the Underworld, as she was picking wild flowers in a meadow. He took her swiftly back to his sunless realm. They mar-ried and she became Goddess of the Underworld. Demeter, not knowing what had happened to her daughter, was mightily dis-traught and searched for her everywhere. Eventually she learned that Persephone was in the Underworld and that Zeus had given Hades permission to marry her. Demeter was inconsolable and could not regain access to her daughter.
>
> Finally an agreement was reached, and Zeus decreed that in the first half of the year, 'While the seed corn is in the earth, growing and ripening, Persephone is with her mother and the earth is glad. But while the seed corn is stored in jars she goes to her husband while the earth remains parched and barren.'
> (*Encyclopaedia Britannica*)
>
> Persephone is the goddess of death and resurrection, shown by her descent into the Underworld and subsequent return to the earth, beautifully symbolized by the annual rotation of the crop of the Barley Mother, the goddess Demeter.

A second influence is needed to bring order into this quickening life, to ground it so to speak, and this comes from the moon. As the sun works through the medium of air and light – the atmosphere – so the medium of the moon is water – the hydrosphere. The moon's influence on tides is well known and its influence upon the wet and dry aspects of the weather is beginning to be taken into consideration. The moon moves through all of the twelve constellations of the zodiac every four weeks.

To sum up: the sun brings movement to water and to life; the moon orders that movement, harmonizes it, impresses a rhythm upon it so that the unique greening life of our planet can find an anchor and establish itself, thereby becoming the basis for all other earthly life.

Now we shall look at each cereal in more detail. On page 106 you will find a table comparing their nutritional content.

Wheat

Wheat is the oldest known cultivated plant. Cultivated emmer wheat dating back to 8000 BC has been found by archaeological and biological research in

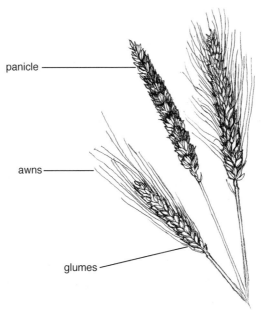

panicle

awns

glumes

Bread wheat, awnless and awned forms

the Middle East, in the area known as the Fertile Crescent, and in Ethiopia where in a small isolated area many varieties of ancient wheat show it had been deliberately selected and grown over a long period. Wheat was also used in the Egyptian, Greek and Roman cultures.

The importance of wheat in world trade, the versatility of its flour (thanks to its high proportion of gluten, higher in summer due to longer hours of sunlight) in baking and confectionery, the fact that it is the main ingredient of our daily bread all speak to its role as 'the sun among the cereals'. Its recent response to chemical fertilizers and hybridization has given rise to yields undreamed of two generations ago. However, the resulting quality of wheat, bred as it has been for high gluten content, has brought with it certain possible health problems and human allergies (see p. 107).

The plant's response to chemical fertilizers was a marked increase in vegetative growth, but the stalks lost their ability to stand erect and the plants fell over before reaching maturity. In modern bread wheat this 'weakness' has been bred out, but although it is able to stand up to the shock of inorganic fertilizers and pesticides, it has lost the finer sensitivity to its surroundings. This can be seen in its lack of awns (see drawing, p. 93), sensitive antennae for a cereal's fine tuning to its environment (reaching, of course, not just to the edge of the field, but as far as the sunlight does).

Varieties of wheat

Types of wheat can be basically divided into hard and soft. Hard wheat contains more gluten and is generally used in bread-making, soft wheat for cakes and biscuits.

Durum wheat has amber coloured grains and is used exclusively in pasta products.

White wheat is low in protein and very starchy, and is used mainly in pastries and breakfast cereals.

Hard red winter wheat has been developed in Canada and takes only 90 days from sowing to harvest. It is used mostly in bread making.

Maris Dove is the most common British wheat. It is a soft winter wheat, high in protein.

Spelt has recently enjoyed a renewed popularity in Europe, partly sparked by the interest in the mystic Hildegard of Bingen (twelfth century) and her nutritional recommendations. People with gluten allergy can often tolerate spelt, richly supplied with nutrients and in general higher in protein, fat and fibre than most wheat varieties.

Kamut is another form of durum-related wheat which had nearly died out but is now grown in Montana. It is growing in popularity because again it can often be tolerated by coeliacs (see p. 107). Its berry is more than twice the size of modern wheat.

Kibbled wheat. The whole grains are cracked in a machine called a 'kibbler' and it is used in granary-type breads.

Wheat was apparently the favoured grain of the Zarathustran period in ancient Persia; he taught his pupils, 'Let us be inspired by the spiritual power of the sun, that the sun will rise in you if you enjoy the fields' – the fields of wheat, which were seen as the earthly embodiment of the sun.

The sun dominates all life on earth and illumines the planets with its light. Its steady movement through the year results in the rhythm of the seasons. As light increases on one half of the earth it decreases on the other.

Rice

A legend from Java

Batara Guru (local name for the god Shiva) decided to create something more beautiful than he had ever created before. He made a most handsome maiden who he called Retna Dumila (sparkling jewel). She was so beautiful that it was not long before Batara Guru fell in love and wanted to marry her. He wooed her as only a divine being can, but Retna Dumila refused him. He persisted in his endeavours but the beautiful maiden remained steadfast.

Eventually Batara Guru could contain his passion no longer. He summoned the gods to a divine council, and thanks to his eloquence and powers of persuasion they decided that he should marry Retna Dumila. The girl could no longer refuse, but she was as shrewd as she was beautiful. When she finally consented she made one demand: that Batara Guru should find a food for the people on earth that would always nourish and satisfy. Thinking that this could easily be done, he set out to find the food of which mankind would never tire. He returned with all sorts of delicacies but sooner or later people became disenchanted with them. He searched on earth and in the heavens but was unable to find the right food. Desperate in his love for Retna Dumila, Batara Guru finally succumbed to his desire and forced her to marry him. The shock was too great for her and she died on her wedding night.

Stricken with grief, Batara Guru arranged a funeral with great pomp and ceremony and ordered her grave to be watched over day and night by his four most loyal guards. The first full moon after her death had passed, when, on visiting the grave, Batara Guru noticed some unusual plants growing in the earth covering the grave. Filled with foreboding, he ordered the plants not to be disturbed and the guards tended them carefully. After four more full moons Batara Guru saw, when visiting the grave again, that ripening grain was swaying gently in the evening breeze and realized with wonder and bewilderment that there it was — the food that Retna Dumila had asked him to find, which mankind would never tire of — Rice.

This great cereal developed in the Far East and is in many ways of greater use to humanity as a whole than wheat. Ninety per cent of the world's production of rice is grown in Asia, where it is the staple diet of nearly half the world's population. Most of it is eaten locally and only 3 per cent enters world trade.

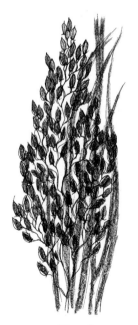

Rice

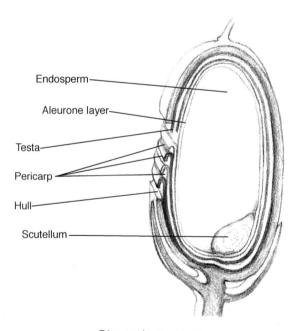

Endosperm

Aleurone layer

Testa

Pericarp

Hull

Scutellum

Rice grain structure

Rice is still the crop requiring the most human labour. Seeds are germinated in a nursery, then each seedling must be painstakingly planted in half-submerged, often terraced, fields. Water prevents weeds from being a problem, but the harvest too must be carried out by hand, the panicles being picked individually after the water has been drained away.

> The song of all songs
> is the farmer's busy hum
> as he plants his rice.
>   Basho

The fact that most rice varieties grow on submerged fields could suggest a relationship of rice to the moon. But we should not forget that the element of water is of less importance than that which the moon imparts through it: the 'anchor', the ability to flourish on earth without completely forgetting its divine origin. No culture based on rice can be completely materialistic. Dr Gerhard Schmidt suggests, 'Rice, unlike the potato, needs very little salt; it is thus especially suited to a low-salt diet. Among the rice-eating peoples of the Far East there is a conspicuously small desire for salt and the high phosphorus content of rice helps to develop the spiritual forces.'[3]

It was through rice that the first clue to vitamin B was found. When the Japanese Navy adopted polished rice on their ships 1000 sailors died of beri-beri. In Java in 1897 Dr Eijkman proved that people eating unpolished rice did not get beri-beri and concluded that something in the outer layers of the grain prevented such malnutrition. An American researcher into vitamin B, Dr Robert Runnels, has said, 'Man commits a crime against nature when he eats the starch from the seed and throws away the mechanism necessary for the metabolism of that starch!'[4] I myself find it difficult to understand how thousands of undernourished Asians still continue to demand polished rice when so much of their nutritional needs would be met by eating the whole grain.

Varieties of rice

Whole rice – only the outer husks have been removed.
White rice – has had the germ, husk and outer layers removed. Often as a finishing process the grains are passed through powerful rollers and

polished with talc. This is sold as 'polished rice' and is little more than pure starch.

Patna and Basmati are traditional Indian rices, with fine pointed grains and a distinctive aroma.

Arborio, from Italy, is bred for risottos so it is sticky and absorbs the cooking flavours.

Wild rice is from a different botanical family and it is harvested by North American Indians where it grows along the low-lying lakes of Minnesota. It has higher levels of protein and minerals. (It is also grown commercially.)

Maize

From the West comes maize, which has become the staple food of the entire American continent. The first boatload of settlers to land in Plymouth colony were most probably saved from starvation by the 'Indian

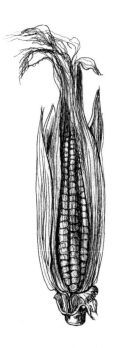

Maize

corne' that they found growing there. Both North and South American Indians worshipped the *Zea mays* plant and called it 'Daughter of Life' and 'Seed of Seeds'. Both the Inca and Aztec civilizations had in their long history impressive city states; these peoples fed on the many varieties of maize. They also brewed maize beer. In the mythologies of the Americas maize always appears suddenly as a gift of the gods. Among the Algonquin tribal groups, for example, the great spirit Manitu sends maize to the earth assisted by his propet Modamin ('Friend of Mankind') in order to overcome hunger there.

Maize grows taller than a man and has the strongest stalk structure of all the grains. A field of dry maize stalks gives the impression of a rather skeletal and fossilized army. No greater contrast to rice can be imagined. There are no light panicles exposing each individual grain to a maximum of light and air. There are not even ears packed tightly onto a central stalk like wheat, held high above the green leaves. Here the ears have sunk down out of the open light-filled air and emerge instead from several of the nodes lower down the stalk. Only the male flowers carrying the pollen appear at the top of the stem, forming the tassel. (Maize has been linked to the planet Saturn.)

Varieties of maize

Flint corn is the successor to the 'Indian corne' of the early settlers. It has a particularly hard endosperm, which makes it difficult to grind. It is now used for cattle feed.

Dent corn is the most widely available corn in the USA. In this type there is a depression at the top of the grain, the 'dent'. Corn meal and flour are made from this. It is used to make polenta (particularly popular in Italy), tacos and tamales in Mexican food.

Blue corn is an open-pollinated variety (not hybridized), indigenous to south-western America. The Hopi and Navajo people use it as a staple. It has a slightly sweet-sour flavour and has a beautiful blue sheen when ground.

Sweetcorn (corn-on-the-cob) – this plant is too sweet and juicy to be dried and is eaten lightly cooked.

Popcorn – the especially hard endosperms are what explode when it is heated. Though very popular, it is nutritionally inferior to the other varieties.

Millet (sorghum)

Millet, possibly the first cereal grain to be used for domestic purposes, was grown in China, before rice was introduced (about 12,000 years ago). It is now an important staple food in Africa, India and Asia. The long-living Hunza people use millet with yoghourt as a staple food combination, and the people of Java grow millet as a border plant around their paddies to activate the growth of the rice plants.

In the many legends around this cereal, its capacity to transmit spiritual energy is often mentioned. The many forms of the panicles and ears of millet might show a relationship with quick-moving Mercury. Its popularity with both captive and wild birds is an indication of the quickness and lightness it embodies. It is also particularly high in silica.

Varieties of millet

Foxtail millet, known as Italian or yellow millet.
Pearl millet, also known as bulrush, or cat tail.
Broomcorn millet.

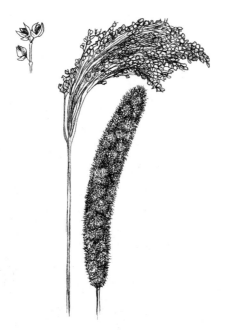

Common and foxtail millet

Barley

Barley was domesticated in the Middle East around 7500 BC. In the Sumerian civilization from about 4000 on it was used as currency. Hammurabi's Code of 1700 BC gives precise instructions as to how many sacks of barley were to be paid for each day's work. For Tibet, barley has been the making of its civilization. Although it lost favour as a food grain, it still has importance for the brewing of beer.

Barley is the humblest of the cereals, not very tall and characterized by the long straight awns which make up the 'beard'. It has the shortest growing season and is harvested while the sun is still high in the summer sky. In Roman times it was used to bake the bread of the poor, as well as being commonly used as animal fodder. John the Evangelist, when describing the miraculous feeding of the multitude by Jesus, mentions twice that the loaves used were barley loaves. The early Greeks too knew of the real value of barley. The name of their goddess of agriculture, and particularly of cereals, was Demeter ('Barley Mother'). The Romans worshipped her under the name of Ceres, from which our word cereal is derived.

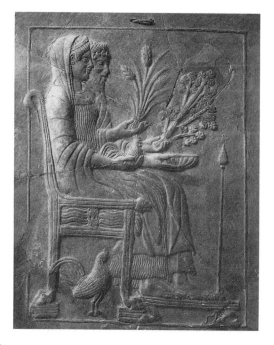

Illustration of the Demeter/Persephone myth; the barley goddess with her consort

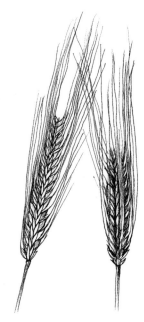

Two and six rowed barley

In some schemes barley has been related to Venus, the last inner planet to consider.

Varieties of barley

Pearl barley. The hull and the two outer layers have been removed. Unfortunately this usually destroys the aleurone part of the endosperm (see drawing, p. 96).

Whole grain brown barley has only had the outer casing removed, leaving the nutritious aleurone intact. It takes longer to cook but is nutritionally superior.

Barley flour is usually made from pearl barley, unless specified. Excellent in breads, it is mixed with wheat flour to give a good rise. It can also be used in mixtures for pancakes.

Oats

Together with rye, a cereal of the north. Its fat content of 4 per cent is twice that of most other cereals, and seven times that of rice, indicating its fiery

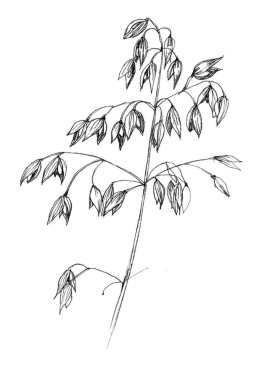

Oats

nature. Its chemical constituents act to protect the heart, balance cholesterol, and help circulation. The Greeks and Romans preferred to use it as animal fodder, though too many oats made their horses hard to handle! The expression 'sowing one's wild oats' refers to the general lustiness and fire attributed to this youngster of the cereals.

Among the Germanic tribes north of the Alps it seems to have been popular as a breakfast cereal eaten as a porridge. Germanic priests conducted spring rituals to celebrate the renewing capacity of the grain, presided over by Nertho, goddess of fertility. It was also adopted enthusiastically by the Scots and taken into cultivation just less than three millennia ago. Oats have been useful in treating mild cases of diabetes. They are easily digestible for young and old alike and are eaten generally as porridge, a basis for muesli and granola, and in some cakes.

Oats in one scheme have been linked with Mars because of their fat content and their fieriness. Mars, the Red Planet, was closely connected with the history of the Romans.

Rye

Rye is also a relative newcomer; it does not have the Neolithic antecedents of wheat or barley. To the ancient Greeks rye was just a vigorous weed, but the Romans tamed the 'weed' and began to grow it as a crop. By the Middle Ages rye had become a staple throughout Europe. In England the basic loaf was made from rye and barley; in Eastern Europe, especially in Germany, Russia and Scandinavia, rye has maintained its popularity.

During the Middle Ages there were several plagues of St Anthony's Fire – ergotism, an illness thought to have afflicted St Anthony in the desert. Ergot is a fungus parasitic on cereal crops, rye in particular, which when eaten affects the central nervous system, producing hallucinations and trances. Ergotism was known as the weird 'dancing sickness', where whole villages danced themselves to death. The active ingredients causing the illness are those of LSD (lysergic acid). Often the sufferers were taken to be witches and tortured and put to death. No one had made the connection at that point.

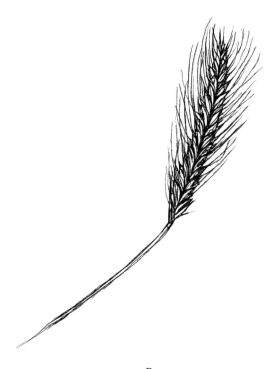

Rye

Rye has been connected to Jupiter, the greatest and brightest planet in the sky. A cereal of central and northern Europe, it is a mountain grain that likes light, air and coolness, and can resist rain and storm, all of which seems to support a particular relationship to Jupiter, the god of light. Known also as the god of wisdom, he ruled the sun and moon and all celestial phenomena. He was also god of wind, rain, thunder and lightning and therefore of great importance to an agricultural population. He was also known as Jupiter Liber, the god of creative force, and as Jupiter Dapalis who presided over sowing.

Varieties of rye

Rye flour is low in gluten, so most rye breads will not rise like wheat bread. But rye bread is more sustaining and has a rich flavour. It can be tolerated by some people who suffer from gluten allergy.
Rye groats can be soaked and cooked like rice, or cracked and kibbled to shorten cooking time.

Other 'grains'

There are 'grains' not belonging to the grass family that have some importance. Amaranth and quinoa (from the chenopod family) are enjoying a new-found popularity, so is buckwheat (from the dock family), which is the beloved kasha of the Russians. Amaranth, used by the Aztecs, is a member of the pigweed family and quinoa comes from the high plains of the Andes; buckwheat belongs to the dock family.

These amazing cereals have been the basis for the emergence of different cultures. To each one their grains were sacred and provided total nourishment. When we look at the composition of cereals we can see some similarity to milk, in that here is a food that nourishes the whole human being. In the starch granules of properly grown cereals a rhythmical concentricity indicates the harmony of their carbohydrate structure. Other vegetables and fruits tend to nourish particular organs, but cereals nourish the totality.

Nutritional content of the main cereals, per 100 g

	Protein	Calcium	Iron	Phosphorus	Potassium	Thiamine	Riboflavin	Niacin
Wheat	14 mg	48 mg	4.6 mg	387 mg	441 mg	0.4 mg	0.12 mg	0.54 mg
Brown rice	11 mg	22 mg	2.0 mg	315 mg	257 mg	0.33 mg	Traces	0.46 mg
Maize*	10–12 mg	20 mg	3.1 mg	294 mg	342 mg	0.4 mg	0.11 mg	Traces
Barley:								
Pearl	8.2 mg	16 mg	2.0 mg	189 mg	160 mg	Traces	Traces	0.31 mg
Whole grain	10–12 mg	52 mg	4.6 mg	240 mg	356 mg	0.44 mg	0.15 mg	0.72 mg
Millet**	7–13 mg	20 mg	6.8 mg	311 mg	430 mg	0.2–0.6 mg	Traces	0.1–0.2 mg
Oats:	11–15 mg							
Whole grain		94 mg	6.2 mg	385 mg	450 mg	0.58 mg	0.13 mg	1.1 mg
Kernel		58 mg	4.3 mg	414 mg	376 mg			
Rye	13 mg	49 mg	4.4 mg	428 mg	524 mg	0.44 mg	0.2 mg	1.2 mg

* traditionally cooked with lime, increasing niacin absorption

** high in silica

Gluten allergy

The coeliac condition is found increasingly today. Sufferers are sensitive to gluten, one of the main constituents of wheat and also present to a lesser extent in barley, rye and oats. Gluten is a non-soluble element in the grain, a complex combination of several different proteins, of which the small fraction known as gliadin is thought to be implicated in the problem, triggering an allergic response.

The healthy immune system of the intestinal wall normally recognizes foods, including gluten, as 'non-self' but acceptable to be metabolized, and triggers the 'safe' immune response – tolerance, in medical parlance. The immune system of the coeliac does not recognize that gluten is harmless, but reacts to it in the same way as it does to infections. Thus antibodies and lymphocytes attack gluten and incidentally cause damage to the wall of the intestine. Also, undigested gluten can combine with other substances and form an intractible layer on the walls of the small intestine, preventing the proper absorption of nutritive materials. When gluten is removed from the diet the health picture improves.

The flours used in modern industrial bakeries come under suspicion as the cause of this allergic condition. The wheat grains have been developed to contain far more gluten than the traditional bread-wheat, and through much hybridization have lost their natural life and light-giving qualities. The addition of chemicals and the need for quick production are also implicated (see pp. 171–2).

Leaves of grass, what about leaves of grass?
Grass blossoms, grass has flowers,
    flowers of grass
dusty pollen of grass, tall grass
    in its midsummer maleness
hayseed and tiny grain of grass, Grammiferae
not far from the lily, the considerable lily.
Even the blue-grass blossoms, even the bison knew it . . .
Leaves of grass, what are leaves of grass
    when at its best grass blossoms.
        From *Leaves of Grass, Flowers of Grass* by D.H. Lawrence

An experiment with grains and the planets

When I was working in the kitchen at Emerson College in the 1970s we began to work with a cereal/planetary menu programme, effectively using specific grains on the different days of the week. Some of this research was done by Dr Udo Renzenbrink at his Nutrition Centre in the Black Forest.

We used the following (there is an alternative progression which reverses oats and barley):

Rice was the grain for	Monday	or Moonday; *lunes* (Spanish); *lundi* (French)
Oats	Tuesday	or Mars day; *martes* (Sp); *mardi* (Fr)
Millet	Wednesday	or Mercury's day ; *miercoles* (Sp); *mercredi* (Fr)
Rye	Thursday	or Jupiter's day; *jueves* (Sp); *jeudi* (Fr)
Barley	Friday	or Venus's day; *viernes* (Sp); *vendredi* (Fr)
Maize	Saturday	or Saturn's day; *sabado* (Sp); *samedi* (Fr)
Wheat	Sunday	or Sun's day; *domingo* (Sp); *dimanche* (Fr)

We worked for several years with the plan presented here. I really came to have a relationship with the rhythm of the days of the week and with those particular grains. It seemed a good way to introduce these cereals to the international student group. It called for inventiveness to make delicious whole grain dishes, particularly with rye (on Thursdays we often used potatoes). Now I do think that it is good to have rhythm in what we eat and it is important that we get back to eating more whole grains, but it is counterproductive to become locked into formulaic practices. Instead of being free and truly creative, one can fall back into empty routine, which is the opposite of nourishing.

I realized that though I had an intuitive relationship with the grains I did not really understand why those planets are connected to each cereal. I asked a friend who is an experienced astronomer/astrosopher and who has researched plant/planet connections. She looked into it for over a year and in all honesty said that apart from the rice/moon and wheat/sun, which were quite pronounced, she could only find tenuous connections. I was naturally a little disappointed, but this is not to say that one cannot bring meaning of one's own into these relationships. It is only dogma that dispels the magic!

PART TWO

5

WHAT HAPPENS IN NUTRITION?

We are linked to our environment in three main processes:

  i) through breathing;
 ii) through sense impressions;
iii) through nutrition.

There was a time when human beings lived more in harmony with the rhythms of the universe; the rhythm of our breathing and the pulse of our blood reflected the greater rhythms of the cosmos. Then the average of 18 breaths per minute would result in an average of 25,920 breaths per day ($18 \times 60 \times 24$) reflecting the 25,920 years of a Platonic Year, the time it takes for the sun to pass through the entire zodiac (the precession of the equinoxes).

Each day of the year is a breathing in and breathing out of the cosmos in our earthly voyage around the sun. People would sleep and wake with sunrise and sunset. In our Western culture we have largely emancipated ourselves from such a rhythm and though we do obviously observe many routines, many of us live somewhat arrhythmical lives. We will return to this question later (pp. 305–7).

Our sense organs receive impressions and stimuli from the environment, which can strongly enhance our well-being or quite the reverse. Sensorial pathways are laid down in the early years of childhood so it is vital that young children are given good quality sense impressions that help to orient them towards the understanding of Truth, Beauty and Goodness, the basic principles of the creative universe. Such principles work on the feeling life of the young child and in time will hopefully inspire the child to act in the world.

The third relationship to our environment takes place through our digestion. Our organs of digestion receive not only sensations but also substances from the outer world. In the process of digestion we divest these substances of all their external properties and then proceed to impress them with our own individual character. Thus the food we eat is submitted to the laws of the living human organism and removed from most outer chemical laws, as Dr Gerhard Schmidt says:

> The complete digestive organization, from the oral cavity to the intestines, represents an everted inner world of the human . . . or an inverted outer world. Activities take place in it which are not yet completely subject to the laws of the inner organization. They represent a field of conflict between inner and outer forces.[1]

Rudolf Steiner spoke of an 'anti-chemistry' and an 'anti-physics' within the organism that must continually control the chemical and physical processes during life.[2] This is the most challenging of the three relationships. It is our food that helps to keep our physical body and the subtler bodies, soul and spirit, together. The quality of our food to some extent determines the kind of relation our body has to our soul, and this in turn influences our relation to the world itself.

The transmutation of food through digestion

All foods are alien substances and if they were to be injected directly into the bloodstream toxaemia would occur. So the complex process of digestion, which in many cases begins in the cooking process, is essential before food can be transmuted into the body of the individual who has eaten it. With each food that we eat – the young child for the first time, with all the wonder of a new experience, or the adult repeatedly enjoying the same foods and never tiring of them – we meet qualities unique to that particular food as it grows in nature. The peculiarities of shape, texture, colour, aroma and taste can never be fully described by chemistry and physics. And although the more obvious qualities can be consciously experienced and perceived through our senses, the finer and subtler qualities are sensed and drawn in by our unconscious powers of digestion.

A cauliflower, for example, has a definite appearance, structure, taste, etc. These properties are not present in the cauliflower's constituent substances, such as its carbohydrates or water. A higher organizing principle gives the constituent parts their unique form and structure. The specific forms of plants are dictated by the species and their etheric (or formative force) bodies. Digesting a piece of cauliflower involves breaking it down, first through cutting and cooking, then with our knives and forks, teeth and, finally, chemically with our digestive enzymes.

When we digest food we have the task of unpacking the formation of the various constituents of the food, since the etheric (form-shaping) bodies of the plant do not correspond to those of the human being. Through digestion the etheric forces of the plant are released and these forces stimulate the human organism. During the process of digestion, information freed into our organism carries the knowledge of the manner in which the plant or animal has previously rearranged lifeless constituents into a structure able to support life.

> The reason why we do not turn into cauliflowers or cornflakes, no matter how much of these foods we eat, is that the substances broken down in our digestive system are not simply put back together again. The profound re-organization and synthesis carried out in the human is due to the stimulating effect of the etheric forces released from the structure of the plant or animal being digested.
>
> *Maarten Ekama*

The Process of Digestion

The process of digestion constitutes such a mighty mystery that it still has not been completely explained by modern science. More and more bio-chemical data become available but little is devoted to the complex links between body, soul or psyche, and spiritual aspects of a human being, or to the transmutation that clearly takes place. I do not for a moment pretend to have grasped the realities of this mystery myself; I merely try to grope my way towards a better understanding through various studies and try to make a synthesis of those that seem to agree with my own experience and sense of truth. What I will attempt to share here will be of necessity a mere thumbnail sketch. I hope, however, to highlight some of the processes that do not often get fully investigated in mainstream traditional nutritional thinking, but which Steiner has brought to our attention and need to be considered.

Most information that we have been given in current nutritional theory is still based on materialistic-mechanistic concepts: the additive and inter-active effects of material properties such as calories, vitamins, proteins and minerals.

Current theory has been based on three – I think – shaky pillars:

i) the applicability of the law of conservation of matter and energy to living systems;
ii) the applicability of the second law of thermodynamics to living systems;
iii) the belief that there is no essential difference in the nature of the interactions of substances inside or outside of the human body.[3]

Digestion usually begins with aroma, linked to taste, and can stimulate our digestive juices before even the visual impact. A lack of aroma is a sure indication that the nutritive value is seriously diminished. When we taste food, the experience permeates our whole body, often to the end of our fingertips and down to our toes within seconds. This tasting activity goes on throughout the digestive process, beginning consciously in our mouth and enhanced by our sense of smell, moving into the unconscious regions after the food has been swallowed. Consciousness only comes into this process if there is a problem, such as indigestion. Normally eating should be accom-panied by a feeling of well-being.

The process of stripping food of all its characteristics begins in the mouth, an exquisitely arranged alchemical laboratory. The aroma, taste, texture and appearance of food all stimulate saliva secretion. In thorough chewing of the food the enzyme ptyalin is secreted which begins the task of breaking down starch into simple sugars; salts are dissolved in this alkaline environment. The composition of the saliva varies to be appropriate to the nutrient. When we eat food we 'surround it'. (The Chinese symbol for chewing is apparently the same as for 'God's work'.) Our chewing in a pleasurable, unhurried way should reduce the food to a paste, opening it up with warmth and water in a process like that of germination. Thus it is lifted out of any gravitational influences and is prepared to be received by the stomach. When the food is then swallowed it passes down the oesophagus into the stomach and hopefully out of our immediate consciousness, though the feeling of well-being should be sustained for some time if the food is good, while the intestines continue to 'taste' the food.

Gastric juices are secreted as a result of two stimuli. The first is a chemical stimulus in the form of hormones, exciting the secretory glands of the stomach. Glands sensitive to the qualities of the incoming food secrete these hormones. The second is a nervous reflex that has its origins in the sensory organs of the tongue and nose and is greatly affected by the setting and atmosphere in which the food is eaten. The secreted digestive juices are mainly hydrochloric acid and peptins, which begin to break down proteins into amino acids. The breakdown of starch continues only in so far as the environment of the stomach is not too acidic. There is virtually no absorption through the stomach wall (alcohol and water are exceptions) and the contents of the stomach pass slowly and rhythmically by peristaltic movements, in a semi-liquid state called chyme, into the small intestine. These rhythmic movements depend for their equilibrium on the automatic nervous system, so the emotional state of the diner will affect all these processes. Different foods require different amounts of time for this to happen. Fruits, for instance, tend to pass through the stomach more quickly whereas concentrated food such as whole cereals, nuts and meat take longest.

In the duodenum of the small intestine under healthy circumstances food is broken down to the extent that the contents are almost sterile. It is here that the activity of the pancreas together with bile from the liver is remarkably intelligent. The breakdown of starches into first complex and then simpler sugars continues with the help of enzymes located in the intestinal lining. Each sugar is split by its own specific enzyme. Thus sucrose is split into glucose and fructose by sucrase. Maltose is split by maltase, and lactose by lactase. Sucrase, maltase and lactase are just three of the host of enzymes that are present in just the right concentration, and it is difficult not to imagine a most subtle and delicate 'tasting' process going on continuously.

The lower part of the small intestine is a critical point in the journey of the chyme. Here in the intestinal mucosa we find millions of villi, tiny finger-shaped excrescences amounting to 2500–3000 per square metre whose total surface area has been estimated at around 40 square metres. Scientist Louis Wolpert described the human being as the 'most intricate and complicated piece of origami', a wonderful image of the complexity of infolded tissue in the human organism. These villi move rhythmically, immersing themselves in the chyme, 'tasting it'. Every villus contracts independently of the others, but all move in a uniform rhythm approximately six times a minute. At this point in the intestinal wall there is not only a 'sucking in' but also a separation of the constituents of food substances destined for fat formation. Some are channelled into the lymph system, others into blood. Says Gerhard Schmidt: 'Only when the stream of nourishment has reached the intestinal villi and appears in the lymph and blood vessels has it reached the stage whereby it can and must follow the laws of that particular human being's inner organization.'[4]

Fats have passed through the mouth and stomach only marginally altered, but now the enzyme lipase, with the help of bile salts, splits them into glycerol and fatty acids. The glycerol and fatty acids are reconstituted within the intestinal wall into fats *with a characteristically human structure.*

Not all the fats need to be broken down before absorption is possible, provided that the fat particles are small enough they may, as we have mentioned, be absorbed directly into the lymphatic system. Only one other food can be absorbed without further breakdown – grape sugar or glucose. Fats, particularly good quality vegetable oils, are amongst the purest of nature's gifts, if taken in their cold-pressed form. Their 'selfless' qualities are an aid to the digestive process.

By this stage, all the carbohydrates have been converted into simple sugars, which can be absorbed into the blood and thence into the liver, where they are converted into glycogen and stored. Glycogen is now a neutral substance, which needs to be enlivened before passing into the blood-stream again in the form of glucose. It is then called blood sugar and fulfils all our energy needs when it is oxidized. The oxygen needed for this process is supplied by the haemoglobin in the red blood corpuscles. The 'ashes' of this process of respiration are water and carbon dioxide, which when breathed out from the lungs re-enter the atmosphere. The green chlorophyll cells of the plants perform the reverse process of photosynthesis and weave the 'ashes' of respiration into new life-giving substances – oxygen and sugar – in a symbiosis full of wisdom (see p. 162).

Protein

Protein is found everywhere in the body as structural material (in muscle, bone, blood and connective tissue, and to some extent in cell walls). Many substances that have an essential function in the body are also types of protein, such as antibodies, all enzymes and some hormones.

Protein, as the universal 'carrier of life', is distinguished from carbohydrates and fats by the presence of nitrogen. Throughout the process of protein breakdown until the creation of the amino acids there is no alteration of the basic elements carbon, oxygen, hydrogen and nitrogen. Protein molecules are the 'giants' of the biochemical world. Each of these macromolecules is composed of a very long chain of building blocks which are amino acids. These display well-defined intermediate breakdown products, characterized by tremendous plasticity. (Protein's nature is half-liquid, half-colloidal.) Thousands of them may be linked together in one chain. Over 20 kinds of amino acids occur in nature.

Until very recently, every standard source of nutritional information emphasized that there were eight essential amino acids that could not be synthesized by the human body and had to be provided by animal products (if not meat and fish, then certainly by eggs, cheese and milk products). Behind such a concern is a belief that plant protein is deficient in certain amino acids and incomplete for the purpose of human nutrition. Much of the research work behind this thesis was conducted on rats. More recent research, and the fact that approximately two-thirds of the world's population live mainly on plant nutrition, indicate that nearly all complex carbohydrates – such as those in whole grain, beans and seeds – have amino acid profiles which are adequate for human needs. In *Healing with Wholefoods* Paul Pitchford says: 'Each human being constructs his own individual protein as the specific forming substance of his bodily nature. This is an expression of his ego.' (p.90)

The question that arises is whether all humans are capable of synthesizing their protein requirements from plant proteins. Much is made of the combination of grains and legumes (see Chapter 6).

Before dietary protein can be absorbed by the body it must be converted by enzymes termed proteases[5] into smaller constituents called polypeptides, and finally into amino acids. Protein digestion begins in the stomach, where it is acted on by the enzyme pepsin. In the duodenum and small intestine it meets several proteases, such as trypsin and chymotrypsin. The final breakdown products – amino acids – pass into the capillary blood vessels of the villi, and are carried via the portal vein to the liver.

When the amino acids arrive at the liver some of them are immediately converted to blood plasma proteins, such as albumin and fibrinogen. Those amino acids not processed by the liver enter the amino acid pool in the blood-stream from where the individual body cells remove them for their needs. In the cells new proteins are constantly being synthesized from amino acids. Scientists are able to tell us that the chemical processes in the various kinds of cell are controlled by a wide variety of enzymes, and that protein synthesis is selectively regulated by the nucleic acids (DNA and RNA) of particular genes. How this is done is extremely complicated, so we shall simply say that the various kinds of body cell select the special amino acids they need for repair and growth.

In living cells not only are proteins being constantly synthesized, but old, damaged proteins are constantly being degraded. Amino acids liberated in the degradation process are mostly 'recycled' by the cell to form new protein or released to the blood to be taken up by the liver where they are broken down into glucose. In the latter case the liver enzymes first remove their nitrogen – a process termed deamination. In this process carbon compounds are liberated for oxidation, and all nitrogenous residues are converted to urea which is removed by the kidneys.

Though the body can store – for future use – carbohydrates (as glycogen) and fats (in adipose tissue), it cannot store amino acids. Instead, they are converted to other compounds. If there happens to be excessive amounts of protein in the diet, amino acids may be taken up by the liver and converted into fat. Though a healthy liver does not store fat, it does release fat droplets in a transportable form into the bloodstream where it is finally deposited in adipose (fat) tissue, and some also in muscle.

A few hours after a meal there is a high level of nutrients in the blood, but these gradually decrease. After a certain number of hours without food, the body begins to break down the protein in tissues such as muscle, releasing amino groups into the blood. Because the liver is a large organ with a rich supply of blood vessels, these circulating amino acids are quickly accessed by it and resynthesized into proteins needed by the liver itself and for maintenance of all the body's tissues and processes. Amino acids liberated during the fasting period may also be converted to additional glucose for use by the central nervous system and other important tissues. This is just one example of how a temporary shortage of one product in the body is compensated for by other available products. Such processes are governed by intricate biochemical feedback mechanisms that keep the whole internal environment as constant as possible.

Rudolf Steiner had something extra to say on the subject of protein digestion. He indicated that there is a second, invisible process *occurring simultaneously* with the digestive process. It can best be described as a *learning* process. The etheric body must overcome the strong individual tendencies of the four basic substances found in protein: carbon, oxygen, hydrogen and nitrogen. For harmonious interaction, every organ has its own relationship to each substance. The organism maintains this harmonious endeavour, keeping these four elements together even in urea, the last stage of protein breakdown. According to Steiner human protein is the expression of the workings of the etheric, astral and ego through the organs.

The importance of the intestinal flora

In a healthy human being we will find a rich and diverse population of micro-flora occupying the lower part of the small intestine; here coliform organisms and the aerobic lactobacilli predominate. The baby receives an 'innoculation' of its own type of *B. coli* bacteria at birth from his mother. In an adult we can find approximately 3 lb of bacteria, yeasts and fungi in the fermentation chamber of the large intestine. These colonies living in symbiosis within the human organism, in a region generally inaccessible to human consciousness, have a tremendous life activity, breaking down fibre (like a compost heap) and producing B vitamins.

What remains is a semi-liquid mass containing a substantial amount of fibre; the water is absorbed from this mass, causing it to become more solidified. Bacteria that inhabit the colon begin to grow in what remains of the food, breaking it down further and helping to convert it into a substance which can be passed as faeces; 30–50 per cent of the dry weight is made up of these bacteria constantly working on fibres and other residues. In the intestinal flora a process is activated once again that was also active in earlier digestive processes: the overcoming of the foreign nature of food, and the liberation of these formative forces in order to achieve an individual build-up of our body substance. Here, in the activity of microflora, a very particular interaction between metabolism and consciousness occurs, and if this is not balanced there can be an excessive growth of bacteria and yeasts, leading to health problems. Or there can be a diminished population due to taking antibiotics or to poor diet. Altogether the flora indicate the health of the person.

Here I would like to touch on the connection Steiner pointed out between the formation and activity of the intestines and that of the brain. He felt there was an intimate connection, with significance for both areas. There must be a proper amount of time taken for faeces to return again to solidity, be subjected to gravity and only then impinge on human consciousness as they arrive in the rectum. When evacuated there is relief for the other pole, that of thinking. We all know how being constipated can impede our feeling of well-being, and people who suffer from headaches may have found a connection here. Just as choice of foods and eating in a balanced way are important, so the proper process of elimination is essential for health.

Breath and sunlight

It is not usually considered as part of nutrition, but the process of breathing is an essential primary interface with our environment and our digestion. As we mentioned at the beginning of this chapter, previously the human being was almost 'palpated' by the breathing of the cosmos, embedded in the breathing of the earth – 29,250 breaths per day, echoing the number of years for the sun's journey around the zodiac. While we breathed 'with the cosmos' we had a deeper, if less conscious, relationship to nature and its effects on our life processes. More recently we have sought to emancipate ourselves from nature, bypassing her rhythms and weathers, altering our own breathing rhythms, individualizing them and often finding ourselves 'out of sync' both with our own intrinsic organic rhythms and with those of the rest of the human family.

How we breathe

The lung's relationship to the air is that of a vessel; in its structure it can be likened to an upside-down tree, whose hollow trunk and roots can be seen as the lung's air passages (bronchi) all directed upwards. The many millions of tiny alveoli (air sacs) form the leafy crown of this inverted tree. In nature the real tree is surrounded by air but in the human the 'lung tree' is the container of air. Whereas the leaves of the tree absorb carbon dioxide and release oxygen, the lung takes in oxygen and releases carbon dioxide. Tree and lung thus complement each other in a beautiful symbiotic fashion.

Oxygen is taken up by haemoglobin in the blood and, combined with the transformed elements of food (now in liquid form), is transported out of the cells. At each cell these nutrients are exchanged for waste products in the form of carbon dioxide. This is then carried back to the lungs by the blood in a never-ending cycle until death. Thus the bright red oxygenated blood vitalizes, strengthens and nourishes the body; on its way back it is blue and filled with waste products. The alveoli are wrapped in a web of blood vessels, and it is here that the cold air coming from outside directly meets the innermost part of the human being, the warm blood, but it is only separated from it by the thinnest of walls (of a four-thousandth millimetre thickness). In this way a real sea of blood surrounds the inhaled air.

During 24 hours we breathe approximately 8000 litres of air and 17.5 litres of blood pass through the lung capillaries. The lung if flattened out would extend to cover an area of around 100 square metres, yet another example of the infolding of fine but strong tissue to maximize the 'internalizing' of the external world.

The effect of the Age of Enlightenment on breathing

With the rise of objective science from the fifteenth century on, a new kind of breathing began to emerge. At first it was confined to those particularly engaged in the new research methods. Intellectual activity had to be confined, separated from any feelings; strict care was taken that nothing of personal experience or emotion should enter into the observation. It was a distanced mode of observation, supposed to guarantee the objectivity of the exchange. However, every human experience is accompanied by feelings, and such distancing in effect bypassed the heart and its natural responses. The philosopher Hans Jonas characterized this basic requirement as follows: 'The transfer of anything of the character of inner experience into our interpretation of the outer world was to be strenuously avoided. Anthropomorphism became the scientific equivalent of high treason.'[6]

It is interesting to note how the use of tobacco coincided with the pursuit of the rational. Smoking tends to throttle down the life of desires and feelings. Here we see the life of feelings being sublimated in order to develop the rational mind. Psychiatrists Sigmund Freud and Carl Gustav Jung made this phenomenon their life's work — the uncovering of these banished soul experiences. Such a detached conception of the world has no relationship to the feeling human soul, since in the search for total objectivity and rationality all inner feelings and experiences are to be strictly avoided. *For centuries in Western culture the feeling soul has been excluded from cognition.* Today, this is leading to a gradual narrowing of human experience.

In a healthy human being *all* experiences are accompanied by feelings. It is important to try to consciously integrate our feeling life with our thought and our actions. To banish it or 'fix it' with taboos leads to a great loss which can be the precursor of mental or physical illness.

Relaxed versus restricted breathing

How we breathe is a real reflection of our psychological condition. To block feeling requires manipulation of the breath. When we have strong emotional experiences we unconsciously tend to restrict our breathing. Part of our body's defence mechanism is orientated towards the shutting out of physically and psychologically painful experiences thus overloading the various systems. Restriction of breathing is one of the main responses in this defensive reaction; breathing becomes shorter and shallower until it almost stops completely, as if one would hope to become completely invisible.

The young child, however, has to learn to breathe. Just as the sea in the incoming tide does not come in evenly, so the little baby begins to unite itself with its body with a certain oscillation in breathing which may take up to seven years to stabilize. We may watch a sleeping baby and see a certain tremulousness, from time to time fluttering through the sensitive little body. The astral body, which moves through the element of air, is thus playing upon something like a stringed instrument with its axis in the spinal column. The child will often pick up his breathing rhythms from those around him and the whole atmosphere of the home or playgroup. If there are constant noises – television, radio or loud music being played – all these will be formative in establishing his breathing, metabolic processes and nervous system. Even car journeys can affect the heart and pulse beat of a small child particularly, but also of adults, through a surrender to passive movement, that is, a lack of active self-movement. Holtzapfel has said, 'During speeds above 60 miles an hour, the pulse beat increases and thereafter takes at least eight minutes to return to normal.'[7] It is very difficult for most of us to conceive of not travelling in cars, buses, trains or planes, but we need to be aware of the effects of things we use often in our daily lives.

As life progresses, 'The lung's capacity for air increases until the middle of life after which it decreases again. This illustrates how during the course of life the soul is membered into the body, a process which intensifies more and more (in a healthy process) during the first half of life, whereas during the second half it gradually lessens.'[8]

Rudolf Steiner concerned himself greatly with the whole question of appropriate breathing in the parenting and education of the child:

> If you regard with an open mind the child who has found his way into earthly life, you will observe that the soul-spirit is as yet disunited from the life-body (physical and etheric). The task of education in the spiritual sense is to bring the soul-spirit into harmony with the life-body. They must be attuned to one another, for when the child is born they do not as yet fit one another ... Amongst all the relationships which the human has to the external world the most important is breathing ... in his breathing there exists already the whole threefold system of the physical human. There is in the first place the digestion and metabolism; but the assimilation process is intimately connected at one end with the breathing. The breathing is also connected with the blood circulation, through metabolism.
>
> The blood circulation receives into the human body the substances of the external world which are introduced by another pathway; so that on the one hand the breathing is connected with the whole digestive system and on the other hand it is also connected to the nerve-sense life of man. As we breathe in we are continually pressing the cerebro-spinal fluid into the brain and as we breathe out we press it back again into the body. Thus we transplant the rhythm of the breathing into the brain.[9]

We know now that brain volume is altered by breathing, being reduced during inhalation and increased during exhalation. 'We only understand because the rhythmical process regulated by heart and lungs proceeds through the brain fluid to the brain.'[10]

Thus in Waldorf schools appropriate rhythms are developed that are chronologically suited to the child. The day, the week and the year are structured in a harmonious way. The children are introduced to the various crafts such as weaving, felt-making, modelling, copper-beating, pottery, basket-making, woodcarving, shoemaking, all of which have their own movement and breathing-related rhythms. The young people also do archery, juggling, javelin and discus throwing as well as art, music and movement, and of course the usual academic subjects. All of this develops not only hand skills (the hand commands a large area in the brain) but helps to bring their consciousness into their physical body parts and therefore allows their soul and mental capacities to develop in a healthy and balanced way. (Each craft has its own gestures and movements, and therefore its own deep-connected breathing.) Relaxed breathing should be one of the outcomes of such an education, which develops confidence in a young person. This is not understood in conventional education, however. Most adults in today's society do not use the total capacity of their lungs; for many people, the upper chest is where blocking of respiration begins.

I was given a tremendous insight into the workings of the breath during my two labours. The first, in a hospital, was without any kind of preparation and I had a very painful and prolonged labour. With my second baby I attended natural childbirth classes where we were taught to work with the breathing and the body as it went through the contractions. The contrast was remarkable, the ability to relax and co-operate with the wisdom of the body through conscious breathing made an incredible difference. At a later date I experienced some re-birthing, which involved conscious breathing, and found this too very revealing and helpful in understanding how I habitually, if unconsciously, manipulated my breath. Many of us would benefit from unlearning age-old habits and integrate our breath with our bodies in a much more healthy and relaxed way. This takes courage, for shallow breathing is fearful breathing and will not irrigate the brain or the body with adequate oxygen supplies.

Breath and brain function

The brain cannot go without oxygen for more than a short time without being irreversibly damaged. Increased depth of breathing gives an increased flow of oxygen-enriched blood to the brain and helps to produce a flushing out of its accumulated waste products. The capillaries expand and, most significantly, the pineal and the pituitary glands are irrigated with oxygen.

The brain is divided into two halves. The right side of the brain is non-verbal and intuitive. It specializes in thinking in images and patterns, and requires *totalities* for comprehension. It has been traditionally viewed as the seat of wisdom and qualitative perceptions. The left side has developed more capacities for rational, linear, deductive thought; information is reduced to component parts before being processed. In a healthy person these two spheres should be fully integrated and there should be free access for the different and complementary types of information to be exchanged.

When there is emotional stress, excessive amounts of adrenalin and related adrenal hormones are released, requiring oxygen for their metabolism. When less oxygen is available for metabolism then there is a build-up of lactic acid and our cellular environment becomes progressively acidic, resulting in the destruction of cellular functions. According to Drs Levine, and Kidd, hypoxia (lack of sufficient oxygen in the tissues) is a fundamental cause of chronic degenerative disease. Low tissue oxygen has been associated with *Candida albicans* and the degenerative disease cancer.[11]

Good breathing is relaxed, connected breathing; if one starts to feel panicky it is important to remember to breathe calmly.

Light metabolism

Although it is known in clinical practice and research that metabolic processes have a clear relationship to light, metabolism of light is infrequently dealt with as such and then only on a calorific basis. Nevertheless, without light we would not have living substance and we would not be healthy. Fairly recently a disorder was identified – SAD or Seasonally Affective Disorder – in which susceptible people become depressed as the days get shorter. The nutrient of sunlight directly affects us in many energizing ways since light is the least dense form of *prana* – life force – in our universe and is all-pervading. Every living thing is combustible, allowing life-energy to be freed once again in heat and light.

Both the skin and the eye receive light. Through the eye light is conducted as impulses to the visual cortex and also to the centre of the autonomic nervous system. From there it travels to the pineal gland (see pp. 126–7) where the neural hormone melatonin is produced – important for affecting our sleep-life and to calm us down. The nerve receptors in the eye translate the full spectrum of light with all the colours of the rainbow into optic nerve impulses which conduct it to the various brain-centres (pineal and pituitary glands and the rest of the endocrine system, called by the Hindus the chakra system[12]). Light from each of the different bands of the spectrum has a different healing effect.[13] This is one of the reasons why colour is so important in food and cooking.

Light is especially important for the anabolic or upbuilding processes governed by the etheric body. The manufacture of vitamin D is a sunlight process. Dr Husemann explains:

> The metamorphosis of life to an 'inner light' process which is the ultimate basis for thought occurs via the agency of iron. Magnesium internalizes the light and brings it into substance, whereas iron again releases the light from a substance through its capacity for spark formation. There is nothing to compare with iron in carrying light into darkness. Thus the complementary reactions with light in plant and human can be summed up by saying that the affinity of chlorophyll and haemoglobin for light is their porphyrin component. Without this, light could not connect itself with a substance. In contrast, the metal determines the direction in which the light is active.[14]

The importance of the pineal gland

The pineal is a small organ about the size of a chickpea situated in the anatomical centre of the brain and intimately connected to the ventricular system. Its existence has been known for a very long time. The ancient Indians thought it was an organ of clairvoyance and meditation, enabling man to remember his past lives. Galen (AD 130–200) made the first extant statements on the pineal gland, which he called *koneiron* (Latin, *conarium*), after its pine-cone shape.

It is an endocrine organ that synthesizes and secretes various compounds, including melatonin (the most well known and best researched at the present time). The pineal has a copious blood supply from a rich capillary network. It receives a sympathetic nerve supply that modulates its secretions. Although it remains an enigmatic organ, it is an ubiquitously acting endocrine gland, modifying directly or indirectly every system in the body.

Modern research implicates the pineal (via melatonin) in reproductive physiology, circadian phase disorders and psychiatric diseases.[15]

Anthroposophically there is more to say:

> The pineal gland is more or less heart-shaped. The calcium carbonate crystals in it are formed like tiny white roses, which form gradually during the years of childhood. They are formed by what I call the 'ash' of the earthly nutrition stream (this is also a basic tenet of the macrobiotic system). In later life the whole of the pineal gland is dotted with these structures and in fact our self-consciousness is intimately connected with them. The more self-aware we become the harder these structures become. If you follow the development of the pineal gland, it starts as a kind of eye, protruding like a lamp. It was the third eye of Polyphemus in mythology, mentioned over 2500 years ago. It was also an organ which sensed warmth. In the course of evolution it has become smaller and smaller, now being minute. Originally the warmth enabled it to receive great imaginations or mythological pictures. But this capacity died out; the head closed, the skull containing the cortex shutting down the clairvoyant powers given by the pineal. So we became thinkers instead of clairvoyants. This is inscribed in our bodies – *each human body is the script of the evolution of the world.* You can read this script if you know how to spell its letters. Although modern science knows that the pineal is one of the endocrine glands, so far it has been unable to determine its function.[16]

Thus we have seen that in the physical process of digestion we are aided by our breathing and by the capacity of the skin and the eye to use sunlight. Now we will briefly consider how our senses are involved with nutrition.

The senses' role in nutrition

The sense of smell is relatively poorly developed in the human being, compared to that of a dog. Humans are not so specialized, we are omnipotential. Nerve cells in the nasal passages are the shortest in the body and lead directly to the brain, so when we encounter a smell it can quickly seem to envelop us. We soon learn to distinguish between good smells and bad smells. Indeed the sense of smell lays the foundation for a developing sense

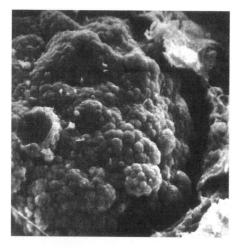

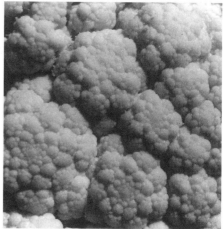

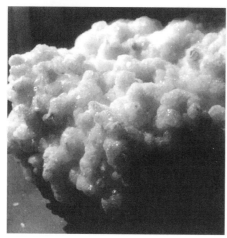

Through her manifold forms Nature shows interesting correspondences: (top left) magnified human pineal from an aged person (actual size is approximately that of a chickpea); (top right) cauliflower; (bottom) calcium carbonate crystal

of morality in the child (demonstrated by expressions like 'I smell a rat!' or 'It stinks!', where there is a strong moral connotation).

Each substance in nature has its own unique and characteristic smell, and for me the quality of a food's aroma is one of the most important indicators of its vitality and authenticity. Smells evoke the deepest of memories, going way back to childhood where the olfactory sense is that first and keenest of sensibilities, enabling the tiny baby to find his way to the nipple before his eyes can properly focus. Sadly it is now difficult in many places to enjoy breathing and smelling the air owing to environmental pollution. People become inured to the fact that they are losing one of the greatest of gifts – the riches available through our sense of smell. We do know that smelling and tasting are inseparable in the way they enhance each other; you only have to suffer from a cold to know that without being able to smell food properly even the best can taste like cotton wool.

With our sense of taste we take in consciously and (often unconsciously) taste a piece of the macrocosm, knowing that it will become the substance of our own body. We may find ourselves asking, 'Is this food compatible with the instrument of my body?' Many allergic reactions arise out of a clear incompatibility between a food and the person eating it, bewildering for both parents and doctors. Children given unnatural foods soon start to lose the capacity to judge the authentic goodness of their food. Lack of real flavours and aromas soon dull the intricate laboratory of our palates.

The tongue is related to the liver, which also 'tastes'. It could be seen as an outpost of the liver, even having a similar shape. The tip of the tongue is particularly sensitive to sweetness, to hot and cold. Much of the tongue is involved in tasting saltiness, the sides sensitized to sour tastes and the back for bitter — taste-buds are grouped all over its surface. It is also of course an important organ in speech. (We speak of 'good taste' and in this sense 'taste' can be applied to our clothes sense, the way we decorate our homes, the kind of books we read and paintings we like. It all points to a gradual refining process, an educating of the sense perceptions.)

Touch is important, especially in gardening or choosing food in the markets, in slicing and chopping and in eating. There are many foods that are best eaten with the fingers (I'm not referring to Kentucky Fried Chicken or hamburgers!) and of course this should all enhance one's sense of enjoyment, for if it's not enjoyable eating is not going to be a nourishing affair. *For Rudolf Steiner, this sense of enjoyment was paramount in nutrition.*

The sense of hearing can also be part of the nutritional process. To hear food bubbling away on the stove or being sautéd, certainly arouses one's interest. Hearing is perhaps a lesser sensibility but nonetheless part of the spectrum of our response to nutrition.

Rudolf Steiner spoke of twelve senses — an important expansion of the rather limiting five senses recognized in current science.[17] We are all multi-sensory beings, a concept that needs to be fostered so children in particular can explore aspects of themselves such as intuition or balance, and give full rein to their wide human potential that sadly is currently being sadly narrowed down.

So, we are nourished through physical food, through our sense perceptions such as seeing a beautiful landscape or listening to a moving piece of music; through breathing in tingling fresh air, or being bathed in spring sunshine. All of these elements can meet in us, being digested in the most varied and subtle of ways, and help to strengthen us to act in life.

However, there have been and still are people who have developed their higher capacities to nourish themselves from a higher nutritional stream, through *prana* – life essence, or the 'cosmic nutritional stream' as described by Steiner. One such person whose extraordinary capacities have been well documented is Theresa Neumann, a young peasant girl from Konnersreuth. One day she fell from a ladder escaping from a fire and was bedridden for a year. She refused to take any nourishment except the eucharistic host which she took at Communion. Every Friday she lived through the crucifixion of Christ and the stigmata would appear on hands and feet. This earned her the reputation of a saint. According to Dr Hauschka, what took place was an activation of the cosmic nutritional stream, also manifested in other sages and yogis, but perhaps not as dramatically as in Theresa. Parahamsa Yogananda speaks of a little grandmother 'who employs a certain yogic technique to recharge her body with cosmic energy from the ether, sun and air ... the technique includes the use of a certain mantra and a breathing exercise. Asked why she would want to live thus she replied "To prove man is spirit. To demonstrate that by divine advancement he can gradually learn to live by the Eternal Light and not earthly food." '[18]

From China comes a Qigong teacher, Yan Xin, who has attracted many students, often from the medical profession. Qigong is an ancient Chinese practice intended to increase the body's stores of 'qi' or 'chi' (universal life energy), to promote its internal circulation and improve healthful vitality. With practice this energy can be directed outwards as a healing benefit to others. Yan Xin is particularly interested in developing an altered physiological state known as *bigu*, meaning 'abstention from food', through Qigong.

These are really interesting phenomena which may give us pause for thought. We are probably only at the beginning of a long journey of understanding the capacities of the human body/soul/spirit. Certainly, in a time when most of us are guilty of eating more than we need it is important to know of the practice of abstention, to have a fast or eat only apples on one day a week, just to give our organism a chance to rest.

After this journey through the digestive system we may ask, 'Do I really need to know all this in order to be nourished?' And the answer is clearly 'no'. But even if we don't understand all that happens in nutrition, I find for my part it gives me such an incredible sense of gratitude that I have all these organs and processes working for me in the darkness of my inner core, selflessly serving me, that it makes me want to do my best for them.

Finally, have you ever considered the 'digestion' of an idea? There is something extraordinary about this process. For instance, you meet an idea, a concept, that may be really difficult at first, requiring you to realign most of the rest of your concepts. Maybe you initially reject it vehemently, but perhaps you find it surfacing again in your consciousness and, as the weeks and months go by, it somehow starts to become more comfortable, more meaningful and enriching to other contexts of your life. Or it can be the opposite, that you are very attracted to an idea, a person, a food, but in due course they are discarded. All this is a digestion process, some of which is conscious and some of which is not. It can be very interesting as an exercise to take a concept that is very dear to you and unravel the process whereby it became embedded in your deepest cosmology. How did it get there? Did it come from your parents? Your teachers? Your partner? Or is it your own synthesis of life's myriad experiences? And has it become rigid?

THE QUESTION OF VEGETARIANISM

In the *Observer* Food Supplement, December 2001, food writer Nigel Slater said:

> Five of the seven people around my table this Christmas will be vegetarians. I haven't planned it that way. That is just the way things have worked out. They know of course that they will be in safe hands; they are aware that I feel the vegetarian diet is best for the long-term future for the planet. I am looking forward to this year's feast more than ever before, and I won't have to do battle with a bird the size of Switzerland!

There are now at least four million vegetarians in the UK according to the Vegetarian Society, a number that is growing steadily, doubling since 1990. Most of these will be lacto-ovarians (eating most things except meat), and a much smaller percentage vegans, who don't eat any animal products (including honey). Following the number of food scandals around the beef industry, many people have given up eating red meat but will eat chicken and fish, and there are 'fishetarians' who will eat fish and not meat.

There is obviously a shift in people's consciousness around the whole subject of feeding themselves. The motives for choosing a vegetarian diet may be manifold: an ethical view and compassion for animals, spiritual discipline, environmental considerations, health and financial reasons. I shall try to look at some of these questions, many of which may be related. It depends on your starting-point.

We in the West must recognize we are at a crossroads as far as the sustainable future of the planet is concerned. Having looked at the historical background of nutrition, it will be clear that the way in which we nourish ourselves in the times to come will have a large impact on both our consciousness and our environment. As followers of a wasteful and extravagant life-style, I feel we have a particular responsibility in reversing some of the trends that have caused this fragility. Unlike many people in the world, we have choices. I would like to make clear from the outset that I am not trying to convert the reader to vegetarianism (personally I favour the 'middle way'). The intention is to air different perspectives, including those arising from Steiner's work.

Support for vegetarianism has come from many sources, traditions and individuals. While I was studying at Cambridge I discovered through Jain friends that whole cultures had embraced vegetarian nutrition for religious, moral-ethical and health reasons. Among these were the Jains (a branch of the Hindu faith particularly sensitive to the sacredness of life, including insects), many Buddhists, the Pythagoreans, the Essenes, the Cathars, Seventh Day Adventists and Zoroastrians. For them life was a whole and food was a gift of the Divine; it was also medicine and, if chosen wisely, an excellent way to stay healthy. Amongst noted vegetarians of the past are Plato, Diogenes, Ovid, Virgil, Plutarch, Leonardo da Vinci, Benjamin Franklin, Gandhi, Albert Schweitzer, George Bernard Shaw, Percy Bysshe Shelley and food reformers Dr John Harvey Kellogg (a Fifth Day Adventist) and Dr Bircher Benner.

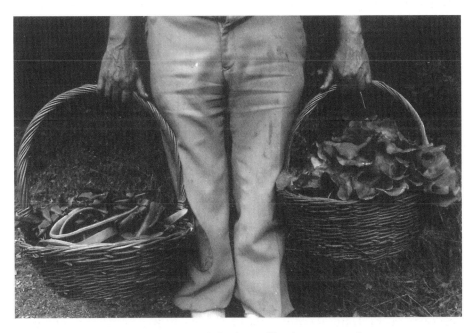

My friend Derek with baskets of biodynamic produce

For acolytes studying the Pythagorean system in the community of Crotona in Italy, vegetarianism was central to their way of life. Pythagoras is deemed by some the 'father of vegetarianism' as well as being well known for his mathematical system:

> O my fellow men, do not defile your bodies with sinful foods. We have corn, we have apples, bending down the branches with their weight, and grapes swelling on the vines. There are sweet flavoured herbs, and vegetables which can be cooked and softened over the fire. Nor are you denied milk, or thyme-scented honey. The earth offers you banquets that involve no bloodshed or slaughter...[1]

The eating of beans was forbidden, not for the obvious reasons that we might conclude, but because during their digestion they disturbed the creative perception of numbers. They were also supposed to have a mystic affinity with the root of sensual and impure desires.[2] (See also Chapter 11 on legumes.)

You will recall the Vedic food categories of *Sattvic*, *Rajasic* and *Tamasic* (see p. 22). In the Sattvic diet the alkaline/acid ratio would be about 70/30. In the Rajasic diet it would be about 50/50 and in the Tamasic the acid pole dominates.

Today most processed or synthetically produced foods fall into the Tamasic category. So do all foods that contain chemicals, preservatives, pesticides, stabilizers, artificial colours and sweeteners. Most fast foods so popular today are Tamasic; they affect the function of the mind as well as the body and tend to irritate the nervous system.

The simple Vedic system is ancient and wise and to my mind does not conflict with Rudolf Steiner's view, or indeed with any wise food philosophies. If we are serious about leading a balanced, harmonious life of inner and outer work that doesn't ravage the environment, we may wish to choose our food under the Sattvic principles. If we wish to be in the competitive thrust of the business world, or do heavy physical work, we may choose Rajasic foods. Or it could be something between the two.

But surely few people would thinkingly choose a Tamasic regime? Yet millions do and millions more succumb as soon as they have the money to make a choice. That this situation has come about through actual choice is difficult to understand. We do appear to be an addictive society – where do these addictions stem from? In general we seem to be experiencing a 'crisis of meaning'; young people particularly are susceptible to fashions and advertising that promote a certain lifestyle of which food is an important part. How can we, in today's culture, find sensible clues to appropriate nutrition amongst all the conflicting information?

Human teeth

If we look at the arrangement of the human teeth and digestive tract we will see that they are intermediate between those of vegetarian and carnivorous creatures. Yet they have a character all their own, allowing the human being the possibility of being an omnivore (eating a mixed diet). When Rudolf Steiner addressed the issue of the human intestine being too short for purely vegetarian nutrition, he said that did not provide proof against the possibility of transformation, although this could take many generations.

Of a total of 32 teeth one quarter are incisors, best suited for cutting and slicing, particularly vegetables and fruits. One eighth are canines, best for dealing with flesh foods, and the remaining five-eighths are molars, including pre-molars ('molar' from Latin *molere* 'to grind'). In the macrobiotic system[3] such a relationship of function to the number of teeth is used as a guideline for a menu that uses grains, vegetables, legumes and a small proportion of animal products if needed. I have noted that many traditional one-pot meals such as paella, cous-cous, polenta pie and cassoulet roughly follow these proportions. They are balanced, nourishing, delicious and satisfying. If prepared properly they show the wisdom and artistry of traditional cooks.

Types of vegetarian

A lacto-ovarian diet is often the preferred diet for vegetarians, though there are those who would dispute this is truly vegetarian. Including milk, dairy products and eggs, it gives a wide variety of foods to choose from. (In Chapter 12 on milk, we shall see how Steiner says it is more 'plantlike' than animal as it is created on the periphery of the animal and does not come into contact with the blood processes.) A certain amount of variety is important for vegetarians, while honouring the seasons and locale as much as possible.

Quality is of the utmost importance and I shall tackle this thorny subject later.

To be a vegan requires a lot of will and a fairly comprehensive knowledge of nutrition, so as to avoid becoming nutritionally deficient. I do think it works better in Mediterranean climates where sun-drenched vegetables and fruits, nuts and olive oil are abundant; but a fuller investigation of veganism goes beyond the scope of this book. The ones who need support are those who may be in transition from a meat-eating diet to one that is more based on fruits, grains, vegetables and dairy foods.

Steiner's perspective

Rudolf Steiner owed his vigour to a vegetarian diet: 'I myself know that I would have been unable to go through the strenuous activities of the last 24 years without vegetarian nutrition.'[4]

Animal protein varies according to the animal. In terms of organization it is closer to human flesh, whereas the plant is further away and the mineral even further. Rudolf Steiner stresses that nourishing ourselves properly should provide a real challenge to the human metabolic system. This system is capable of transforming substance and reorganizing it through processes of catabolism (destruction) and anabolism (upbuilding). Human digestion can transform plant material into human flesh — something we are not used to thinking of.

Biological transmutations take place within the human digestive system, a vital activity that demonstrates how in living matter higher levels of organization are able to completely transform lower or simpler levels. Animals and plants can change one element into another. Stones do indeed become bread!

What the plant does in the sphere of life (the etheric), the animal does in the sphere of sentience (the astral). This world of inner experience includes the dim awareness of the earthworm, the myopic dreaminess of the cow as she ruminates, or the nervous awareness of the stag. The plant enlivens substances from the mineral world and transforms sunlight into a living starch; the animal 'ensouls' living plants. We have said earlier that these substances must be reorganized and reformed. It is not just the chlorophyll greenness but life itself (from the etheric perspective) which is sacrificed to a higher power – the soul of the animal. It is the soul that transforms living substances from the plant kingdom into a body suitable for the expression of its particular awareness.

When the human being eats animal protein he has to break it down into amino acids, urea and glucose. However, the 'cosmic images' revealed to him in this process are quite different from when he eats plants. The information carried in the plant has been absorbed by the animal. We are confronted with information about the building up of a body suitable for the manifestation of the animal soul, as expressed in behaviour and instincts. Is this information of use to us in building up our own human bodies? In so far as our bodies are the instruments of instincts and inherited behaviour, yes, it can be, but if we wish to fine-tune this instrument to become sensitive for soul/spiritual work, requiring the most subtle configuration of nervous tissue, it may be a burden. So there is a question of how flesh-eating may affect the consciousness of the human being as well as his metabolism.

Hunters such as American Indians, who ate the flesh of animals, maintained a state of health and alertness greater than is seen commonly in our sedentary societies. They had insight and respect for the animals they hunted and in eating them knew that they were transforming the animal onto a higher level of existence. Thus there was a kind of pact between hunter and prey. The hunters took only according to their needs. However, hunting and eating an animal that has foraged in a natural environment cannot be compared to eating the flesh of animals that have been commercially reared. Those who eat a mainly meat diet without having to hunt, kill their prey or even do much in the way of physical labour may well suffer from pent-up aggression. One anthropologist has suggested that warfare in prehistoric Europe became 'an everlasting proclivity' only after livestock breeding became common in rural communities.[5]

Herodotus noticed similar effects:

Among our humanity there are those who lead wars against one another, who relate through anger, antipathy and sensual passions. They draw this out of animal nutrition. They have, however, developed bravery, courage and boldness. Other cultures, occupied with more spiritual pursuits, customarily used mostly plant nutrition.[6]

And Rudolf Steiner says that, if we look at the physical processes which result from meat-eating,

[...] we find that red blood corpuscles become darker and heavier and the blood has a greater tendency to clot. Phosphates and salts are produced more easily; with predominantly vegetarian food the sedimentation rate of the blood corpuscles is much lower. Connection with the plant world strengthens the human inwardly. Meat introduces something which gradually becomes something of 'a foreign substance' in humans, and goes its own independent way in him. Because the nervous system is thus influenced from outside it may become susceptible to various nervous diseases. So we see that in a certain sense, 'man is what he eats'.[7]

A diet too centred on meat products also tends to cause deposits of uric acids which in excess become toxic in bodily tissues, particularly in the joints. Gout – caused by these deposits – was once considered to be the illness of the rich and idle, but it is still with us. Excess uric acid is also implicated in arthritis. Our bodies are able to excrete only eight grains of uric acid per day, but eating 1lb of meat would leave a residue of 18 grains of uric acid.[8] Uric acid initially has a stimulating effect on the human being as its structure is similar to that of caffeine. It is also low in oxygen.

In 1923 Rudolf Steiner made what amounts to a prediction of BSE:

Now these salts of uric acid have their own special habits. They have a liking for the nervous system and the brain and if the cow were to eat meat, enormous quantities of uric acid salts would be deposited; they would be deposited in the brain and the cow would become deranged. If we could make the experiment of suddenly feeding a herd of cows on doves [pigeons] the result would be a completely mad herd. This is how it would be, in spite of the gentleness of the doves, the cows would become mad.[9]

Plant material, however, leaves the human nervous system free of those extraneous astral products from the animal whose sentient life is imprinted upon its tissues and in its blood. So a nervous system built up of mainly plant substances allows a person to be more sensitive to subtle spiritual impressions and to become aware of the wider interconnectedness of all things. Steiner felt that 'plant food will take an ever larger place in human nutrition'.[10]

Years ago Professor Erwin Schrödinger, Nobel prize-winning physicist, asked: 'What is this precious something in our food that protects us from death? Our organization is maintained by removing order from the environment.'[11] In other words, the mark of a living organism – order and regulation – can only be effected by order itself, which gives us a powerful hint about quality in foods.

Food quality

Now we may move on to explore the question of quality, particularly in plant food, for there is a great deal of variation. As I see it, for those who are going to use mostly plant-derived nutrition it is of utmost importance that they seek out really freshly harvested and properly grown organic or biodynamic produce. We now find many vegetarians taking mineral supplements because they don't seem to be able to manage on conventionally grown food. However, there is a problem in accessing the missing nutrients taken out of context as dietary supplements, even if they are chelated (see Chapter 15 on minerals). Swamping the system with non-food state minerals does not necessarily mean they will be absorbed by the body.

Nutrition is concerned with the assimilation into the human body of orders of energy; the higher and finer they are the closer they are to sun energy. Rhythm and order are usually the hallmarks of well-grown plants, the carriers of transformed sunlight, and nutrition from them would work against entropy and death forces. This gives us a powerful hint as to where the best quality is to be found.

Where do these higher forces exist?

Of the bodily [and plant] substances, sugars (in the form of starch) and protein show a special relationship to light in that they are optically active. [...] In the same way as living substances can only arise from a living body, an optically active substance can be produced only by another such substance.[12]

This process is primarily responsible for the fact that light in substance can be 'life'; that is, the 'life body' is a 'light body'. These are thoughts echoed by Rudolf Steiner:

Sunlight has the task of stimulating the etheric body to build up the plant organism out of inorganic substances. [...] The inner light [the astral body] initiates the partial destructive processes through which alone consciousness and inner soul life are possible.[13]

There is dispute and debate whether organic food is healthier. It is in the interests of the food industry to have people believe it is impossible to prove this. But most good cooks don't need scientific proof, they know only too well the importance of aroma (which greatly affects flavour), of texture, of the weight/size ratio, and of colour – all indications of the vitality of a fruit, vegetable or herb. A good cook has developed over years an attuned sense perception regarding such qualities; he or she doesn't need to know a food's chemical composition. That, after all, is only part of the picture, but one that the food chemists spend a great deal of time and energy on. More honest labelling regarding the origins of foods will also help.

Methods of illustrating the vitality of food and water have been researched within the biodynamic system.[14] (See pictures, p. 141.) The pictures from these methods show rhythmic and integrated structures in plants grown organically and biodynamically, whereas conventionally grown plants show a denaturing, with gaps in their organization, spaces which can fill up with water causing weak cell structure and weak nuclei. Such plants generally have poor keeping quality compared to biodynamic and organic produce.

The German physicist Popp believes it is impossible to measure by conventional means the energies necessary for the maintenance of life processes.[15] He has demonstrated that food of the highest quality shows the highest photon transmission, compared with average quality food of identical caloric value. (Photons are stored in the DNA during photosynthesis and transmitted continuously by living cells.) His work might also cast some light on the essential nature of vitamins and minerals.

Dr Popp's current research has demonstrated a difference of up to 98 per cent in the amount of low-level luminescence in plant foods from biological farming systems over that from conventional systems. Another quality-testing method uses forced storage, and shows loss of nutrients in differing degrees during storage.

The fluids present in living material show important differences too. Water has many important properties. Well-grown plants have a 'structured-water' content that is dynamic and contains well-distributed solutions of specific minerals, just as our bodies contain fluids with crystal qualities. In its essential (Platonic) form of a tetrahedron, a water molecule contains the potential forms of all crystals. Water can bring all different forms of ions into a crystalline state and hold them in solution. In addition, the more structured the water is the higher concentration of ions it

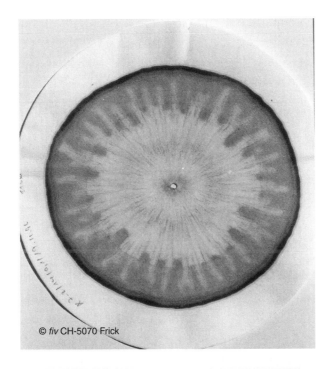

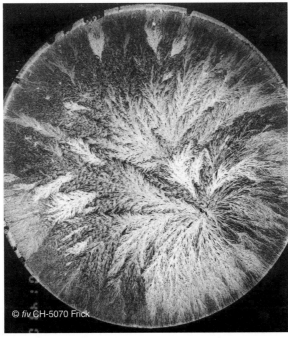

Illustrations of plant vitality: the sensitive crystallization process as developed by E. Pfeiffer demonstrating plant vitality: (bottom) copper chloride crystallization; (top) circular chromatogram

can hold, one of the most important of these ion solutions being dissolved cell salts.[16]

The finer energies held in plants can now be measured. But we can also develop our own sensitivities to this level of energetic activity and recognize it when choosing one item over another. The more aware we are when we select our food, the more likely we are to be drawn to the best.

The question of slaughter

Dr Marthe Kiley-Worthington[17] asks:

> Is it acceptable to slaughter animals at all, even if the conditions of transport and at the slaughterhouse will cause them no distress and pain? The major problem with maintaining that it is not right to slaughter animals at all for food is the consequence.
>
> What would happen if animals were never slaughtered?
>
> - In a short time their numbers would be unsustainable. As a result they would gradually be got rid of.
> - Would there be any animals around at all? Would we not (as I fear) just descend into a totally anthropocentric world, with a few precious nature reserves where we could go and 'view' nature like going to the Tate Gallery, and where one would have to queue for tickets?
> - How would their roles in the farm ecosystems be fulfilled without them? Animals use areas not suitable for food production and their manure gradually upgrades the whole system.
> - We stand to lose so much. If there are no animals around we would not be able to learn from exposure to different sentient beings.

She suggests that even if we had animals for milk, wool, energy or any other product without causing death or suffering on their part, we would still have to kill some of them. For example, if we want milk we must have young born every year. What happens to the spare males? If we never kill old or decrepit animals we shall end up with very large populations to be supported on the farms. There is a case for raising some animals for meat provided their lives are happy and joyful.

It is relatively easy to fulfil the majority of the ecological and ethological criteria when keeping suckler cattle outdoors. However, fattening feedlots where animals or birds are kept indoors in crowded conditions, fed low-fibre diets, given no bedding and very restricted behavioural opportunities make for conditions highly inappropriate both environmentally and etho-logically.

Domesticated animals are no longer self-regulating as most wild animals are and so we should take full and conscious responsibility for the welfare of farm animals; if it is necessary to cull them in the production of milk products or wool, we should develop the most humane way of dealing with this. That some farmers have lost their traditional ways in animal husbandry and only perceive their animals as units of profit shows the high degree of spiritual deterioration in our fundamental attitude to agricultural practices.

Michael Schmundt, who used to be a farmer and herdsman at Ringwood Camphill Community, has said:

> It is not so long ago that the bullock which was to be slaughtered on the farm for the winter's meat supply was the most venerated animal there. He had his own name and was handed the best scraps. The slaughtering day became a festival and the animal's exit was accompanied by antici-pation. The butcher would be local. They were proud of the animal and remembered for years its character and good meat. They were grateful.
>
> In this characterization there was not a moment when there was the occasion of fear or terror for the animal because the people around it kept its soul in an atmosphere of human warmth. Today this has largely changed. It is not death that terrifies the animal, but the being left alone by his keeper, the farmer. It is the large slaughterhouses with so little of this human warmth, the clanging of metal, the cold concrete floors and walls, the bright lights, the being beaten, being too close to other animals. It is the apparent lack of humanity in the people around them. It is a terrifying nothingness into which they are plunged; the hurry to dismember the animal's body. This is what causes the fear in the eyes of the animal, a fear that causes suffering in the whole soul existence of the species. Because domestic animals have kept as we have seen, throughout evolution, close to human beings they continue to need this closeness particularly in death.[18]

Animals that have obligingly provided us with milk, meat, wool and leather are innocents. How can we have become so alienated from the warm and intimate relationship that used to be the stamp of the herdsman or shep-herd, the feeling of care and responsibility? Of course, there are farmers who still maintain such a relationship and I am glad to say this has been my experience with biodynamic stockmen, who create special events involving people and animals, such as singing carols to the cows in their stalls at Christmas (marked by a special attentiveness from the cows). Domesticated animals need us as we need them. It is a question of balance and proportion and of responsibility.

A statistic used popularly today to illustrate the wastefulness of cattle-breeding for meat is that one animal needs to eat 20 lb of vegetable protein to produce 1 lb of meat, resulting in dairy herds being fed high protein con-centrates. Another even more alarming statistic is that 1 hectare of cleared tropical forest is said to yield meat enough for 1850 beefburgers, meat worth at the site not more than $40, especially unsustainable in the tropics, of course, where the forests are so much more valuable to us than we seem to have grasped. Breeding beef cattle is wasteful on many counts, but cows and steers were designed to convert rough pastures and there are still areas of rough pasture ideal for grazing and not for growing vegetables.

As I said in the chapter on agriculture, biodynamic farms ideally operate according to the character of their own land and will only keep the appro-priate number of animals that can be fed comfortably on that area. It all sounds so simple and obvious, and practical, but the kind of thinking that has created our present-day situation is divorced from what is obvious and practical, and it will take some very strong minds to recreate a healthy, balanced agriculture – a 'culture' rather than an industry.

The protein question – which sort should we eat?

Not long ago nutritional scientists were convinced that in order for a human being to thrive it was necessary to eat protein from meat, fish, eggs or milk. When they were confronted with the phenomenon of two-thirds of the world surviving with little or none of these proteins they assumed it was because such people were genetically different from Western people. It could have been partially true, as we shall see in a moment, but it also shows how inadequately the whole question of protein has been understood.

Amino acids are the building blocks of protein. The antibodies of the immune system, most hormones, the haemoglobin of the red blood cells and all enzymes have protein at their centre. It is now commonly accepted that an adult person needs only eight essential amino acids in the diet, but virtually every unrefined food from the vegetable or animal kingdom has not only these eight but all the non-essential amino acids.[19]

To obtain vegetable protein equivalent to that of meat one can eat a diet of two parts grain to one part legume (see p. 193). Adding nuts or seeds will also increase the amino acid spectrum and with the inclusion of seed oils, fruits and vegetables an almost complete spectrum of nutrition can be obtained.

Vitamin B_{12} is often cited as the vitamin likely to be deficient in vegetarian diets, but in healthy people B_{12} is manufactured in large amounts in the colon through the action of beneficial bacteria. Small amounts appear in mouth enzymes also, and in the gastro-intestinal tract. Foods that contain B_{12} are live yoghourt, miso, algae and yeast products. However, the conditions for healthy gut flora need to be encouraged by our nutritional habits. (See Chapter 5 on the processes of nutrition.)

Despite the obvious potential for humans to nourish themselves entirely from plant sources, there are still those who find themselves unable to thrive on a vegetarian diet and appear to have a physiological need for meat. Perhaps the recent research by Peter J. d'Adamo may shed some light on this:

> The story of human survival is reflected in our digestive and immune systems. It is in these two areas that most of the distinctions in blood types are found. Blood provides a keystone for humanity – a looking-glass through which we can trace the faint tracks of humanity.[20]

It might appear an overly simplistic explanation of differences, but blood is certainly an indicator of our genetic heritage and the study is a very interesting one with many implications. Here is a brief outline of Peter d'Adamo's groupings:

Type O reflects a human being whose ancestors have experienced the entire spectrum of human nutrition, going back to the Cro-Magnons who were skilful hunters around 30,000 BC. By 20,000 BC these people, now in Europe, are thought to have quickly become omnivorous (hunter/gatherers). The Arabic population around the location of biblical Babylon is primarily Type O, with some frequency of Type A.

Type A reflects a more domesticated agrarian lifestyle, emerging in the Middle East around 15,000 BC. Planning ahead and networking became important: seeds had to be kept, so storage and distribution meant co-operation with others. Blood type A is still found concentrated mainly around the Mediterranean – the Aegean, the Adriatic, in Spain, Corsica, Turkey, the Balkans, and also in Japan.

Type B is for 'Balance' and also developed 15,000–10,000 BC in the Hima-layan highlands, now India and Pakistan. This new blood type was soon characteristic of the great tribes of steppe dwellers, inhabiting the vast Eurasian plains. The Jewish peoples also show a high pre-ponderance of blood type B, particularly the Ashkenazin and the Sephar-dim. And so do the modern sub-continental Indians, northern Chinese and Koreans.

Type AB represents the most modern evolution of blood type, emerging from the intermingling of Type A Caucasians with Type B Mongolians. It has been identified as only occurring in the last thousand years and is found in less than 5 per cent of the world's population. It is the first blood type to manifest a synthesis of immune characteristics and may present a fitting metaphor for modern life: complex and unsettled.

Hence blood type is other than race, more fundamentally revealing than our ethnicity and shows we are all potentially brothers and sisters – in blood. Peter d'Adamo goes on to explore what combinations of food might be appropriate for different blood groups, which you may choose to follow up for yourself. There could also be a link to what Rudolf Steiner meant when he said, 'Not everyone can become a vegetarian in one lifetime' (both blood type and hereditary conditions may make that difficult). The theory may also explain why certain groups (e.g. many Africans) cannot digest milk and milk products.

We acknowledge that few people live from an exclusively meat diet. However, we in the West seem to be excessive consumers of animal prod-ucts; the average Western diet contains more than 50 per cent animal products, and the diets of Americans generally exceed the Federal Govern-ment's recommended daily allowance of protein by 100 per cent for men and 40 per cent for women. Paul Pitchford in *Healing with Whole Foods* says: 'The mega-protein mania symbolizes the consciousness of a society based on continuous growth, as protein is the body's builder.'[21]

Steiner stated: 'By eating too much protein one calls forth the dominance of the reproductive forces. The control of the sexual passions is therefore made very difficult. [...] It is actually impossible for a person to eat too little protein.'[22]

The modern vegetarian is faced with many choices. Each has to find their way through this labyrinth of options, according to their ethical position, linking to issues of conservation, animal welfare, health, food miles and finance.

PART THREE

THE THREEFOLD PLANT

Let us look at the nature of the plant, its threefoldness — root, stem and leaves — and its relationship to the human being. We can see in the plant a correspondence to the organization of the human being. The human being experiences himself as a centre of being in the universe; the plant experiences the universe as streaming in from the periphery of the cosmos and from the earth. This is a significant distinction. Plato expresses it when he declares that the human being is a plant turned upside down with the roots reaching to the heavens and the branches to the ground.

A biodynamic horticulturist describes the cosmic context of the plant as follows:

> The plant depends on the day and night cycle of the sun for its rhythm; transpiration is directly linked to the sun. The yearly solar rhythm affects weather and precipitation and thus the annual rhythm of the plant growth. Its warmth is that of the sun. Its 'blood' the green sap, which is a mirror image of the red blood of the human, even to its chemical formula. The molecule for chlorophyll is the exact mirror of haemoglobin, except that the chlorophyll has a magnesium ion where the haemoglobin has an iron ion. No chlorophyll can be formed, however, without iron being present, just as no blood can be formed without magnesium being present. Red and green are complementary colours, and if one stares at one too long the retina compensates by producing its opposite.[1]

Thus the plant stands as a mirror to the human being and the animal. The act of respiration provides another instance of this. The human being breathes in oxygen and breathes out carbon dioxide, whereas the plant reverses that process, absorbing carbon and breathing out oxygen. So we are in a symbiotic indebtedness to the plant world; we are in a stream through which life moves as water moves through the bed of a stream, ebbing and flowing.

> By means of the plants the rays of the sun are transformed into flesh. Alone of all the life forms plants can not only catch sunlight, but by a unique alchemy (the porphyrin ring) compound it with terrestrial in-gredients to make the basis of food and substance of all living things.[2]

In the lily and the rose we have the archetypes of all food plants, which derive from the two main groups – the monocotyledons and dicotyledons. Later we shall be looking at some of the plant families of the principal food crops.

If vegetables, grains, fruits and nuts come to play an increasingly impor-tant role in our diets, it is important that they are grown organically (with compost and no artificial additions), or, even better, biodynamically (these crops are likely to have a higher proportion of trace minerals and vitamins, reflecting the etheric qualities of life that I am trying to emphasize).

Threefold plant – threefold human being

The plant manifests a threefold nature corresponding to the threefold nature of the human body, so that particular parts of the plant nourish and strengthen particular parts of the human being.

When as a result of sunlight starch has been formed in the plant's green leaves, further changes take place as more warmth and other environmental factors bring the plant into blossom. Here starches are refined into sugars, sugars become glycosides and contribute to the plant's fragrance and colour, and later the fruiting process develops. In contrast to this upwards refining process we find plant tissues usually more condensed the closer we get to the root. Here the substance of starch is hardened to become cellulose, which is an excellent structural material. We find it throughout the plant as a framework and it is a much valued structural part of man's diet. In the root and the stalk this material can harden and become quite woody. In root, leaf (and stem) and fruit (including seeds, nuts and cereal grains), the corre-sponding polarities in the human being can be seen in the nervous system (centred in the head), rhythmic system (heart and lungs, centred in the chest), and metabolic-limb system (intestines and limbs):

Human being	Plant
Nervous system (head)	Root
Rhythmic, breathing system (heart and lungs)	Leaf and stem
Metabolic and limb system (intestines and limbs)	Fruit, seeds, nuts, blossoms

The root of the plant is most sensitive to the earth (so 'geotropic'). It often spreads out over wide distances, its fine lateral roots seeking out and selecting minerals, salts and water in the cool depths of the earth. These are then lifted up and vitalized through fine capillary systems out of the dark and towards the light. As we have seen, the root is the most dense, mineralized, ligneous part of the plant.

The human nervous system, centred in the head, also seeks out, selects and vitalizes ideas, thoughts and concepts. It depends on fine amounts of trace minerals such as phosphorus to carry out its activities. It also functions best when it is slightly cooler than the rest of the body. These characteristics it shares with the root vegetable.

The leafy part of the plant, with its large surface area for assimilating sunlight, is where respiration occurs. It unfolds rhythmically, node by node. Rudolf Steiner compared this to the human heart/lung or rhythmic system. The spine with the ribs enclosing the chest cavity is where the human organs of respiration are found, giving the gesture that gives a clue to the particular efficacy of plant leaves to stimulate this breathing part of the human being.

In the part of the plant where blossom, fruit and seed are created we have warmth and sugar formation. In human metabolic activity we also find a greater degree of warmth and activity. So we may say that the fruiting part of the plant particularly nourishes the metabolic, digestive processes.

The middle system, which is to do with feelings and emotions, mediates between the other two poles of the human being – the nervous system and the digestive system – bringing balance. Illness can occur when the two poles are out of balance and the middle – respiratory – system is unable to correct it.

I have given you here a larger picture to provide an insight into the nutritional values of various plant parts, rather than a rigid formula. Let us now look at some specific families of vegetables and other food plants.

Umbelliferae (carrot family)

This family is noted for dense and bulky roots and, above ground, for fine, feathery leaves and heads of delicate flowers (the umbels), which in some cases produce aromatic seeds. Members of the *Umbelliferae* are highly developed in attracting and transforming the forces of light, and provide us with many of our most nutritious foods, herbs and medicinal plants. The foods include the carrot, parsnip, Hamburg or root parsley, celeriac, Florence fennel and celery. The herbs are lovage, sweet fennel, chervil, dill, coriander and parsley. Aromatic seeds containing essential oils are produced by coriander, cumin, aniseed, dill, fennel and caraway. The poisonous hemlock and fool's parsley belong to this family too.

The carrot particularly deserves our attention. The blossoming process that produces colour in the plant has penetrated the root, giving it a rich colour, fragrance and sweetness. Many minerals are to be found here: magnesium, iron, calcium, potassium, phosphorus, arsenic, nickel, cobalt, copper, iodine and manganese. Furthermore, in the carrot there are considerable quantities of silicic acid with its relationship to light (perhaps supporting the old saying 'carrots help you to see in the dark'). Carotene (a yellow pigment), too, lies in the root in crystalline form and thus has a 'salt' character.[3]

The young child will benefit greatly from having carrots in his diet, which will help to stimulate his 'silica building processes', since his sensory organs and brain are still developing. He needs a proper 'salt' process (not to be confused with table salt) in order to build a sensitive nervous system. Carrots, either grated or in the form of juice, strengthen children's teeth, brittle nails or hair. They are also helpful in cleansing and detoxifying. In the cooked form where the cellulose is softened and starches become sweeter, it is more gently cleansing and nourishing. The quality of the carrot is of course important; if it becomes weak, for instance it is infested with carrot fly, then it cannot be nearly so effective. When using carrot for juice it is critical to avail yourself of organic vegetables as any residues will be concentrated even more in the juice.

The *Umbelliferae* generally help with the breakdown of the products of digestion and with the excretory processes (sweat and urine). The aromatic seeds of certain members of the Umbelliferae such as coriander, caraway, fennel and aniseed act medicinally in cases of poor carbohydrate digestion where there may be blockages of gas. Dill, chervil and parsley are used in aromatic sauces and salad dressings; they help stimulate digestion.

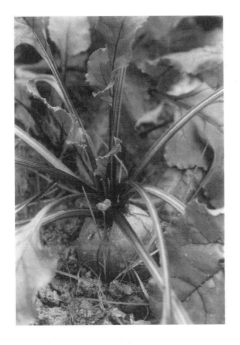

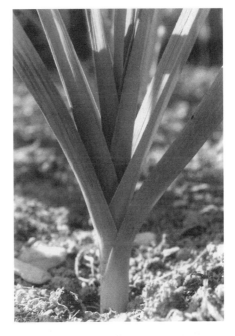

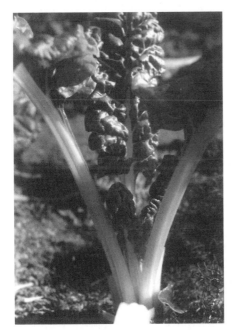

*Edible root: beetroot (top left). Edible
stem: leek (top right). Edible leaf: chard*

Cruciferae (cabbage family)

This family includes the brassicas, recognizable at the flowering stage by the four petals forming a cross. The cabbage and its relatives spring from the wild *Brassica maritima*, a native of Mediterranean coasts, which can tolerate salty soil. Sulphur is a characteristic element of the crucifers; it has a warming quality and through its plasticity of form makes an enormous variety of shapes possible in the different plants of the cabbage group. They form swollen heads in all areas of a plant from top to bottom. Here are some examples:

turnip	root
kohlrabi	swollen base of stem
white cabbage	solid leaf head
red cabbage	sweet leaf head
savoy cabbage	curly leaf head
kale/spring greens	curly open leaves
brussels sprouts	compact buds borne along the stems
cauliflower	single large swollen blossom head
broccoli	several swollen flowerheads
calabrese	loose, green terminal head

The various brassicas have the same thin blue-green wax layer on their leaves and stems, and contain oils midway between fats and resins. All crucifer seeds are rich in oil; rapeseed, for example, is 40 per cent oil. Other crucifers that are particularly rich in sulphur, are cress, radish and horseradish. Their penetrative capacities quicken slow digestion and horseradish particularly stimulates the liver and its activity in gall-secretion, relieving the head pole in the process. The sulphur quality in the brassica family activates a fermentation process which can cause flatulence (it can be tempered by adding a very small quantity of caraway or fennel seed during the cooking process). Kale and cabbages can also harmonize the rhythmic system.

Chenopodiaceae

Also known as the Goosefoot family. Here we find the beetroot, which has similar properties to the carrot, sugar beet, the mangel, spinach beet, seakale beet, Swiss chard and fat hen. They are strong in sugars and mineral salts.

Compositae
This family, which includes the daisies, has many contributions in both the culinary and medicinal sphere. The complex flowerheads show a really harmonious and rhythmical structure. Food plants include the lettuces, endive, chicory, salsify, both the Jerusalem and globe artichokes and their relative, the sunflower. Medicinal plants are chamomile and dandelion (both used in biodynamic preparations), arnica, mugwort, wormwood, marigold and tarragon. Globe Artichokes are particularly good in stimulating liver processes, arnica for bruising (both internally and externally). Marigold petals are lovely in salads and in rice puddings.

Leguminosae
See Chapter 11 on Legumes, p. 188.

Cucurbitaceae (gourd family)
This family includes cucumbers, marrows and courgettes, pumpkins, summer and winter squashes, melons, water melons and gourds. With their high water content they tend towards having a cooling effect on the metabolism. The large flowers of marrow plants are delicious stuffed with a mixture of rice, herbs and nuts. All members of this family need warmth and a rich soil for healthy growth.

Polygonaceae
A family that features buckwheat (traditionally used in the Balkans and often mistaken for one of the seven cereals), as well as sorrel and rhubarb, whose oxalic acid content gives purgative properties.

Convolvulaceae
This family, to which the bindwind belongs, provides the exquisite blue flowers of the morning glory. And it supplies us with sweet potatoes, which were first cultivated in Peru and have now spread round the world. In America they are often called yams, but the true yams belong to the *Dioscoreaceae* family, whereas the *Malvaceae* or mallow family provide the vegetables okra and gumbo as well as the mallows and hollyhocks.

Dioscoriaceae
In this family are several species of yam, which have underground tubers.

Many varieties of yam are cultivated as an important food crop, mainly in the tropics.

Solanaceae
See Chapter 10 on the nightshade family, p. 178.

Labiatae
Members of this family are noted for their gesture of offering themselves; through their leaves or flowers they exude powerful fragrances that help both assimilation and purification of the blood. Examples are the various mints, melissa (lemon balm), marjoram, rosemary, sage, summer savoury and thyme, revealing a very rhythmical growth process connected with warmth and mineral salt formation. (See Chapter 16.)

All the families mentioned above belong to the Dicotyledons. The Mono-cotyledons include the grasses and cereals (*Gramineae*) and the lily family (*Liliaceae*) symbolized by the Madonna, epitome of purity and grace. Closely related to the lily family are the onions (*Alliaceae*), which also include leeks, garlic and chives. Onions aid digestion, stimulate appetite and excretion, and add flavour to food.

Fruits

So many fruits come from roses
From the rose of all roses
From the unfolded rose
Rose of all the world.
Admit that apples and strawberries and peaches and pears
and blackberries
Are all Rosaceae
Issue of the explicit Rose,
The open-countenanced skyward smiling rose.
[...]
Ours is the universe of the unfolded rose,
The explicit, the Candid revelation ...

From *Grapes* by D.H. Lawrence[4]

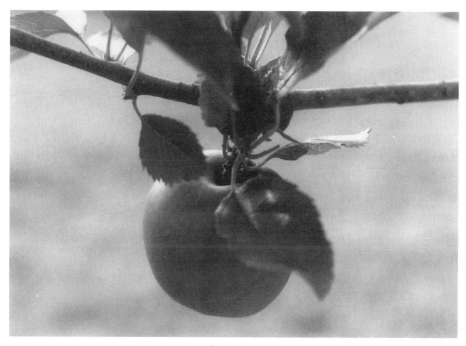

Apple (Roseacae)

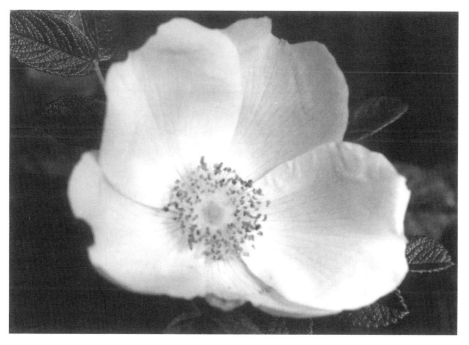

Briar rose

How could this gift of the rose family of fruits be more lovingly described?

Fruits are important in our diet not only because when ripe and well grown they are delicious, but because they act particularly on the blood and circulatory system. They act to cleanse and stimulate; sometimes they warm, sometimes they cool (as melons do). They bring in the most natural way that element of sweetness into our lives that we all crave, so are incredibly important, especially for children.

Fruits are good sources of vitamins, particularly vitamin C, beta carotene, potassium, magnesium, and many other micro-nutrients. According to their season fruits come with specific nutritional tasks. For instance, in late summer, blackberries, damsons, sloes, rich in iron (absorbed from the finely dispersed meteoric iron from meteor showers), give us that special Michaelmas energy to face the winter.

Recent research has begun to uncover the amazing complexity of substances that give the particular colour to fruits and vegetables. Their colours are so important both physically and aesthetically:

> Another class of antioxidant polyphenols found in many plants are red and purple pigments called anthocyanins and proanthocyanidins (found to have powerful and varied anti-cancer activity and also protect against coronary heart disease). They give colour to berries, cherries, red grapes, plums and, pomegranates.[5]

And, according to Dr Gabriel Cousins, each coloured food particularly energizes, cleanses, builds, heals and rebalances the glands, organs and nerve centres associated with its colour-related chakra.[6] (For instance wild strawberries are used as a cure for anaemia.) So we must become more and more aware of the importance of colours in foods; they are by no means arbitrary but part of the plant's unique signature.

Dried fruits are also an important adjunct to the diet. If sun-dried, which is preferable of course, they will be full of sun forces and vitamins A, B and C. They have warming and often laxative properties (figs and prunes), and are rich sources of proteins and of the minerals iron and calcium.

CARBOHYDRATES AND SWEETENERS

Carbohydrates are built through the agency of warmth and the light of the sun. We find carbohydrates in roots, stems, leaves and fruit of the plants in varying forms and they constitute the physical bulk of our nutrition. Carbon, oxygen and hydrogen form the carbohydrates.

Carbon is the most universal building block of creation and its presence in the universe is special. Though carbon forms less than a millionth of the earth's volume, it forms the basis of all organic compounds. From it are built sea urchins, brown bears and operatic divas! The carbon atom is composed of six protons, six neutrons and six electrons and was formed in the centre of stars. In the carbon atom is contained a storm of electricity – that whirling presence which apart from its structural role makes it essential for the thinking process. If we burn a plant in a test-tube we will be left with a skeleton of carbon.

Green plants synthesize carbohydrates from water and carbon dioxide, in the presence of chlorophyll and the light of the sun. The carbohydrate molecules are formed from the elements carbon, hydrogen and oxygen, and the process is known as photosynthesis, or carbon assimilation. We find carbohydrates in roots, stems, leaves and the fruits of plants as starches and sugars; they serve as a store of energy. From the simpler carbohydrates, such as glucose, the plant synthesizes more complex substances, such as cellulose, fats and oils and – together with nitrogen – proteins. The plant is thus able to build up new living substance from these complex compounds. The animal kingdom, on the other hand, has to obtain food substances ready-made from the plants or, indirectly, from other animals.

Chlorophyll is necessary for the capture and utilization of the energy in sunlight. The process takes place through the porphyrin ring,

[...] one of the greatest acts of creativity in the four billion years of the living earth. [...] It proved to have the delicate ability to handle individual electrons – twisted it in conjunction with other chemicals and discovered a molecular net with the power to capture photons in flight. This mutation had the ability to convert the energy of a particle rifling through the air at the speed of light into the molecular structures of food![1]

Sugars and starches play an important part in human nutrition. Says Dr Schmidt, 'The metabolism of carbohydrates in the human organism proceeds in a direction exactly opposite to that of plants. Thus there is clearly a polarity between these two.'[2] All these arrangements are the result of the incomparable achievement of the plant world producing life on earth – with the help of the cosmic sun forces.

The human ego is particularly strengthened by the ability to create sugars from complex carbohydrates, according to Rudolf Steiner. The complex carbon chains are broken down slowly, particularly in cereals, and release their energy in a rhythmical and sustained fashion, bringing their characteristic warmth to the human organism.

In Chapter 5 we saw the complexity of the breakdown process, through to the storage of glycogen in the liver. In human blood, under healthy circumstances, glucose flows with great consistency and its concentration can only vary within very narrow limits (between 60 and 120 mg %).[3] However, people are increasingly taking much of their carbohydrate nutrition in the form of refined sugar, particularly in Western countries.

Cane sugar, which used to be very costly, is now relatively cheap but has been produced at the cost of great hardship to those who are involved in the growing and harvesting of it. The use of sugar has increased and statistics seem to indicate that refined sugar consumption is in direct ratio to the per capita income of a nation. Therefore, in developed countries the average consumption is 45 kilos per person per annum compared to China which is 6.1 kilos per person per annum.[4]

Such a high consumption of refined carbohydrate in the form of pure refined sugar places a heavy burden on the liver which has to regulate the sugar concentration in the blood. Refined sugar passes quickly into the blood-stream in large amounts, giving the stomach and pancreas a shock. An acid condition then forms whereby the body's minerals are consumed (notably calcium), since eating anything refined requires the body to compensate what has been stripped away.

So too little or too much sugar can make a person sick. A low blood sugar level causes tiredness and hunger, but if refined sugar is taken the blood sugar levels rise dramatically. High energy is released for a while, but the final effect is one of depletion of energy. Diabetes and hypoglycaemia are two conditions steadily increasing in the West. The most common form of diabetes is diabetes mellitus (sugar diabetes). The hormone insulin, which is produced by the pancreas, is necessary for the utilization of sugar in the body and its conversion into glycogen. If there is insufficient insulin, or if the body is not able to respond to it normally, the normal metabolism of glucose cannot take place and a high level of blood sugar results. In addition, fats are imperfectly broken down, leading to an acid condition of the blood that could end in coma in severe cases.

Many diabetics require insulin or drugs to control their condition, but a proportion need only dietary management. Different types of food differ in their effect on blood sugar levels. For example, fruits and fruit sugar (fructose), legumes and wholegrains produce a relatively low rise in blood sugar. Eating refined white sugar and other simple sugars also contributes to diabetes because excess sugars convert to fat in the body. Also, it has been found that there is a higher incidence of diabetes in people who are overweight, especially the very obese.

> When a low-fat diet based on complex carbohydrates such as unrefined grains, vegetables and legumes is followed for several weeks, approximately 80 per cent of diabetics can stop taking insulin and diabetic pills and the remaining 20 per cent can reduce their intake.[5]

Hypoglycaemia (low blood sugar) can also be the result of the body producing too much insulin, which can happen if too much refined carbohydrate, such as foods containing sugar, is consumed. The pancreas reacts to the rapid increase of blood sugar by producing excessive amounts of insulin, followed in turn by low blood sugar.

The brain in particular needs glucose to function normally, so common symptoms of hypoglycaemia include headaches, weakness, tiredness, and mental conditions such as mood swings.

Hypoglycaemia has also been linked to young people with behavioural problems, with records of vandalism and violence. In such a situation the real 'I' or ego of the person is just not in the body, the person is not conscious of what they are doing. Alexander Schauss, author of *Diet, Crime and Delinquency*, researched the effects of diet on probationers, whose usual diet was lots of refined sugars, fats and carbohydrates. When introduced to a diet of wholegrain breads, fruits and salads tremendous improvement in mood and behaviour was noted.

So we can see refined sugar as a 'stripped carbohydrate' consisting of empty calories. The correct metabolism of sugar will only proceed through the use of all the accessory nutrients that are involved in its digestion. Vitamins, minerals and even some proteins and fat molecules are all necessary for this; when they are not present they will inevitably be pulled from the tissues to support metabolism. It is thus, as we have already said, that sugar can be stored as fat, resulting in people who suffer from both obesity and malnutrition at the same time.

So what is this world-wide search for sweetness? For a quick fix that just as quickly fades? As mentioned above, the human brain uses the greatest amount of sugar (approximately 110–120 gm of glucose a day according to Dr Schmidt), so we need sugar for our thinking, for our feeling (the heart requires 30–40g per day) and for our limb activity. It has been shown in Chapter 1 that in particular the forces of the intellect have been developing since Renaissance times. (It is interesting to note that the wonders of the Renaissance were achieved on one teaspoonful of sugar per person per year!) Sugar has also the capacity, in the appropriate quality and quantity, to awaken the potential individuality in the human being, and to develop the necessary forces for physical work. Like salt and spices, sugar then was being added to the diet in greater and greater quantities.

Now perhaps we can also see the quality of sweetness as symbolizing the 'heavenly pole' (as opposed to salt, representing the 'earthly pole'). The tiny baby who has just descended from the heavenly spheres takes as his first food his mother's milk (more than 7 per cent sugar) and we must not deny this real need for a certain amount of sweetness in nutrition, particularly for young children. In fact Steiner indicates in *The Study of Man* that children deprived of sweetness – he was not referring to refined sugar and candies – may well begin to steal little things, because of a lack or sense of deprivation of this quality. Perhaps sweetness is a deep memory of paradise lost? (Dr Schmidt suggests that there could be a connection with the liver function if sugar or sweets are craved.)

When we look to history for the evolution of the main sweeteners, we note that wild honey was held as a sacred substance. An Egyptian myth tells how the tears of the sun god Re fell to the earth and became bees, and honey and beeswax arose from these divine tears. As well as eating honey they made healing poultices of it to treat burns and wounds. The patriarchs and the people of Israel used it too (it is mentioned more than 50 times in the Old Testament). For the Greeks it was used in honey cakes in religious ritual. Druidic England was known as 'the isle of honey'; honey was an important ingredient in the making of mead. In the Americas the Indians had a long tradition of extracting maple syrup from the maple trees and corn syrup from maize.

Arabian culture developed a way of refining and crystallizing sugar sap from sugar cane (*Saccharum officinarum*, originating in Malaysia, according to recent findings) and they kept the process to themselves. They created those beautiful original cone-shaped sugar loaves, wrapped in palm leaves. It was only at the time of the Crusades that news of 'a reed that brings forth honey, unaided by bees' came to Europe. An order of German knights took over the sugar plantations and refineries from the defeated Arabs and thus a new agricultural product began to be exploited. Increasing desire for sugar in Europe significantly contributed to the increase in demand for African slaves to work in plantations and so the history of sugar has a painful legacy. Alexander the Great, Columbus, Charlemagne and Frederick the Great all played their parts in the popularization of sugar. It is said that Elizabeth I was a sugar addict.

In England there was a heavier consumption of sugar, earlier than any other country. The first sugar arrived in 1319. By 1799 there had been large-scale experiments in creating sugars from a root – the sugar beet. This research was first piloted in Germany, so when Napoleon blockaded Europe in 1806, stopping the sugar cane trade, the new kind of sugar was already in production. The sugar content from beets was increased and by the turn of the century 50 per cent of the sugar produced in the world came from beets. This progression shows how sugar was first used from the blossom in the form of honey, then down to the stem, where we find sugar in the sugar cane, and then further down into the root, from the sugar beet.

When eaten, the root of the plant is particularly effective in nourishing the brain and nervous system. The stem/leaf nourishes the feeling/breathing/middle part of the human being, and the blossom stimulates the metabolic and regenerative powers. (See p. 153, 'The Threefold Plant'.)

Let us look briefly at how some of the different kinds of sweeteners are produced. Sugar is made by first crushing the cane in a press, then impurities are removed from the juice which is then boiled down until it begins to crystallize. The liquid is separated by centrifuging, leaving a raw sugar, then further refined using steam to clean it. Brown sugar is made by pouring some molasses over granulated white sugar, so it will have a few of the trace minerals returned but is still 98 per cent sucrose. Beet sugar is manufactured in a similar way.

Honey

Honey — a very special substance — comes from the nectar stored in flower blossoms, which themselves arise out of the refining powers of sunlight, culminating in scent, colour, pollen and sweetness. It is the bees' special life within the hive which really is an embodiment of love in action, for the quality of this product rests upon the fact that the bees work so completely together, arranging their lives so that everything is in an intricate harmony. The warmth (a hive operates specifically at the same temperature as the human blood), the sweetness and the cooperation make it a healing substance willingly shared with humans, if the bees are not exploited. I have been told by a beekeeper that he estimated it takes something like 2000 hours of work on the part of the bee to make one teaspoon of honey! This was an amazing thought. The only thing is that for the bee there is no difference between work or play — she is wedded to her activity and to the rhythms of the sun.

So bees collect the nectar from flowers, herbs and orchard blossoms. The nectar begins as a weak solution of sugars and is then carried to the hive in the honey stomach of the bee. Here enzymes convert the sucrose into the pre-digested sugars fructose and dextrose. In the honeycombs, constructed of perfect hexagons, the conversion process continues. Water evaporates in the warmth of the hive; the bees then cap the full cell with wax when it is 'ripe'. The honey for our use is extracted by centrifuge.

Honey is easily assimilated; it has a gentle and sedative effect, and also a laxative action. It contains ingredients that have defied laboratory analysis, so mysterious a substance it is. There are many different qualities of honey now available. The cheaper ones tend to come from bees that have been sugar-fed through the winters (long here in Europe), but this is harmful to the bees and means that the sensitive enzymatic processes are diminished, as are often the traces of pollen, minerals and vitamins and more spiritual qualities found in the honey from the bees of a caring beekeeper. Most imported honeys are pasteurized, of course destroying many of their vital properties. Perhaps the exception is manuka honey from a very limited source in New Zealand. This product has received a lot of publicity for its efficiency at healing bed-sores where allopathic applications have failed.

Steiner recommended honey in particular for the very young and very old. In the days of sugar rejection I would often makes cakes with honey. But I realized this was very wasteful of such a highly sensitive product; many of the special qualities would be lost when exposed to high temperatures. Today I will use a good quality muscovado sugar if I want to bake a cake and sometimes non-refined organic sugar. (Cakes and puddings only appear now and then so I don't think this leads to sugar addiction.) Alternatively, I use as sweeteners malt syrup, rice syrup, maple syrup, dried fruits and fruit sugar.

'The story is now so well known,' says Henry Hobhouse, ' that there is little need to repeat that refined sugar, after illegal drugs, tobacco and alcohol, is the most damaging, addictive substance consumed by rich white mankind.'[6] And Dr Schmidt feels artificial sweeteners are definitely not substitutes for sugar – they only deceive one with their sweet taste. The best sugar, says Steiner, is that which the human being produces himself from complex carbohydrates.

> Eating complex carbohydrates maximises the concentration in the bloodstream of the amino acid L-tryptophan which is manufactured in the brain into the 'calming' chemical serotonin. Most people feel calmer within half an hour of a carbohydrate snack.
>
> Paul Pitchford[7]

BREAD AND BREAD MAKING

Bread making in history

Bread is an archetype of the earth, holding all the elements necessary for life; it is primarily made from seeds, each an entity at the start and capable of new life. I covered the cereals in more detail in Chapter 4.

The word for bread in Homer's time, *sitos,* was also the generic term for food. Not only a nourishing staple, it was the staff of life. Sharing bread formed a sacred bond between companions (from the Latin *cum panis,* 'with bread'). Bread was an important step in the human nutritional journey, but it was preceded by grain pastes and porridges, still cooked widely today. One of the earliest communities to have pioneered agriculture and primitive breadmaking was Çatal Hüyük.

In Çatal Hüyük, the extraordinary Neolithic city in Turkey still being excavated, bread wheat (*Triticum aestivum*) has been found at levels IV, V and VI.[1] Such a discovery was a revelation, as this variety is a hybrid (no wild form is known), making this one of the earliest incidences of bread wheat. It shows that wheat was being cultivated together with six-rowed barley as early as 7800 BC. Most of the houses in Çatal Hüyük had a saddle quern for grinding grains and a central hearth for cooking. (This method of grinding is likely to have given very gritty bread.)

The typical bread then would be in the form of flat-bread, quite appetizing when freshly cooked and hot but somewhat heavy and indigestible when cold. However, improvements continued to be made but flat-bread has survived in numerous forms to become a staple in many cultures today. We know it as the Mexican *tortilla,* the Indian *chapati,* the Chinese *pao ping,* the American Johnnycake, the Scottish oatcake, and the Ethiopian *injera,* to name some varieties. These are all traditionally unleavened breads, simple and sustaining.

By the time the New Kingdom in Egypt had developed (1400 BC), there were more than 40 varieties of baked breads. There were still unleavened cakes of barley, the chewing of which left its mark, as shown by the worn teeth of surviving Egyptian skulls. But the Egyptians developed raised breads, a tremendous advance in the history of cooking. As the brewing of beer was by now established, perhaps it was 'by accident' that the barm from fermenting beer found its way into the grain paste causing a spontaneous fermentation that could be controlled with temperature. The results led to a much lighter loaf and made possible various shaped breads, baked in different moulds, some even like pyramids.

In Exodus xii we read: 'When they left Egypt they took their dough before it was leavened and their kneading troughs bound up in their clothes upon their shoulders, because they were thrust out of Egypt and could not tarry.' The Israelites were given the order, 'Seven days shalt there be no leaven found in your houses, in all your habitations ye shall eat unleavened bread.' Leaven represents the sin of pride, of being puffed up, so the special wheat used for the Matzah (unleavened dough for Pesach) is called *Shemurah* – 'watched'. Once it is sown it is watched to make sure that no yeasts invade growing, harvesting or milling. The whole question of leaven is very interesting and complex, but we shall investigate it in more depth later (pp. 170–1), noting that the Jewish people have a long tradition of making sourdough bread, the main method of leavening until the eighteenth century.

Barley is enshrined in classical Greek rituals of sacrifice. Barley cakes in special shapes were offered to Demeter and Persephone at Syracuse with flavourings of sesame, coriander, cumin and marjoram. It was barley loaves that were used to feed the multitudes at Christ's miraculous feeding of the five thousand. Meanwhile the Thessalonians made oven-bread, brazier bread, 'spit' bread (a speciality of travelling armies), and *artos* baked on hot coals.

Galen, the venerated Greek physician, made recommendations that were to underpin dietary habits for the next 1500 years:

Bread baked in the ashes is heavy and hard to digest because the baking is uneven. That which comes from a small oven or stove causes dyspepsia and is hard to digest. But bread made over a brazier or in a pan, owing to the admixture of oil, is easier to excrete. [Note the addition of oil at this point.] Bread baked in larger ovens, however, excel in all good qualities, for it is well-flavoured, evenly cooked and good for the stomach, easily digested and very readily assimilated.[2]

The Roman writer Pliny remarked on the fact that there were no public bakeries in Rome before the war against Perseus in Macedonia (171–168 BC). This innovation marked, says Phyllis Pray Bober, 'the transformation from simple home baking in ashes on a hearth by a basically rural population to the need to serve the burgeoning proletariat of the capital, urban folk living in multi-level apartments without any more than a brazier on which to cook.'[3] Thus urban life created the need for commercial bakeries. In cities bread was no longer made at home (for the wealthy at least), clearly a defining moment in the development of a culture now relying on specialist skills of others. Roman bakeries produced myriad breads – with honey and oil, suet bread, mushroom-shaped loaves covered with poppy seeds, griddle cakes, and wafer bread, thin and crisp. Pepper, wine and milk were amongst the ingredients. 'Dice', for instance, were square loaves flavoured with anise, cheese and oil.

Bread ovens

Galen and Pliny recommended larger ovens. There was, however, an intermediate step whereby a pot was inverted over the bread and surrounded with hot embers (a method still quite commonly used in England less than a century ago according to Elizabeth David). In cities at least, beehive shaped clay ovens gave way to more sophisticated, brick-built ones (a good example was found in the ruins of Pompeii). Meanwhile the poor continued to eat grain pastes and hearth bread bristling with chaff.

Yeast

The precise nature of yeast had been a mystery for millennia, but it was the invention of the microscope around 1600 and the science of microscopy that later enabled Louis Pasteur to establish beyond doubt that yeasts are unicellular fungi. Brewer's yeast converts starches and sugars into alcohol and carbon dioxide at an optimum temperature of 36°F, which is close to that of human blood.

The discovery of this new world of burgeoning microscopic life brought about controversy in seventeenth century France. (All these developments were happening in the atmosphere that led up to the French Revolution in 1789.) The Paris Faculty of Medicine spent months debating the question of 'beer leaven' and whether bakers should be permitted to use it, eventually coming up with the solemn decision that it was injurious to health and should be forbidden.

The ancient spontaneous leaven and sourdough systems worked well for bread made from wholemeal flour, but more and more the refined white loaf was being produced, requiring a more reliable and stable yeast. So an ancient system where a piece of the mother dough is always kept for subsequent baking was deposed by a new development. The keeping of the starter had provided continuity down the millennia, weaving communities together in companionship. Now each batch of dough could be started afresh with no reliance on past endeavour – a change of significant symbolic and practical importance. Flour began to be sifted and sold separately, so there was also more money involved, with higher profits to miller and baker.

We should be aware that today many yeasts are genetically modified.

Developments in bread making to the present day

During the past 150 years all aspects of bread production, from the sowing of the seed to the finished loaf, have undergone even greater changes. The complete mechanization of all stages of the grain's journey from the farm via the baker to the table began in this country in Glasgow in 1850 when bread was kneaded by a machine for the first time. (Strictly speaking, not all the stages have been mechanized. In an age where time means money, several stages are simply left out.)

One of these stages is the binding of the reaped grain in sheaves, which used to be allowed to stand on the fields for some time longer in the maturing warmth of the late summer sun. After several weeks the sheaves were brought in and threshing could begin. Today's harvesting and threshing is done in the same mechanical operation. Another such stage is allowing the milled flour to 'rest' to improve its baking qualities. Quite early in the last century it was discovered that certain chemicals achieve almost the same results artificially. A commonly used substance is potassium bromate (proposed E number 625), saving enormously on the cost of storage and reducing risks of spoilage from insect infestation.

More recently a third stage, possibly the most crucial of the entire journey, has been severely curtailed. This is the process of fermentation, or leavening. The first step towards this was taken early in the twentieth century with the elimination of the sponge-dough process. The discontinuation of the old method, with its 12-hour sponge followed by a two-hour fermentation period, was made possible by the production of a monoculture – strains of fast-fermenting yeasts that require only 3–4 hours before the dough can be divided, moulded, proofed in tins and baked. The processes of transformation occurring in a sourdough fermentation which play such an important part in the taste and digestibility of bread are missing. A pure white airy loaf was now produced, no more than a convenient carrier of whatever you wanted to put on it. In order to hold the airy pockets in the bread, wheat strains were developed with higher and higher proportions of gluten (see p. 107).

In 1958 the second step was taken with the discovery of a completely new method of dough-conditioning, the Chorleywood bread process, named after the Hertfordshire town where the British Bakers Industrial Research Association is based. One of the main objects of fermentation is to condition the dough. When wetted, the gluten in the flour is sticky and elastic. This allows the dough to stretch as it rises, giving the loaf, when baked, the desired texture and 'crumb'. During the 1960s the Chorleywood bread process began to be widely used in Britain and today about 85 per cent of British bread is made using this method.

Using huge machines, a batch of dough, which may be as large as 600 lb, is violently mixed for just five minutes, with the addition of a chemical oxidizing agent, after which it can be moulded, proofed and baked. Smaller machines taking as little as 10 lb of dough are available for the increasingly popular hot bread shops. Whether large machines and chemical additives are really necessary in the production of our daily bread is a question for many of us. To alter this trend now would require an unimaginable change in the thinking of the large producers, whose aim is to produce cheap bread and make a profit. But there is no doubt that the short cuts taken in this industrial process do away with one of bread's most vital ingredients, that of time.

Time is one of the most important elements in the journey from field to

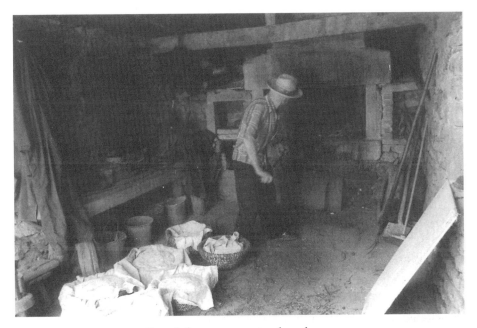

French farmer preparing bread oven

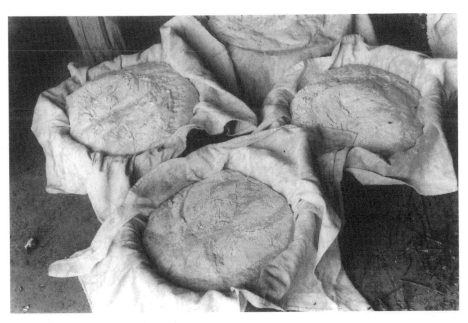

Rising dough

table, quite simply because the journey is one of transformation. Real transformation requires time, and a pause for 'breathing' between each stage. The grain requires a pause for breath after reaping, a pause after milling, a pause after the mixing of the flour and leaven, another pause after kneading and a pause after baking. Sheaves are almost a thing of the past (though I was very excited to see some in rural Ireland). The small baker and the home baker, however, still have control over flour quality and the time allowed for fermentation.

When we had our farm project in northern Majorca we made our own natural-rise bread. Our Spanish partners had developed a real genius for this and passed on their skills to others. We used stone-ground flour milled locally, damp, grey, mineral-rich sea salt, green-gold local olive oil and water from our spring. The warmth of the Mediterranean climate provided ideal conditions for fermentation and from each batch of dough a portion was kept wrapped up snugly and placed in a warm cupboard as a starter for the next batch. The dough started in the evening rose during the night and in the morning looked like a plump cushion, all taut and speckled with wheat bran. It was kneaded until it was silky, and divided usually into seven fat cushions which sat warmly swelling for another hour. Firing the stone bread-oven using pine brushwood was a real art and, managed by Felix, became a rhythmic alchemical process demanding experience and con-centration. The bread came out golden and sweet with a suggestion of wood-ash. All our visitors remembered the fragrance and flavour of this bread. Slices scrubbed with tomato, drizzled with olive oil and sprinkled with sea salt were as sustaining a breakfast as you could wish for. Along with a handful of home-cured olives, this constitutes the famous *pa'amb oli* (bread with oil) that has sustained the sons and daughters of Majorca for aeons.

Steiner's view

A small group of farmers and millers concerned about the denaturing of the daily bread approached Rudolf Steiner for some advice on the questions of milling and baking.[4] According to Steiner the aim of baking bread is to produce something that by itself constitutes a complete food for the human being. In his opinion 'Rainer' bread, a country loaf, met this requirement. The flour had been milled by a water-driven mill and the wood used for the fire had been felled at the time of a waxing moon the previous winter. These were but some of the sensitive processes involved.

Steiner's recommendations were to guard against loss of life-forces in the grain during the process of milling. This advice has led to experimentation in the design and construction of mills where the grain is not crushed violently as it is with steel rollers but converted into flour by friction between itself and the lightly resting millstones. Water-mills were favoured, because one is working with natural rhythms dictated by the water, rather than mechanical ones. He also stressed the importance of cleanliness in the mill and bakery.

Several of our friends confirm Steiner's insistence[5] that rye bread is particularly important for Central Europeans. For Steiner himself, the preferred bread to eat with soup was white bread. This is interesting but controversial (presumably the white bread of those days was still nutritious).

A bread was developed known as Burkhardt bread, made of a combination of four grains — wheat, barley, oats and rye — with the addition of roasted walnuts or hazelnuts, and flavoured with fennel, caraway or aniseed. Yeast or leaven was not used but instead a raising agent that works with the polar opposites of honey and salt. It is possible this method may have originated in Persia. Early in the twentieth century the European followers of an ancient Persian teaching known as Mazdaism made their bread with honey, salt and oil, believing this method to date back to the time of Zarathustra. Honey contains several strains of yeast, which are gathered by the bees together with nectar. Whenever honey is diluted with a sufficient quantity of water and allowed to stand in a warm place, spontaneous fermentation will occur. Under favourable conditions the honey fermentation can be used to leaven bread. These conditions are exacting and include correct kneading and firmness of the dough, accurate timing of all the processes and a strict temperature control. The bakers and millers mentioned above (p. 174) investigated these methods.

The idea of using the field of forces existing between honey (blossom) and salt (root) by using honey and salt to initiate fermentation is discussed by Dr Rudolf Hauschka in his book *Nutrition*.[6] Whether the leavening of honey-salt bread, as it came to be called, is the result of spontaneous honey fermentation under controlled conditions or whether it is set into motion by an alchemical field of force must remain an open question. The difficulties of producing consistently a honey-salt bread acceptable to a larger public led to further investigation into how to reduce the stringency and uncertainties of the conditions. In this research attention was focused on the honey fermentation process and not the honey-salt polarity. Work on this was carried out in the 1930s by Hugo Erbe in Ulm, Germany, where he was proprietor of a large commercial bakery. He succeeded in developing a consistent honey fermentation process using wheat flour, water, honey and pea-flour. The process was allowed to come to a natural conclusion and the resulting product could be dried. It could be easily reactivated for use in baking. His method although patented was lost, but in 1965 workers in the grain laboratory of the Research Centre for Biodynamic Agriculture in Darmstadt, Germany, rediscovered it. The baking ferment available today on the Continent is a result of their work.

Bread as a sacred symbol

At the Last Supper, Jesus Christ made bread a sacred symbol, together with wine. He took a decisive step away from blood offerings of the past into this bloodless offering of bread and wine. According to Emil Bock:

> Externally, blood-sacrifices were carried out in the Temple in the presence of the people, but in hidden sanctuaries esoteric Sun Mysteries had always been preserved, where bread and wine were the symbols of the Sun God. On the very spot where the circle were gathered at the Last Supper, the sanctuary of Melchizedek had stood. From there he had taken bread and wine, and carried them down to the Valley of Kedron to dispense them to Abraham. Now bread and wine become more than symbols; as Christ distributes the bread he can say, 'This is my body,' and in handing the disciples the chalice, 'This is my blood.' In the twilight of the room bread and wine are enveloped with a shining sun-aura.[7]

A new meal is created where all share the same substances. (On the Passover meal, see Chapter 1, Note 17.)

We have taken a rather swift journey through the fascinating biography of bread, a product that unites the four elements of Earth, Fire, Air and Water. It is a process reflected in the human being: the ferment, the soul/spirit rising, swelling, expanding; the fire that helps the process but firms it up, stamping its impress on the mineral/physical body.

How different human consciousness will be within a culture that eats a good bread rather than a poor one, or a porridge! The act of chewing, apart from helping digestion, strengthens memory and the capacity to reflect, according to Steiner.

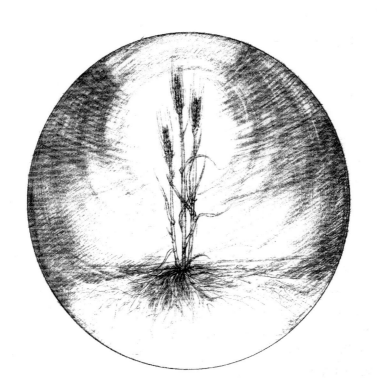

THE NIGHTSHADE FAMILY (*SOLANACEAE*)

The nightshade family includes the potato, tomato, eggplant or aubergine, the capsicums, chilli, cape gooseberry and tomatillo, tobacco, henbane and deadly nightshade (belladonna). Excepting the potato, which originates on the cool slopes of the Andes, the plants all favour warmth and fertile soil. With their strong flowering processes, bright colours and enclosed pockets of air (capsicums), or wateriness (potato and tomato), the family contains amongst its members species with strong psychotropic poisons such as belladonna, thornapple and henbane, used in former times by witches to induce hallucinations, and tobacco with its nicotine. It is quite difficult to understand what part the poisons play in the plant's life; they do not protect it from being devoured (rabbits eat nightshades with impunity). All the plants of the nightshade family, particularly capsicums, emit the chemical pyrazine which can be smelled at a concentration in the air as low as one part in a trillion.

These poisons are alkaloids in the process of becoming amino acids. Amino acids are the building blocks of proteins, which as we know contain nitrogen. But this plant family shows an above average nitrogen content. Normal protein-forming activity is found in seeds which usually only contain a limited amount of nitrogen. Above the seed-buds of the nightshade family we see a deeply carved cavity, echoing the inward-turning gesture of the 'gastrula', the beginnings of interiorization in the animal kingdom. The anabolic or upbuilding forces shown in the chlorophyll process are distorted, and the poisons come about through an unusually strong 'down-building' or catabolic process. The potato – not a root but a tuber or swollen stem – tries to grow towards the light. When it succeeds it becomes green and produces the poison solanine, which is bitter and acrid to the taste.

The story of the potato

The potato was cultivated by the peoples of Peru, the Incas. In its indigenous state it can survive in conditions that most cereals could not, growing in the poorest of soils. The hardiest species can grow at 15,000 feet and there are 230 wild varieties. The Peruvians must have realized its poisonous nature because they developed a treatment of potatoes that not only made them easy to store but rendered them more digestible. They used a kind of freeze-drying process giving a result known as *chuno*. I mention this because, as we will see with the soya bean for example, preparation and cooking of certain plants can substantially alter their predominant features.

After harvesting, the potatoes were sliced and spread out and left over-night in often freezing conditions. The next day large numbers of families came to tread out the moisture, the process continuing for several days till the potato, freed of its liquid content, could be stored as *chuno*. (These potatoes were smaller and had more dry weight nutrients than our present highly fertilized, watery varieties.) The *chuno* was eaten with squash, maize and beans with a little chilli and tomatoes, giving a better balance than, say, eating meat with potatoes (acid/alkaline).

The discovery of the Americas marked the beginning of a new phase of consciousness. With improved boat-building techniques came the ability to sail into all corners of the world, bringing new foods, precious metals and minerals, and new ideas through an extension of the human search for knowledge.

The Spanish *conquistadores* found the potato to be a very cheap staple to feed their gold and silver mine slaves. It could yield a huge amount of bulky starch on little arable land and thin soils. The potato was first grown in Europe in 1588 by the botanist Clusius. However, it was treated with a great deal of suspicion in Europe where the peasants saw the plant as evil, with its angular bluish-purple, five-pointed flowers, crimson stamens and mysterious underground workings. Surely the devil had crafted such a plant! If planted again the tubers would divide and proliferate. The people of Burgundy were convinced that too frequent use of them caused leprosy and in Switzerland where potato was taken up it was blamed for scrofula. Despite poverty and malnutrition the people of Munich in the 1790s, two hundred years after those first plantings, were convinced that potatoes were poisonous and refused to eat them. The Scots resisted them for two hundred years because no mention of potatoes could be found in the Bible.

It took 40 years of preaching on the part of pharmacist and agriculturist Antoine-Auguste Parmentier to turn the tide of French public opinion. The peasantry had hitherto trusted nothing but grain before the Revolution, but after it *millions of Europeans abandoned tradition to take up potato nutrition at roughly the same time*. How could people be persuaded to make food plants of the potato (and tomato), every part of which is to a lesser or greater degree poisonous? Was it through trying various cooking methods that they found them palatable?

By 1600 the potato had entered Spain, Italy, Austria, Belgium, Holland, France, Switzerland, England, Germany, Portugal and Ireland. William Salmon (in the seventeenth century) claimed that potatoes were good boiled, baked or roasted, eaten with good butter, salt, orange juice or lemon juice and a little sugar, saying, 'They increase seed and provoke lust, causing fruitfulness in both sexes!' (possibly deducing this from the underground proliferation of their tubers).

By the nineteenth century Ireland had become an almost one-crop state, proving to be a tragedy of short-sighted monoculture. The potato blight of 1845 that struck potato crops of northern Europe was devastating to the peoples of Ireland, who were the worst to suffer on their subsistence diet of milk and potatoes. Grain prices rocketed, milk ran out, cattle were slaughtered for their meat. Over a million people died of starvation; a further million who could manage the fare embarked for America from whence the potato had come. It is intriguing to think that the Irish vote of the eastern states could therefore be attributed in no small way to the failure of the potato crop.

John Ruskin, the social theorist, was convinced that the use of potatoes and tobacco made people lazy. Today the potato has become the fourth most important food crop in the world, after wheat, rice and maize. Today's annual world potato crop is valued at more than 100 billion dollars and in Britain each of us on average consumes annually over 100 kg. Approximately 30 per cent of the crop is made into convenience forms of potato such as instant mashed potato, crisps and frozen chips and it is also used in the making of Swedish schnapps and some vodkas.

The potato is often extolled as an excellent foodstuff, containing vitamins (especially C) and protein as well as large quantities of starch. The relatively small amount of protein is found mainly just under the skin where it is lost by peeling. Iron, potassium and vitamins B and C, although present, are not found in high concentration. Nonetheless, potatoes do not compare favourably with cereals —

Potato: Carbohydrates 18%   Proteins 1.5%   Fats 0.1%   Water 80%
Wheat: Carbohydrates 75%   Proteins 10%   Fats 1.0%   Water 10%

These are interesting indications of quantity and relationship, but what they do not reveal is quality, one of our main concerns in this book. Starch originating in a well-grown cereal — a seed with new potential for life — is going to be significantly differently organized from the starch in a potato.

The starch granule of wheat tends to be organized in a series of rhythmical concentric circles whereas the structure of potato starch is more lopsided and off-centre.

Rudolf Steiner spoke often about the effects of eating potatoes:

The potato was introduced into Europe in comparatively recent times. And now I will tell you something about which you can laugh as much as you like. Nevertheless it is the truth.

One can study the development of human intellectual faculties from the time when there were no potatoes to the time after their introduction. Potatoes at a certain time began to play a particular role in Western development. If you compare the increasing use of the potato with the curve of the development of intelligence, you will find that in comparison with today, people in the pre-potato era grasped things less quickly and readily, but what they grasped they really knew. Their nature was more conservative, profound and reflective. After the introduction of the potato people became quicker in taking up ideas, but what they take up is not retained and does not sink in very deeply.

The potato makes great demands on the digestion. Very small, almost homoeopathic doses find their way into the brain, but these tiny quantities are very potent, they spur on the forces of abstract intelligence.[1]

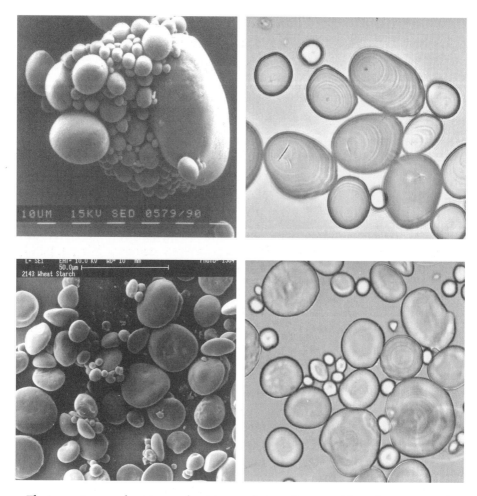

Electron-micrograph pictures of potato starch (top, from outside and cross-section); wheat starch (from outside and cross-section). The wheat starch granules demonstrate a centred organization with concentric circles. The potato starch is off-centre and does not display the orderliness of the cereal starches

Dr Rudolf Hauschka also explains how the brain is involved in the digestion of potatoes:

We described how carbohydrate foods are used chiefly to nourish the middle portion of the brain. This is the brain area that supports creative, artistic and imaginative thinking. If the middle brain is made to serve digestive functions, as it has to do after a meal of potatoes, it cannot do its proper work and the forebrain has to substitute for it; but this part of the brain is very differently constituted, both as to cellular structure and what might be called a localized capacity. These fit it for an entirely different function: that of serving the more materialistic thinking and conscious-ness of the present day, with their tendency to dry scientific abstraction. Creative thinking has declined in Europe since the potato was introduced and became so popular.[2]

A child who is fed too many potatoes may have problems with his memory and become 'scattered' (especially if potatoes and high sugar consumption occur together), according to Steiner. The parents should try to reduce the amount, substituting grains, fruits and leafy vegetables.

Of course the whole metabolism of foods can differ enormously from person to person, so we should beware of making blanket statements. We can ponder on such phenomena and in so doing begin to observe for ourselves some of these correspondences between diet and behaviour or mental processes.

Nevertheless I think most people enjoy potatoes, including myself. They give a feeling of being comfortably 'weighed down', replete. However they are often used just as a vehicle for some other tastier food, as when baked and served with cheese or chilli, in much the same way as we have seen with white bread as a filler. They don't need as much chewing as whole grains do and pass through the intestines easily but sometimes lead to post-prandial headaches, as can tomatoes, and perhaps in view of the earlier quotes, we can now see why. We may realize that sun-ripened, wind-pollinated cereals have a superior quality of carbohydrate to the cold underground swollen stem of the potato, and balance our diet accordingly.

In Japanese macrobiotic tradition the potato is seen as extremely 'yin' (cold, expanded, watery, dark); it needs to be balanced in cooking by fire, sea salt, oil, butter, horseradish, fennel or cumin seeds. Baked in their jackets potatoes give more nutritional value as the nutrients lie just under the skin. They are also good roasted and served with lots of chopped parsley, garlic, chives and basil or served with a good crispy green salad. If some apple is included in the menu it helps to lift the quality of the starch.

The tomato

Tomatoes are now so widely used — children will eat most things if liber-ally covered with tomato sauce — and it's difficult to imagine Mediterra-

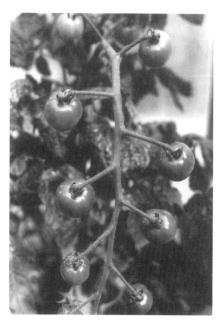

Tomato plant, which does not have the strength in its stem to support itself

nean cooking without tomatoes, or indeed peppers, potatoes and aubergine.

Apparently the original tomatoes appeared as weeds in the maize fields of South America. The first to be introduced into Europe in the sixteenth century were yellow in colour; they were named 'golden apples' and thought to have aphrodisiac powers. Looking at the way the tomato plant grows may yield some clues as to its nutritional qualities.

Tomatoes do not have much strength in their stems and therefore have to be artificially supported with canes; the foliage grows in an almost chaotic profusion and the plant likes best to grow on raw compost by itself, or even on its own compost. The tension between the shiny tough skin and the sweet watery contents is quite interesting. Rotting tomatoes, potatoes, aubergines or peppers have an incredibly foul characteristic smell and tend to decompose very quickly, supporting a host of interesting fungi. There is also the very characteristic smell perceptible when entering a greenhouse growing any of the nightshade crops, quite pleasant and with a soporific effect.

The word 'solanum' is believed to come from the Latin *solamen* meaning 'quieting' (or dumbing down). If so, the meaning was appropriate, since the potato's more infamous siblings were poisons, narcotics and witches' potions. (In the Mediterranean area and the Middle East the nightshade plant datura with its heavily scented hanging flowers was used to make women drowsy if a suitor sought her favours.)

Tomatoes, according to Steiner, could be helpful in stimulating a sluggish liver but people suffering from carcinomas should not eat them 'because carcinoma is itself something that has made itself independent within the organism', a characteristic tendency of the tomato plant. From this stems its power to influence any independent organization within a human or animal organism.[3]

I don't think that we are likely yet to give up eating tomatoes, but a few points here will make sure that we are not more burdened by them than we need be. They should be organically grown and *ripe*, preferably sun-ripened, when they make lovely salads with warming basil, olive oil and fine slices of red onion. If they are not ripe, no amount of cooking will make them thoroughly digestible, and they should *never* be eaten if starting to decompose.

Aubergines and peppers

Most Mediterranean cooking also calls for aubergines and peppers. Aubergines need to be sliced and salted and left to 'weep' for one hour (to reduce the 'yin', watery/airy condition), then rinsed, dried and fried in hot olive oil to balance them or they can be roasted on a griddle, then skinned and mashed with seasonings and oil. I tend to see these fruits (which they are) as stimulants or flavourings and not as staple everyday foods. Raw peppers — unless they are the fine sweet salad variety, not available here — are extremely indigestible. They are best roasted with rosemary, garlic and olive oil, or sautéd until they are soft and sweet.

Tobacco

Nicotiana tabacum is a hybrid of two wild South American plants. The main producers of tobacco are the USA, China, India, Russia and Brazil. After being harvested and dried, the tobacco leaf is heated and put through a fermentation process for a month or more, reducing starches and proteins.

The active ingredient is nicotine, which interferes with the nervous system, quickens the blood and in the long term may raise the blood pressure. Smoking increases the incidence of free radicals, which tend to use up the body's supply of vitamin C. Nicotine and carbon monoxide are introduced into the blood vessels. Carbon monoxide encourages blood clotting and reduces oxygen levels in body tissues.[4] Unfortunately, nicotine is a substance that can lead to addiction.

The American Indians used it in rituals where they wanted to contact the spirits of their ancestors; they also offered it as a pipe of peace. Christopher Columbus learned the habit of smoking in Cuba in 1492 and within decades the habit had more Spanish converts than Christianity. Sir Walter Raleigh is credited with bringing the first tobacco plants to England. The king, James I, wrote a diatribe against smoking but, despite this, smoking or the taking of tobacco as snuff increased in popularity, though it was confined to the male population on the whole. Soon great forests in America were being cleared to grow tobacco, and slaves were sent over from Africa for its cultivation.

Why did people start smoking in Europe and the USA in the sixteenth century? It seems to have caught on at a time when a new type of consciousness arose, beset with anxieties. Tobacco screens the anxiety within, quietening to a certain extent an astral restlessness. It acts as a depressant, rather than a stimulant. The person who is an occasional smoker will often light up a cigarette when he is in a group, but would also, perhaps unconsciously, like to withdraw or hide behind a smokescreen where he can hide his inmost thoughts. In contrast, a person who in a fit of anger reaches for a cigarette finds he regains his composure; smoking temporarily 'throttles down' the life of cravings and desires but also his anxiety.

With chain smokers there can be a real danger of isolation. Often they appear to be unaware of how they disturb non-smokers by polluting the air, and of course they are in danger of causing themselves serious health problems. Nicotine attacks the breathing and rhythmic system of the body. It alters the relationship between pulse and breathing; the heartbeat becomes irregular and blood needs more oxygen than breathing can supply because the alveoli have become coated with tar resulting in shortness of breath. Smoking in public places is more and more restricted by law, but despite health warnings and high taxes many people still are heavy smokers, including many schoolchildren. Smoking often goes hand in hand with the consumption of coffee, tea or alcohol – all stimulants and expansive, whereas smoking brings a contractive gesture. I was interested to see the smoking of cigarettes by Muslim and Chinese women in some recent films. What is this saying?

LEGUMES

In Steiner's cosmology all of creation is striving for ascendancy – the humans to become angelic, the animals to eventually become human and the plants to become sentient. Nitrogen is the element needed to create protein and in the legume and nightshade families there are unusually high levels of nitrogen, so we can say they display a 'striving for sentiency'.

The legume family (*Papilionaceae*) includes beans, peas, lentils, clovers and vetches. We know that two species of bean[1] were independently domesticated in Middle and South America, and together with maize and squash became staple foods. Beans, and particularly the fava bean or broad bean, were used extensively in the ancient world, but only as food for peasants. Egyptian priests or any high-ranking person would not touch them, so there is no depiction of the plant on either tomb paintings or frescoes from that time.

Later, Pythagoras, who had studied the lore of the Egyptians, also forbade his adherents to eat beans, not for the reasons that we might suspect but more interestingly because the eating of beans interfered with the ability to perceive the subtleties of number. Pythagoras apparently met his death at the edge of a field of flowering broad beans where a group of enemies had pursued him from the town of Croton. Rather than run through the beans, Pythagoras allowed himself to be captured and killed. One theory about this violent end suggests that he suffered from a little known disease called 'favism' where high temperature, anaemia and jaundice follow inhalation of the pollen or eating the beans (only people from certain Mediterranean areas are afflicted). There are other schools of spiritual discipline that also avoid beans as they are thought to interfere with meditative practices. Nowadays, however, the legumes are an important plant family and millions of people would be even poorer nutritionally without them. So how can we understand this story better?

Rudolf Steiner had some interesting things to say about the legumes:

> The *Papilionaceae* or *Leguminosae* — all those plants which are well known in farming as the 'nitrogen-collectors' — indeed have the function of drawing in nitrogen and thus to communicate it to what is beneath them. Observe these leguminosae. We may truly say, down there in the earth something is athirst for nitrogen; something is there that needs it, even as the human lung needs oxygen. It is the limestone principle which is dependent on a form of nitrogen 'in-breathing'. These plants represent something akin to what takes place in our own epithelial cells [...]
>
> Broadly speaking the *Papilionaceae* are the only plants of this kind, so they have specific functions. [However, we must learn to see each plant species in relation to the total organism of the plant-world, so that we understand the role of each one in balance.] If we lose sight of this the danger is very great that in the near future, when still more of the old ways of agriculture are lost, humans will adopt false paths in the application of the new.[2]

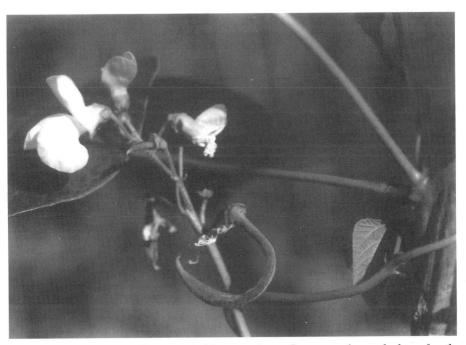

French bean plant, whose flower resembles a tiny butterfly at rest — hence the bean family name, Papilionacae

We have described nitrogen activity in the nightshade family, and here we see another form of exaggerated nitrogen production in the legumes. It too has corresponding signatures in its flowers pointing to the world of butterflies – *Papilionaceae* means 'butterfly family'. The flowers look like stationary butterflies, indicating a kinship with the animal world, also shown in the plant's high protein content.

> There is a deep inner connection between the insects and the plants. Insects are really a repetition in the animal kingdom of the flowering plants. The mutual correspondence between insects and plants – as for example those between butterflies and bees on the one hand and blossoms on another – can easily be understood when we know that the blossom is a butterfly which has no locomotion, and the butterfly is a flying blossom. The idea may seem strange, but if we consider that most flowers cannot be fertilized without the help of certain insects, it becomes evident that these insects must be considered as part of the plant kingdom.[3]

The germinating time for the bean family is relatively short, as we see when we make beansprouts with their almost miraculous speed of growth, and we all know the story of 'Jack and the Beanstalk'. The plant shoots up rapidly, and the flowers develop while it is still vigorously growing both above and below ground, fixing gaseous nitrogen in the soil with the aid of captive bacteria in its roots. Because of this nitrogen-fixing process, the bean family needs to be used in a balanced way – in agriculture with other crops and in diet in a healthy proportion with the grains and other starches. (Nitrogen, according to Steiner, is the carrier of sentient life, the life of feeling.)

Traditionally legumes were used in a three-year rotation with another crop, leaving the soil fallow for a year to regenerate. This no longer happens where soya production occurs. Soya has become such a big agribusiness (like potatoes) that we need to reflect a little upon just what is happening with this 'panacea' plant.

The soya bean

This bean fruits closer to the earth than the cereals. On germination, instead of a vertical shoot to seek the free air it produces a bent neck, both ends of which – the root and cotyledon poles – stay in the soil. The plant somehow seems reluctant to leave the earth. Its seeds only retain their germinating power for a short term and find it hard to compete with weeds. The high protein content in the soya bean is its chief attraction to food producers and it is a fact that most people in our culture, regardless of whether they wish it or not, will be using soya beans in some product or other.

In China and Japan the soya bean was seen as 'the vegetable cow', and has traditionally been used as a rotation crop. However, raw soya beans are highly indigestible. They contain toxic substances that interfere with the action of trypsin, a protein-digesting enzyme in the intestinal tract.[4] So the Japanese cleverly devised ways of transforming them into something highly nutritious, through processes that involved salt, time (up to three years for miso) or a bacillus fermentation (to produce miso and tamari, tempeh and natto). Tofu, a cheeselike protein, is made by adding a curdling agent, e.g. nigari, vinegar, lemon juice, to hot soymilk. These foods have become familiar to many.

With its properties of mimicking other substances and holding them fast, soya is now used in medicines (plant oestrogens), cosmetics, paints, milk substitutes, ice cream, sausages and pet food. It is the chief source of lecithin, which 'smoothes the way', giving the silky smoothness of chocolate and sauces; it also hinders the crystallization of sugars, and fatty substances are made lighter (e.g. margarine is made to contain 20 per cent water). Soya flour mixed with wheat flour prevents shrinkage in baking. It has this useful capacity to expand and hold water and thus volume can be increased, literally by a watering down of quality. Most of all soya is used as oil and as oil-cake for cattle fodder. Tunisia, amongst other countries, dilutes most of its olive oil with imported American soya oil.

A recent book has this warning about soya formula for babies:

> Infants on soy formula may receive the equivalent amount of oestrogen to that found in 5–10 birth control pills each day. Boys on soy-based formula are also ingesting oestrogen and manufacturing large amounts of testosterone. Receiving these confusing hormonal messages can wreak havoc with a child's emotionality.[5]

The production of soya is proliferating worldwide, but it is largely controlled by the American Soyabean Association which unites industrialists, soya bean producers and scientists and gives farmers incentives in the form of subsidies. The USA convinced the Japanese that their efforts should go into the industrialized side of production, into the construction of oil mills, so the Japanese import their soya for fodder largely from the USA. Europe, despite producing oil-cake made from rapeseed, sunflower, cotton-seed and peanuts, imports soya oil-cake to meet 70 per cent of their needs. In these trends we can see developing a fragile lack of choice and co-dependency on this one crop. Everywhere the temptation is to gain wealth by means of the soya bean. America currently has the strongest position, with some competition from Brazil and Venezuela. The possibility of self-sufficiency diminishes yearly with such a powerful co-dependency founded on the exploitation of this one crop. The production of soya, like that of potatoes and tomatoes, has changed agricultural practice, nutritional habits and human and soil biochemistry.

The meatlike aroma of soya protein has been exploited by the modern food industry. Soya is 'spun' to resemble meat and sold as a TVP – textured vegetable protein. Dr Gerhard Schmidt comments: 'The vegetarian has here a pure plant product which affords him the pleasure that others have in eating meat.' But Dr Schmidt also remarks that in TVP, 'Western materialism here celebrates a calamitous triumph with an ancient Eastern agricultural plant.'[6] The kind of thinking that produces such a product misses the point of people embracing vegetarianism. Steiner implied it is better to *eat* meat than to *think* meat.

Genetic modification

Soya with its incapacity to tolerate weeds became a natural target for bio-technology and Monsanto's Round-up-Ready soya beans have come onto the market to a very mixed reception. Monsanto genetically engineered this bean to make it resistant to a glyphosate herbicide produced by the same company under the brand name Round-Up. An incident of genetically manipulated soybeans entering the commercial supply unlabelled has given consumers even more cause for concern.

Rudolf Steiner warned of the increasing development of a deep materialism, when humanity would rely too much on these bulky foodplants, so arrhythmic in their structure. As we grow away from being a cereal-centred culture we need to be awake to these imbalances.

Soya is a legume quite 'out on a limb'. But I do not want to seem dismissive towards all legumes. I use them. The dried ones are very warming and comforting in casseroles (vegetarian cassoulet is a favourite of mine). Cous-cous with chick peas is delightful, hummus and falafel, also made from chick peas, can be wonderful with a crisp salad and some black olives. Lentil soups are versatile, studded with bright vegetables and fresh green beans, and peas are a delight in the summer. Dried beans need to be soaked overnight and the soaking water thrown away before cooking them. A piece of kombu seaweed (kelp) added to the cooking water will help soften the beans. Salt tends to harden the skins, so it should be added towards the end of the cooking process.

Lentils

Lentils have a much finer structure than beans and are usually therefore more easily digested. They are diuretic. India produces more than 50 varieties of different colours and sizes; they are an ingredient of the traditional dhal. My favourites are the Le Puy lentils, grown on mineral-rich volcanic soils in the Auvergne region of France.

Protein complementarity

One of the reasons vegetarians often eat legumes with grains is that it is thought that with the combination one can obtain all the necessary essential amino acids, in the required proportions. The protein in legumes is deficient in the amino acid methione. The proteins in grains, on the other hand, contain ample amounts of methione but are limited instead by a low amount of lysine, another of the essential amino acids. Lysine, however, is abundant in legumes, so grains and legumes mesh perfectly as nutritional comple-ments.[7] For the body to absorb them as 'complete protein', they must be present simultaneously, i.e., eaten at the same meal.

But Paul Pitchford says, 'The idea of complementing the protein of legumes with other foods to make it more complete and like that of animal protein is an idea that gains unquestioned acceptance only in a society *obsessed with protein.*'[8]

What a labyrinth of seemingly conflicting information we have to work our way through, in order to feel secure in our nutrition. We can but experiment and find out what suits us; everyone has a different response. There are people who can digest beans and pulses without difficulty and there are those who suffer enormously from gas and a general heavy feeling. The problem may be with the quality of the beans, the cooking of them, the person's constitution, or it may simply not be an appropriate food for them. As we have seen, beans were not encouraged for people doing meditative work and creative thinking. We must choose, and moderation in all things is my motto!

MILK AND DAIRY PRODUCTS

Looking at milk in the context of human nutritional evolution we see that mankind has been using animal milk for food as far back as records go. The Aryans of central Asia, some of the first herdsmen, were using milk as food certainly by 5000 BC. Milk mixed with honey from wild bees was their prized drink, even before it was extolled in biblical times. The Bible records the use of milk throughout the history of that area; it was often looked upon as the ultimate in desirability. When God promised the land of Canaan to the children of Israel, he described it to Moses as a land 'flowing with milk and honey'.

Steiner connects milk with the moon principle of rhythm, associated with aiding a person to incarnate rightly and to develop a feeling of the oneness of the human race, and of the continuity of the generations. An ancient custom may illustrate this. It was permissible in some Germanic tribes for fathers to expose, and thus put to death, a newborn baby – but only up to the moment when it drank its first drop of milk. Taking milk signified its reception into the tribal community and the baby's exposure after this event was considered murder.[1] (Milk was seen as a bridge between heavenly and earthly principles; the word 'galaxy' comes from the Greek *galacto*, milk.)

In various parts of the world the milk of different animals has been used, depending on climate and geographical location. Camel's milk is drunk in the Middle East and North Africa, mare's milk in Russia and Asia (as well as cow's milk). Sheep's milk is very commonly used in Bulgaria and other Balkan countries and goat's milk has been widely used in the east of Europe and around the Mediterranean. The last major food animal to be domesticated appears to have been the cow, *c.* 6100 BC. Remains of cows have been found in Çatal Hüyük and Nicomedia in Macedonia.[2] But it was the ancient

Indians who had special intuitions about the sacredness of the cow. Observing it as it chewed its cud, a picture of perfect contentment, the cow became for the Indian a model of the development of inner spiritual life. She illustrated how the forces of earth and cosmos weave together, properly digested and totally transformed. In legends cattle are often described as rising up out of rivers and later disappearing once more. Only later, in the Iron Age, were oxen used for ploughing.

The production of milk is a very special process. Rudolf Steiner said milk has a more 'plantlike' than animal nature. For many this may seem a puzzling statement, I myself have puzzled over it for some time. Let us consider where and how milk appears. It is produced by the lacteal glands on the outside of the organism, but its formation is dependent upon the blood system. 'For every pint of milk produced 300 pints of blood must pass through the cow's udder.'[3] It never comes into contact with the blood and therefore, according to Steiner, it is thus completely 'emancipated' from the soul life (or astral principle) of the animal.

Milk, as part of the mother principle, shows a polarity to that other important fluid, blood. Milk streams freely out of the organism, a symbol of the willingness to give ('the milk of human kindness', 'a sacrificial gift'), whereas blood is manufactured deep in the most mineralized part of the human being – the bones – and coagulates immediately upon contact with the air, having no life outside the organism. Milk is closer to cosmic terrestrial forces, whereas blood is related to the process of individualization. Rudolf Steiner from his special insight said that the substance milk can only be found on earth, nowhere else in the galaxy.[4]

Breast milk and cow's milk

For aeons mothers have known that breast milk was the best beginning in life for their infant and hence breast-feeding was honoured. In cases of illness or if you were an aristocrat a 'wet nurse' might be employed. During my lifetime scientists have endeavoured to produce a formula milk that would liberate the mother who could then go back to the workplace, so in industrialized societies bottle-fed babies have been common. This is a relatively recent development and the disadvantages of bottle-feeding over breast-feeding are now coming to light.

Perhaps we can consider some of the issues. Rudolf Steiner in *A Study of Man* says:

> As a child is given his mother's milk, it works upon the sleeping spirit and awakens it ... the only substance, essentially, which can do this. Here the spiritual principle that dwells in all matter asserts itself in its rightful place. Mother's milk bears its own spirit within it, and this spirit has the task of awakening the sleeping spirit of the child. This is no mere picture, it is a profound scientific truth that the genius in nature, which creates the substance milk [...] is the awakener of the human spirit in the child. We must learn to penetrate into these deep and secret relationships in the world, for only then shall we understand the wonderful laws that hold sway in the universe. Only then do we come to see what horrible ignoramuses we are when we theorize about matter as though it were some uniform mass that could be divided into atoms and molecules ... from this

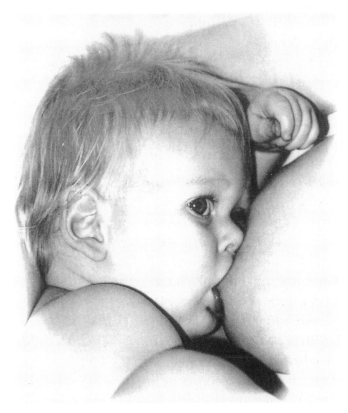

Breast feeding: Daena and baby Ethan

you will see that nature educates in a natural way and this is her genius. In the milk of the infant's mother lies this educative bridge to the world.[5]

How are we to interpret this very powerful statement? Many baby-milk formulas have been produced to mimic breast milk. None of them are as effective as the real thing, which is hardly surprising. Each mother indeed produces her own unique version, and it is in the organization of the various elements that this 'spirit-awakening' food shows its vitality and appropriateness for the human child. In looking at the proportional arrangement of the constituents in human milk we may begin to understand some of the genius of nature:

Water – 80% (in a dynamized state, see Water, Chapter 18)
Proteins – made up of whey proteins (1.2%), vitamin B_{12}, enzymes, hormones, immunoglobins, lactoferrin, folates and casein.

By contrast cow's milk has 3.3% protein, which the calf needs as it grows quickly, doubling its birth weight in 50 days. When cow's milk enters the human baby's stomach it becomes curds and whey, with casein-forming curds that are bulkier and more rubbery than those formed when taking breast milk. Human milk forms finely separated curds in the stomach that pass quickly into the small intestine where they are broken down.

Sugars/carbohydrates
Breast milk contains more than 25 sugars, in particular lactose, which is very sweet and is perceived by the taste-buds on the tip of the tongue (human milk has 7 g sugars per 100 g; cow's milk 4.8 g per 100 g). This sweetness is significant in human development and consciousness (see p. 164). Some of the lactose is split into two simple sugars: galactose and glucose. The rest travels through the intestine undigested, where, interestingly, undigested lactose improves calcium absorption and encourages a healthy balance of micro-organisms in the gut. Galactose is an important part of the myelin coating of nerves, and besides getting it from breast milk a baby makes it from glucose in the liver.

Minerals
There is no milk formula that has as low a mineral content as breast milk. (This is taken as an indication of the slower process of mineralization in the

human skeleton, as compared to the animal skeleton. Through this longer period of relatively helpless dependency on the mother in the human infant the foundations are laid for the unfolding of consciousness and human intelligence.)

Sodium
The amount of sodium in breast milk is ideal for human babies. It is higher in cow's milk and most formula milks. Sodium is closely linked with water in the body and an imbalance of either can be serious or even fatal.

Calcium and magnesium
Higher levels of both of these are found in cow's milk. Babies absorb calcium better in breast milk than in formula milk. The infant is always assured of an adequate supply even if the mother herself is malnourished; her own bones and teeth will be demineralized before she would provide her infant with incomplete milk. Hence the image of milk as a gift, and sometimes a sacrifice.

Phosphorus
Less in breast milk than in cow's.

Iron
Present in human milk in higher proportions than in a cow's (twice as much) and also a significant element in the human constitution. Iron has a manifold task:

> The spiral tendency [shown in the 'iron process' ...] always arises when time enters space and develops towards the centre. The function of iron is to help 'cosmic' and 'weightless' elements to enter the sphere of gravity. [...] Iron then conforms to the force patterns of the earth's magnetism [and its presence in our blood helps us to orient in space]. It also helps to anchor us in our personalities and in our bodily processes. Without iron, we would literally lack 'presence of mind'. It serves as a mediator, relating the ego to the spatial dynamics of the earth. It provides a basis for our earthly activity and creativity.[6]

Iron works rhythmically and is influenced by its contact with light, air and oxygen. Our breathing depends on iron's activity to bring air into motion, and its close bond with carbon, which combines with it, dissolving or otherwise transforming it.

Trace elements

These minerals include copper, zinc, manganese, chromium, cobalt, molybdenum, selenium, silicon and boron.

Vitamins

A – Carotenoids can be used as antioxidants to protect cells from damage.

C – Concentrated in breast milk. A mother who eats a healthy diet of fresh organic or biodynamically grown fruit, vegetables and cereals should not need extra supplementation.

D – Helps minerals such as calcium to enter and strengthen bones. Oily fish, eggs and butter are also rich in vitamin D. Sunlight is an excellent source; when it shines onto the skin the body produces vitamin D in response. The body stores vitamin D.

It is extraordinary to look at the composition of breast milk and to see how finely-tuned are the relationships within its structure. The indications of high sweetness, high iron and low protein speak particularly of the human organism. Sweetness can be seen as representing the 'heavenly pole', where the spiritual aspect of the child originated, and nothing can compare with the unique sweetness of mother's milk. The 'earthly pole' is represented by the salts and mineral content. Steiner speaks of the particular need for sugars and complex carbohydrates to form the ego, or individuality of the human.

Thus we can see the potential in mother's milk for awakening the spirit and building a healthy physical body, and providing the best possible help to *slowly* 'awaken' the child without a too mineralizing action. Of course, quite apart from the milk itself, the activity of breast feeding is also very therapeutic for both mother and child. Michel Odent, the obstetrician and pioneer of water-births, has said:

> The effect of breast feeding on the emotional development of the mother-child pair is explained by the recent discoveries in endocrinology. Secretion in the mammary gland is triggered by hypophysial prolaction [an action of the pituitary gland], and there is a reason to believe that this same hormone also triggers mothering behaviour in a more general way.[7]

Perhaps mothers do not need to know this! It is simply that more and more scientific findings reaffirm the exquisite and complementary wisdom of nature, which we cannot possibly better in this case. The mood created by the unhurried mother, who is healthy and enjoying the task of feeding and caressing her infant is an archetypal blessing. All newborn babies regardless of nationality produce the enzyme lactase, which allows them to digest the milk-sugar lactose from their mother's milk. After being weaned, babies in hot climates, where there are few milk-giving animals, appear to stop manufacturing lactase and can no longer digest milk. This was discovered when aid in the form of milk-powder was given to Africans and many had strong allergic reactions. The milk powder was more useful for painting their houses than nourishing themselves. And they are not the only ones.

Colostrum

Colostrum, the very first milk to come into the breast after delivery, is rich in anti-infective, iron-binding whey protein. It mops up potentially harmful excesses of iron and inhibits the growth of many potentially harmful organisms, including E. coli.[8]

Problems with cow's milk

There appears to be a growing incidence of people, often children, who are unable to thrive on cow's milk or milk products. Here is a food that has nourished people down the ages, particularly valuable at times of crop failure, being rejected by the human constitution. I believe we must ask ourselves whether it is the way that milk is now produced that is the main source of the problem. When we look at the intensive management of dairy animals in conventional farming systems, the kind of pasture they feed upon and then what happens to this living food before it gets to our doorstep, we can see that usually the public is being sold a very denatured product, bearing little resemblance to that original substance we spoke of earlier on.

The cow has been intensively bred to increase her milk yields beyond all natural capacity, resulting in a high incidence of mastitis and a shorter life span. Until the end of the nineteenth century cows gave about as much milk per day as their calf could drink, around two gallons (16 pints). This has been multiplied by three or four times today. Rudolf Steiner describes how the exhaustion caused by over-production of milk would debilitate cows. Last summer I watched the sad sight of a newly born calf unsuccessfully trying to suckle. The mother's udders were so distended as to almost touch the ground.

The cow is injected as a matter of course with antibiotics to combat mastitis, notably penicillin and aureomycin, traces of which can often be found in the milk. More and more the cow's feed is supplemented with concentrates made from grain and soya to increase the milk yields. Traces of detergent used in sterilizing milking equipment also add to the unnatural content of our milk. Yet another problem that has also been increasing is the taking up of radioactive iodine into the thyroid of the cow. Added to this there is increasing use of artificial fertilizers and pesticides on pastures for grazing.

Traditionally the cow, designed to convert large quantities of forage material (see Chapter 2 on agriculture), would find all her necessary nutrients in a mixed pasture with a variety of grasses, clovers and herbs. Alas, such meadows are a rarity today. The cow, apart from giving her milk, contributes the best manure (when properly managed) so soil fertility is her realm too.

> The whole art of husbandry (not farming) is connected with the life of the cow. In the human collaboration with cows we create meadows and fields. In some countries it seems that husbandry has come to an end. This can only be because cows are separated from meadows and fields. In this separation neither the meadows nor the fields can really thrive any more. To carry such an image further, we may see, in the green, fully sprouting leafy meadows and fields with hedgerows, and in the herds of cows ... the powers which stream down from the 'Bull' forces.[9]

Human use of cow's milk and milk products has become somewhat controversial in our times, and it is not difficult to see that what we buy in supermarkets (when not labelled organic) is liable to be a highly denatured substance. However, it is still possible to find good quality milk and dairy products, so let us not forget its role in human nutrition. Milk is the body builder *par excellence*, building *kapha* in Ayurvedic terms – the solid, substantial part of the human being (see Chapter 1, Note 4). Milk protein is more complete than other kinds of animal protein.

Lactose appears only in milk and there is no other way to obtain this form of sugar. It is transported undigested into the large intestine where it is used as food for the beneficial acidophilus bacteria. In addition, to help establish a healthy bacterial balance it aids the assimilation of important minerals — calcium, phosphorus and magnesium.

In the case of lactose intolerance, the cause can be a definite allergy or a deficiency in the enzyme lactase. When this enzyme is lacking the unabsorbed lactose remains in the intestinal tract, feeding certain bacteria which then begin to grow and multiply there. The result can be abdominal pain, diarrhoea and gas. In such situations yoghourt may be more easily digested, as the lactose has already been converted.

Dairy products get blamed for being mucus-forming. Yes, this is true, but again it is a matter of quality and quantity. Let us not forget that we do need mucus, as we do need cholesterol. Unfortunately these have both become threatening elements and, for many, things to avoid. Mucus keeps the stomach and all the internal membranes in good health; in the stomach it protects from the corrosive effects of strong acids.

All commercially sold milk has been heat treated (except 'green-top', which has to be bought directly from a licensed dairy farmer). The pasteurization of milk was introduced to protect the consumer from any possible disease-causing bacteria. But pasteurization also destroys the nutritive value of the milk; it not only fails to kill all the harmful bacteria, but also destroys many of the beneficial bacteria. It destroys some of the heat-sensitive vitamins and changes the chemical structure of the protein, rendering it and the mineral content less digestible.

The pasteurization process involves heating to 72°C for 15 seconds. There are some bacteria that remain, and the very important question of viral growth is still a subject for study. Pasteurized milk tends to coagulate in a tight mass when exposed to stomach acid. Boiling the milk quickly is a much more effective way of sterilizing it. In India, with thousands of years of experience, milk is never taken without first boiling.[10]

It is noteworthy that the peoples we have always associated with remarkable health and longevity (Swedes, Bulgarians, Russians and Hunzas) have dairy products as central to their diet. The long-living Bulgarians use very little meat but consume large quantities of milk and dairy products. The Dutch, too, are noted for their dairy products and energetic lifestyle.

Deep down our enjoyment of dairy products is clearly linked to the archetypal nurturing experience of nursing which usually brings a sense of comfort and security. Perhaps with the diminishing presence of dairy herds and lush meadows we are being weaned away from this comfort and security. I personally hope not.

Varieties of cow's milk

To summarize the varieties of cow's milk that are available to us now in Britain:

Untreated: sold only from a small number of licensed farms and over a small local area. It has an obvious cream line and will last 2–3 days refrigerated.

All the remaining varieties are pasteurized and usually homogenized (warmed and forced through a fine aperture to break up the fat globules so they remain evenly suspended throughout the milk, leaving no cream line). Almost all milk sold in UK supermarkets is homogenized. The fat globules are reduced to a thousandth of their natural size, fundamentally changing the milk's make-up. This is possibly linked to rising levels of heart and circulatory disease and has also been linked to milk allergies and arthritis.

Semi-skimmed: Half the cream has been removed. Fat content about $1\frac{1}{2}$%.
Skimmed: Cream is removed, leaving milk that is thin and bluish in colour.
UHT: Heat treated to 132°C for 1 second then cooled. Will last four months without refrigeration, unopened.
Sterilized: Bottled, sealed, then heated to above boiling point for 30 minutes, and cooled. All micro-organisms are destroyed. It is a dead product and has a cooked flavour.

The proteins in milk are of high biological value and contain the essential amino acids. The principal milk proteins are casein, lactalbumin and lactoglobin (which only occurs in milk).

Other animal milks

Sheep's milk
The fat globules are smaller than those in cow's milk and are closer to human milk. It is higher in protein than human milk.

Goat's milk
Contains less protein than cow's or sheep's milk and has a higher sugar content, 3.7%–4.6%. But its slightly sharp and acid flavour is not liked by many people. The flavour is modified in goat's cheese, which has become very popular.

Donkeys' or asses' milk
This was recommended by Steiner as the closest to human milk (1.9% protein, 6.6% lactose). By the end of the nineteenth century there were in Europe a number of donkey herds milked for the children of wealthy parents.

Yoghourt

Yoghourt can be a very nutritious and delicious food with helpful properties, particularly if it has been made from milk from a biodynamic farm, or at least from cows who have grazed on organic, chemical-free pastures. It can also be made from goat's or sheep's milk. It contains high-quality proteins, minerals, vitamins and enzymes, including vitamins that are otherwise hard to get: D and B_{12}. It is a food which has been partly digested, changed to this state by the action of a special culture of bacteria, *Lactobacillus bulgaricus* (originating in Bulgaria), added to warmed milk at 43°C and left overnight. This process of pre-digestion enables yoghourt to be digested and utilized in the body even more readily than milk.

Lactobacillus bulgaricus destroys putrefactive bacteria and promotes the growth of necessary acidophilus bacteria, which help in the manufacture of vitamins B and K in the intestines, and it also assists in the assimilation of nutrients from food. It helps to prevent constipation and is a natural anti-biotic. It has been reported that an 8 oz pot (450 g) of yoghourt, refrigerated for one week, provides an antibiotic value equal to 14 units of penicillin.[11] Yoghourt can digest such virulent micro-organisms as certain amoebae, streptococcus and staphylococcus bacteria. It also can assist in restoring helpful intestinal flora after a course of antibiotics, which tend to diminish them.

Yoghourt is such a versatile food, it can be used with fruit, in sauces and salad dressings or just plain by itself.

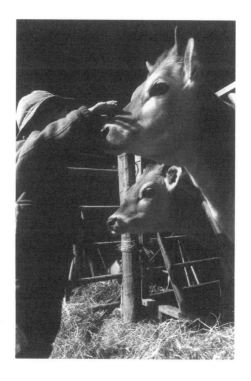

Other dairy products

Other milk products are butter, cream, skimmed milk, buttermilk, whey, quark, cottage cheese, soured cream, crème fraîche, soft cheeses and hard cheeses. Of these, hard cheeses, butter and cream can be difficult to digest, particularly cooked hard cheese; here again the significant questions will be about quality, and the health of the animals. We can also assist the digestion of these fats by doing physical work and exercise, otherwise fatty deposits accumulate and our cholesterol levels become too high.

The formation of butter is based on a unique property of milk fat, its globular structure, coming from the natural emulsion of the milk globules. To evaluate butter it is important to look at its fatty acid content. Up to date 75 fatty acids have been identified in butter, so in this respect milk fat bears a qualitative resemblance to olive oil.[12] (See also Chapter 13 on fats and oils.)

Many further questions may spring to your mind concerning dairy products – there are so many perspectives to explore. I would not try to deny that some people do better without certain dairy products in their diets; this was true of my daughter Daisy for a period, but now she can happily digest most forms of dairy foods in moderation.

Quality testing

Nothing is more revealing to us than what our own senses tell us. We don't have to have a Ph.D in chemistry to do some experiments in our own kitchens. The kitchen is indeed potentially a true research laboratory. Just study milk: what other food has this colour, consistency and smell? Nothing else, for instance, can be compared with the smell of burnt milk. How would you characterize that smell? When we heat milk a skin forms that is really strong and resilient. It can hold bubbles of air for a short time. What kind of properties does this signify?

Only when we can trust our own sense reactions to perceptible and obvious information shall we develop our inner authority on matters such as nutrition and quality.

Here is an interesting experiment to try —

If you have access to milk from a biodynamic or organic farm, take equal samples of milk from as many differing qualities of milk, such as raw, ultra-heat treated, ordinary pasteurized, as you can find. Put them in labelled jars with a piece of muslin to cover and keep on a warm shelf in the kitchen for up to a month (*do not refrigerate*). Then observe smell, proportions of milk solids to whey, which ones grow moulds and what colours and textures they are. This is enormously revealing and children find it very interesting, when they get over the 'urghhh' response!

13

FATS AND OILS

In the human being and the warm-blooded animals the fat substances are the carriers of warmth and therefore are mediators for the soul, which needs this warmth. The temperature at which the human body operates is very specific (37°C) and it is one of the function of the fats to insulate us and maintain this crucial temperature. Fat acts as a store of energy if other food supplies fail, and although fats are important constituents of food, conversion of carbohydrates to fat does occur in the body.

What are the properties of fats and oils? The first important observation is that they are not water-soluble, unlike the salts and carbohydrates. They form themselves into fine, globular droplets and work as an emulsion which plays a special role in the absorption of fats.

All fats and oils are made up of substances called tri-glycerides and each of these is made up of three fatty acids plus one unit of glycerol. The differences in fats are due to the different fatty acids in their molecules. Although there are many different fatty acids in nature, they are divided into two groups: saturated and unsaturated. Saturated fats (e.g. animal fats, cocoa butter) tend to be solid at room temperature. Unsaturated fats, which tend to be liquid at room temperature (oils), can be subdivided into mono-saturated and polyunsaturated.

In digestion it is notable that the body accepts fats and oils readily and they are able to proceed to the small intestine without substantial alteration. Here they are acted upon by bile acids and lipase in the intestinal fluids and enter the lymph system. In the body, the closer we find a fat to the skin the more saturated it will be, and therefore more insulating. For example, the fat in the cheeks is more saturated, whereas the fats that lubricate the deepest interior have a more plastic structure and are unsaturated.

Oil facilitates cooking and makes things that might be incompatible compatible; it lubricates and so has a special place in nutrition.

Where fat is found

All living cells contain traces of fatty substances such as oils, fats or waxes. Even in minute amounts they play an important role in the processes that relate individual cells to each other to form a unified organism. Fat has its origins in the barrier (the cell membrane) that protects the delicate chemical organization of life within from the forces of dilution and disorder (entropy) without. In the central nervous system, the cerebrospinal nerve fibres (axons) are protected by a fatty sheath known as the myelin sheath. Myelin has a high electrical resistance and its presence (rather like insulating tape around wire) makes possible the rapid and efficient conduction of impulses. So fat provides both a barrier to acute external impressions and a smooth transmitter of information.

Oils in plants

Oils are produced in quantities large enough to warrant extraction in only one plant organ – the seed. In tropical countries the coconut palm, the oil palm, sesame, soybeans, cottonseeds and peanuts are grown for their oil content. In more temperate climates, the olive, rape, maize, flax, sunflower and safflower seeds yield most of the oils suitable for human consumption. The fat content of plant tissue ranges from about 0.1% in potatoes to about 70% in nut kernels. Green leaves contain about 1% fatty substances, the cereal crops between 2% and 4%.

Such a concentration of oil in plant seeds is usually explained on the basis that it is a food reserve in the embryo. However, such large quantities are found in the olive and the avocado that they become rancid and break down well before germination (again, these plants have been developed for their oil content). With the exception of the olive tree and the coconut and oil palms, most oil-yielding plants are annuals. It should be noted, though, that *a significant part of our dietary fat actually comes from food without it having been separated from the plant material.*

For most annual plants the growth period draws to a close as the fruit and seed mature. The leaves begin to wither and vitality seems to withdraw. The remaining life-processes are all directed towards the maturation of the seed. The seed serves as a kind of earthly anchor that allows the plant a first point of contact in the following spring and thereby it makes its appearance again. Within the seed itself oil is found mainly in the embryo or germ.

Composition of oils and fats

Vegetable oils are amongst the most perfect substances provided by nature. From the food chemist's point of view, however, fats and oils are made up of the same two materials as carbohydrates, i.e. carbon and water. It is the degree of saturation, or hardening, which determines whether we are dealing with a solid fat or a liquid oil (saturation is dependent on the amount of hydrogen it holds).

Most fats are derived from the animal world and they are solid at room temperature. Oils are derived from plants or fish, and are liquid at room temperature. The nature of both fats and oils is however very different from that of carbohydrates, for they have undergone a complete transformation. The most important difference is in what is called the 'energy value', that of fats and oils being more than two times greater than that of starch and sugar.

If we look at the origin of this energy we see that plant oils have absorbed more than twice the amount of sunlight than other substances, this absorption of light and warmth occurring during the ripening stage. In unripe seeds sugars and starches predominate, becoming first the building blocks of oil (fatty acids and glycerol), then the oil specific to the plant with its characteristic aroma and taste. These subtle characteristics are based upon a unique blend of small quantities of oil-like substances. They include phospholipids (lecithin for example), chlorophyll-like and carotene-like pigments and the vitamins A, D and E. Physiologists often refer to them as 'growth factor lipids'.

So, because of the unique process of photosynthesis (the miracle by which sunlight is turned into food), plants are an abundant source of poly-unsaturated fatty acids. In fact the most abundant fatty acid on the planet may be tri-unsaturated linoleic acid, since it is the predominant fatty acid surrounding plant chloroplasts.[1] This membrane is packed so tightly in the chloroplast, maximizing the amount of surface that can intercept sunlight and convert it into energy, that a square inch of spinach leaf contains nearly four feet of membrane!

Fatty acids

Fatty acids are called saturated if they cannot absorb any more hydrogen. The process of saturating a liquid oil by forcing it to absorb hydrogen results in a solid fat (see later, on margarine, p. 216). By technological means we have found a way to mimic artificially what the normal metabolism of animals achieves: hardening a vegetable product and changing its inherent nature. The degree of saturation determines the temperature at which an oil solidifies. For example, oleic acid is more saturated than linoleic acid and as olive oil contains about 80% oleic acid it easily solidifies in very cold weather.

The fatty acid composition of vegetable oils is strongly influenced by ambient temperatures during the period of maturation. Sunflower seed oil from plants grown in cool climates contains about 70% linoleic acid but oils from the same seed variety grown in warmer climates contain only about half as much, with a corresponding increase in oleic acid. Animals show a similar response to environmental temperature. Tallow from Indian cattle contains as much as 70% saturated fatty acids, compared with the usual 50–55% range for tallows in Europe, North America and Argentina.

From a nutritional point of view there are only three fatty acids usually labelled as essential, that is, essential in the structure of human fat. With the possible exception of linoleic acid there is no evidence that the human being is unable to synthesize them, but a deficiency in one or more of the growth factor lipids mentioned above manifests primarily as skin lesions, and retarded growth in children.

Fats in the human diet

The recommended amount of dietary fats is around 20%. However the diet of Americans is said to contain 30–40% fats; arteriosclerosis is one of their most fatal disorders. In Japan only 10% of the diet consists of fats and arteriosclerosis is relatively infrequent.

Cholesterol

Cholesterol is a waxy, fatlike compound that serves a multitude of purposes in the body. It is a complex molecule with the same ring structure as many hormones and it is the base from which oestrogen, cortisone and testosterone are made. It is also a component of nerve tissue.

One end of the molecule can form a salt, which is soluble in water, while the other end combines readily with fat. The salts are known as bile salts since they constitute a major part of the bile and promote the mixing of fats in the small intestine with water, so that they can be broken down and absorbed through the intestinal wall.

It is important that the amount of cholesterol derived from our food is less than that synthesized by our liver. Too much dietary cholesterol can bring about an imbalance in the whole cholesterol metabolism. When it accumulates it develops a kind of hard plaque on the walls of blood vessels and can cause arteriosclerosis.

Dr Schmidt has pointed out, 'When we realize, for example, that the excretion of cholesterol is inhibited by animal foods while it is stimulated by plant foods, this raises important nutritional questions.'[2]

Foods which are helpful in reducing cholesterol build-up are wholegrains, flax seeds, almonds and hazel nuts, omega 3 fish oils, dark green vegetables such as kale and collards, mustard greens, spinach, chard, parsley, indeed all chlorophyll-rich foods that are also rich in alpha-linoleic acid. Pungent foods such as horseradish, onion, leek, shallot, chives, together with celery, beetroot and a little cayenne all can assist with the blood-cleansing process.

In the Ayurvedic system, fats, including milk and butter, build up *kapha*.[3] This category of foods helps the gentle anchoring of the human being to the earth, developing solidity, muscle and a certain feeling of well-being. Butter fat consists of 81% milk fat, 18% water and 1% milk solids. The fat is in the form of globules containing phospholipids, cholesterol, glycerides and protein. It is made by churning cream and melts at human blood temperature, which allows it — taken in moderation — to have a protective effect on the heart. In contrast to milk and butter, other animal fats have a higher melting point, being saturated, and are therefore less easy to metabolize.

Some people need more fats than others, particularly if they live in cold climates. Those who benefit most from fats are the thin, wiry types with a nervous constitution, as the lubricating quality of fat acts as a barrier to harsh external stimuli. The original desire for fats can be developed in childhood and that desire stored as memory in the liver. The most important element in the metabolism of fats is physical movement. If a person is active in a healthy, balanced way, they will have a greater chance of maintaining an equilibrium in their cholesterol levels.

Olive Oil

It appears that cultivation of the olive began six thousand years ago at the eastern end of the Mediterranean. The original spiny, straggly plant, poor in oil, was already found in many places but it was the agricultural genius of the Syrians and Palestinians that bred a more compact, thornless, oil-rich variety and spread it all along the shores of the Mediterranean. Oil was everywhere in demand in the ancient world, for food, lighting and medicine. It was used in the anointing of the heads of kings, priests and others with important missions.

This perfect, natural substance was not only used to signify the highest esteem, but it was believed to allow a divine influence to slip into a mortal person. However this did not stop the Egyptians, for example, from using oil for more down to earth purposes. They used olive oil to move heavy loads in construction work, and a mixture of animal fat and lime as axle grease. In Crete the olive was under cultivation at least as early as 2500 BC and the island soon flourished on the export of the smooth green oil, stored in great earthenware stirrup jars and perfumed with wild herbs.

Olive oil is the oil of 'the middle', of balance and mildness, soothing in quality. Pressing should be mechanical rather than chemical, and filtration either natural or by decanting. A good extra virgin olive oil has an acid content ranging from 0.2% to no more than 0.4%. It should be yellow-gold with greenish highlights and have a fresh smell (clean and vegetal). It is thought to be a contributing factor to the low rate from heart disease in Mediterranean countries.[4] It contains mono-unsaturated fatty acids which

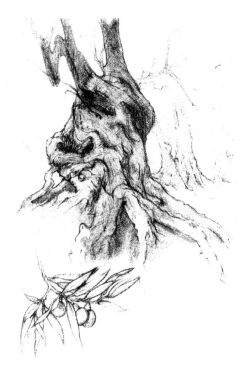

Olive tree and branch

help to keep blood cholesterol at healthy levels; it also assists bone growth and digestion and helps to increase the absorption of the fat-soluble vitamins, A, D, E and K. It has 80% oleic acid content.

Olive oil is an essential in Mediterranean cuisine, but there are many varieties and qualities, the most delicious and nutritious being the cold-pressed virgin olive oil. It should be kept in a dark glass bottle in a cool place to avoid oxidation. Dressing a salad with a thin coating of olive oil renders it more digestible and prevents oxidation of nutrients. Tomas Graves (son of the poet Robert) speaks of the Majorcan culture that he had been born into:

> I have no Majorcan blood or surnames and if I consider myself a local lad it's not so much for having been born in Guillem Massot Street in Palma or attending the village school, as for having been suckled from the same breast as the majority of islanders: the 'setrill', the olive cruet. If children who share the same wet-nurse are known as 'brothers in milk', then consider me your 'brother in oil'![5]

Such is the binding intensity of the Mediterranean folk-soul, steeped in the tradition of olive oil.

'We consider the olive tree to be a symbol of our Mediterranean culture, and in our diet there's no substitute for its fruit,' declares Antoni Pinya. 'There is hardly any part of our culinary heritage in which olive oil doesn't play a major part – seasonings, dressings and sauces. Now we know how healthy it is other cultures want to copy our diet.'[6]

Some other vegetable oils

Corn oil
The 'softest', most unsaturated oil of all the grains. Source of phosphorus and vitamins A, D and E.

Hazelnut oil
Deep rich flavour, which is at the same time light. Use it in salad dressings and sauces.

Linseed oil
Has recently become known as a dietary help in cases of skin disease such as eczema and cradle cap. Also stimulates the digestion. One tablespoon of soaked linseeds drunk daily is extremely efficacious for regulating good bowel function. It is high in linoleic acid.

Sunflower oil
Particularly rich in vitamin E. Diuretic.

Sesame oil
Does not easily turn rancid. Contains 40% linoleic acid, 50% oleic acid and lecithin. Among other vegetable oils, sesame seed oil is used predominantly in Japanese, Thai and other oriental cuisines, although the Mesopotamians used it too.

The Egyptians list two unusual sources of culinary oil: the seeds of radish and lettuce!

Refined oils

Refined oils are mostly produced by using a solvent and high temperatures, often exceeding 230°C. Trans-fatty acid formation starts around 180°C. This denatured compound can interfere with the normal transformation of fats in the body into immunity-building fatty-acids and prostaglandins.

Margarine and hydrogenation

The process of hydrogenation was developed about a hundred years ago to provide raw material for the manufacture of soap. The waste products of inedible fish and vegetable oils were hardened, i.e., rendered solid at room temperature, and could be substituted for the more expensive lard. Some decades later the US cotton industry sought a market outlet for increasing excesses of cotton-seed oil. The answer was to hydrogenate it and to turn it into a cheap substitute for butter, which came to be called margarine. In Britain, waste beef and mutton fats no longer needed for candle making provided some of the raw material. With increasing popularity, other fats and oils came to be used in the production of margarine, mainly soya and safflower.

Basic production methods have not changed greatly. The oil is made odourless and tasteless by passing steam through it at temperatures of 205–250°C and at a very low pressure. The oil is then placed under pressures of up to 60 lb per square inch and kept hot at 100–200°C. Hydrogen is bubbled through it in the presence of a copper, nickel or platinum catalyst. The result is a dark, malodorous product which is then filtered, bleached and deodorized to produce a pure white, odourless and tasteless fat. (Greek *margaron* means 'pearly white'.) The selective addition of preservatives, flavourings and colouring agents, emulsifier, water, liquid oils, vitamins and flavour protectors results in the variety of margarines available today.

Since artificially hydrogenated fats are a fairly recent addition to the diet of the human being and since the body had no previous experience of it, it is reasonable to question whether the human being has the capacity to deal effectively with such a synthetic product. Clever marketing has given the strong impression that margarine is less cholesterol-raising than butter, but to know the truth of things we need to know what has gone into their manufacture. The further away from natural processes products are, the more burdensome on the digestion.

Summing all this up, we can say that oil mediates wherever two opposing tendencies meet and it lubricates surfaces, stopping friction. 'Pouring oil upon troubled waters' signifies the healing role of sun-charged, unsaturated oils that have a vital part in both form and function in plant, animal and human.

Rudolf Steiner suggests that the person who can manufacture his own fats from plant material has a distinct advantage over those who take their fats from an animal source.[7] From this discussion you will gather what those advantages are.

14

SALT

The story of salt

Salt was used as a preservative in early Egyptian times. We know that the Egyptians traded salted fish for Phoenician cedar, glass and purple dye. It was also an important ingredient in the mummification process. *Natrum*, a substance containing sodium chloride, was used for preserving the bodies of wealthier Egyptians and regular salt for the poorer ones.

At the same time it was a sacrificial substance, being offered to those gods responsible for providing the fruits of the earth, and covenants were made over a sacrificial meal in which salt was present, its preservative qualities symbolizing an enduring pact. The Arabic phrase 'There is salt between us' is reminiscent of the power of such a bond. Salt had connotations of esteem and honour, as illustrated by the Hebrew phrase 'to eat the salt of the palace'. The most honoured guests were seated 'above the salt' at table, in those early times reserved for the leaders of the people. Even today we still have an expression referring to people as being 'worth, or not worth, their salt'. Later, salt was used more widely as a condiment by the ancient Greeks and Homer called it divine. The Romans paid their soldiers with salt-money (salary from *sal* = salt), showing its increasing importance. This was the time in history when philosophy, debate and logic were developing. Rudolf Steiner said in 1923, 'Salt is an extremely important nutrient. We salt our meals so that we can think. Salt and the minerals have a relationship to the human being's life of consciousness.'[1]

Salt was also associated with fertility, probably from the saline oceans teeming with fish. Celibate Egyptian priests had abstained from salt, because it was thought to excite sexual desire. The Romans called a man in love *salax* – in a 'salted state' (our salacious). The Gauls or Galli (so named by the

Romans meaning 'the salt people') sacked Rome in 390 BC and ruled it for the following 40 years. So highly prized was salt that many battles were fought over the possession of salt-mines and taxes were levied on salt trading, often financing more wars. The Chinese maintained that excessive salt taking encouraged greed. By the first millennium BC the management of salt mines and pans was an administrative tool in China, and similarly exploited later by the Seleucid dynasty of Persia.

Venice built her original trade supremacy on salt, and more recently in the twentieth century salt was still a government monopoly in British India. Indeed it stimulated one of the greatest political demonstrations of modern times, when in 1930 Mahatma Gandhi marched with a great number of followers on a pilgrimage to the seashore at Dandi, there to make salt illegally. Gandhi's idea was to focus the independence movement on the issue of salt monopoly and taxation. He argued that it was an example of British misrule that touched the lives of all castes of Indians. Everyone ate salt, except for Gandhi, who renounced it for six years as a non-violent means of protest.

Nevertheless, there are few places on the earth that do not have access to salt and, as Cassiodorus, the fifth-century Goth, said, 'It may be well that some seek not gold, but there lives not a man who does not need salt.' So what is it about salt that became so universally important?

The properties of salt

A salt crystal has the structure and form of a cube, so salt symbolizes the mineral world; in Steiner's system it also symbolizes the 'fourfoldness' of the human being. The use of salt in food shows we are now taking nourishment not only from the plant and animal kingdoms but also directly from the mineral kingdom. Most minerals should be contained in the plants that we eat but sodium chloride (table salt) is an exception, so we have to seek it out and add it to our food.

In the Eastern system salt is said to have a dual nature, being both 'yang' (contracted, assertive, masculine, active and hot) and 'yin' (expansive, fluidic, receptive and feminine). In its crystalline form we can see the 'yang' qualities, but when dissolved it becomes more 'yin'. Chemically, salt is a compound of sodium and chlorine.

Sodium reacts violently when placed in water; it raises the temperature to near boiling and behaves in a most unruly manner, dashing about, fizzing and releasing hydrogen in an explosive way until it dissolves and turns into sodium hydroxide. Chlorine is a very nasty, lethal gas which was used to devastating effect in the First World War. Dissolved in water, it turns into hydrochloric acid, one of the strongest burning acids. Yet when sodium and chlorine are combined its duality is contained, making an important nutritional catalyst. In this we see that in chemistry the totality is never the same as the sum of its parts.[2]

Steiner's view

Old alchemical teachings involved the processes of *sal-mercur-sulfur* (salt-mercury-sulphur) and Rudolf Steiner pointed out that salt appears as the earthly principle, in contrast to sulphur, which represents the fire- and light-carrying properties of substance. Salt, then, reminds us of the relationship of life processes to the soul-spiritual in the human being. The saltlike processes that result in the 'lifeless' (lacking the capacity to regenerate), i.e., nervous tissue, brain and skeleton, become the matrix for the unfolding of the soul-spiritual. 'Life becomes frozen thought.'[3]

The behaviour of salt has inspired an interesting metaphor:

> When salt crystals are put into water we see a constantly changing flow of transparent forms emerging from their planar surfaces and merging with the solvent [...] the 'sleeping' crystals have now 'awakened' and become chemically active [...] [They] now exert osmotic pressure and behave exactly like a gas [...] A gradual dematerialization happens which finally reaches a condition of pure warmth.

Might this be seen as an image of our thought processes – a fluid, dissolving, translucent activity, constantly in flux, which can be warmed by interest and enthusiasm?

In *Seasalt and Your Life*, Jacques de Langre says: 'Salt is a grounding crystal that takes us down into the body/mind, where well-centred concentration of matter attracts a clear perception of its opposite: Spirit (non-matter).'[5] Whereas, Dr Schmidt suggests, salt, 'because it is lifeless and has forsaken all that was once its own, has become especially permeable for extra-terrestrial activities. When we metabolize salt, dissolving this mineral substance within us, we are in effect battling against the mineralizing tendencies within us.'[6]

The sodium and potassium balance in the human being

In the human being sodium is related to potassium. These two substances are 'earth metals' of fundamental importance for the functioning of human processes and responsible for the electrolytic balance in the body cells and fluids. Their atoms each have a single electric charge as opposed to the two of most other minerals. This means that they are less tenacious in their hold on other structures and can therefore move easily through solutions, especially water. They are termed 'electrolytes' and exist in an important ratio on either side of the cell membrane, establishing a dynamic tension. It is this tension that lies behind the ability of living cells to respond to a stimulus.

Potassium is necessary for normal growth, healthy skin, regulation of the heartbeat, muscular activity and stimulation of the kidneys to eliminate waste, together with the transmission of nerve impulses. It helps to prevent both constipation and diarrhoea by maintaining a normal contraction and relaxation of the muscles and has a beneficial effect on the excretion of hormones. Sodium acts in partnership with potassium to regulate the pH (acid/alkaline) balance of the blood, and is also involved in transmission of nerve impulses. In addition, it helps to keep other minerals in suspension, especially calcium.

Potassium is concentrated within the cell membrane, whereas sodium is to be found in greater quantity in the fluid surrounding the cells. The ratio between them is important and reflects the balance of these two vital substances as found in nature – the seas surrounding the land are high in sodium, and potassium is abundant in the vegetation of the land. Similarly, in the evolutionary processes sodium predominated in the earliest forms of life in the great oceans; as more complicated forms evolved, sodium was gradually excluded from within the cell walls, to be replaced by potassium. The amniotic fluid in which human and animal foetuses float before birth contains salt, like seawater, as well as sugar and protein and can be seen as a remnant of this primordial process. The replacement of sodium by potassium within the cell has been the physiological basis for the development of much more complicated biochemical processes, helping the unfolding of individual consciousness.

Our need for salt

Salt, though a very crucial substance, is needed only in small doses – approximately 5 gm per day (a salt-spoonful). This is an average and can vary somewhat according to season and climate, between child and adult, and even temperament or constitution. The daily amount, however, is known to be constantly abused, Europeans often taking an average of 20 gm and Americans 30 gm.

The desire for salt is physiologically related to the amount already in the body and this desire can become a real craving. As more sodium is taken in, the level in the blood rises and the sodium 'pump' has difficulty in keeping a healthy sodium/potassium balance. The problem is often exacerbated by the fact that most people use commercial salt, a highly refined, chemically made variety which is 99.5 per cent sodium chloride, containing anti-caking chemicals, potassium iodide and sugar (dextrose) to stabilize the iodine. Refined salt has been stripped of all the 60 trace minerals that can be found in true sea-salt, which has a similar profile to our own blood. It is the unbalanced nature of refined salt that contributes to salt craving.

The balance may be quite successfully maintained by a person with a lively constitution who has plenty of physical activity. But others may experience difficulties, with symptoms such as heaviness, lethargy and a tendency towards fluid retention (which can eventually lead to high blood pressure). Excess sodium is also irritating to the nervous system.

The incidence of excessive salt intake in our 'minerally-awakened' society is widespread. It could be seen as a sign of mankind's grappling with this earthly pole. There is in this a danger of a materialism that prevents the spirit getting the upper hand, but at the same time we may observe a wrestling with a new kind of consciousness – one that may be trying to 'dissolve out' the inherent wisdom in these crystalline forms.

Some people have taken to salt-free diets, and for many of us there is certainly room for some reduction. However, a person on a salt-free diet will automatically decrease his fluid intake, showing that the organism needs to retain the salt present in the bodily fluids. In a healthy situation the salt in the blood, and that in the tissue fluids, is continually being exchanged, and in this process, by which new salt is regularly introduced into the system, lies one of the most important biological functions connected with digestion and nutrition. The crucial importance of salt and its underlying health hazards are today widely discussed but its true function is still little understood.

Salt and consciousness

The total withdrawal of salt often results in the person becoming tired and apathetic, and the ability to think clearly is impaired. These phenomena are connected with the other side of his life – his consciousness. It is interesting to note what Walter Cloos has to say about the link between salt and consciousness:

> In order to appreciate what far-reaching significance salt has for a person's whole constitution, one only has to deprive them completely of the salt they would usually use for seasoning. The first symptom is lack of appetite. This is due to the fact that salt has this peculiarity of bringing out the individual tastes of all foods, and through the experience of taste in the area of mouth and tongue it works deeply into the unconscious function of the inner glands, connected with the stomach and intestinal digestion. Thus through salt, something becomes conscious that works unconsciously in digestion and nutrition. The 'inner' taste is stimulated, which according to Rudolf Steiner extends right into the liver. This 'inner' taste, which only consciously appears as appetite, is linked with another peculiarity of salt: it guides the individual nutritive substances to the appropriate places in the organism.[7]

So we see the action of salt is catalytic, enhancing our capacity to taste (when taken in the right proportions), not only in the mouth but also right down to the liver. Digestion and nutrition provide material up-building (anabolic) processes whilst certain aspects of consciousness arise as a result of breakdown processes (catabolic). These two are in their nature diametrically opposite, but both essential.

Physiologically, consciousness and self-awareness destroy what is built up, and the breaking down process takes place almost entirely in our nerves and our brain. In this 'nerve-sense' system, as it is described by Rudolf Steiner, the human is able to concentrate nutritional substances to the point of mineral density and lifelessness, but he is also able to dissolve them again and cast them out of his system. Physicians such as Paracelsus referred to this as the 'salt-process'. It signified that out of something in solution, particularly a saturated one, a hard substance could be precipitated. In this sense one could even call the forming of all rocks and minerals of the earth a 'salt-process', but one should note that most rocks and minerals are not soluble in water – at any rate not to the extent of real salts. Only true salts are soluble in water.

> Thus in the human we find salt in two conditions: first in solution in the blood, and then as a process in the brain and nervous system, which leads to a sort of depositing and which is the physiological basis for consciousness. The most well-known example of this is the 'brain-sand' (crystals of calcium carbonate) in the pineal gland which if it is absent or abnormal causes idiocy or feeble-mindedness.[8]

Alchemists and cooks therefore make themselves familiar with the activity of salts and their mysterious qualities. We know from our own experience that it only takes a pinch of salt to bring out a deeper quality in something like porridge, or when whipping egg whites to create a firmness, and we know that salt has the capacity of enhancing – 'bringing out' – other flavours in a subtle way. We need to know for instance that because salt helps with the digestion of starches it is best cooked *in with* grains rather than being added on the plate.

So it is important to know something of the story of salt and its crucial importance in the human nutritional journey. Not too little, not too much! Sesame salt (*gomasio* in Japan) as a condiment is a good way to have salt on the table. Small children need very little salt, as it will cause the 'awakening' process prematurely. It can easily develop into a craving for salted snacks. We only too frequently see small children clamouring for potato crisps or peanuts, which can lead to health problems in later life as well as encouraging the desire for sugar (the other polarity).

As cooks we can try to bear in mind the true wisdom-carrying properties of this once sacred substance in its whole, unadulterated state, and try to use it with our own proper wisdom and discretion.

MINERALS AND THE QUESTION OF DIETARY SUPPLEMENTS

In Chapter 1 we followed the various stages of human nutrition through those early 'milk and honey' times, when nomadic peoples lived from the milk of their animals and gathered wild foods, to the more settled agrarian communities with their creative innovation. Later, during the Graeco-Roman period, we saw the beginning of a more mineral nutrition – using the roots of plants, the most dense and mineralized part hitherto not commonly eaten, along with salt as a seasoning. Further exploration to greater distances later brought us spices and sugar, which also have a mineral quality. Today, at the beginning of the twenty-first century, in Western society we witness a new phenomenon – many people adding mineral supplements to their diet. What lies behind this seemingly strange practice? To begin to answer the question we may ask: what has been our conscious involvement with this world of minerals so far?

The old alchemists worked with three elements of the mineral kingdom: salt, mercury and sulphur. Salt (or *sal*) to them was the 'ponderable' matter subject to the forces of the earth, whereas sulphur (*sulfur*) represented the substances which were permeated by the 'imponderables' – the forces streaming in from the world's circumference. Mercury (or *mercur*) stood between these two, harmonizing the rhythmic forces, one radiating out from the earth, the other radiating in from the cosmos. These processes were relegated to different parts of the human physiology: the *sal* processes were the hardening forces of form that worked more strongly in the head and nervous system; the *mercur* was mediated through the breathing/rhythmic system; and *sulfur* through the heat of the metabolism, the dissolving forces of fire.

According to Paracelsus, in the human being are contained all the substances that exist in the universe including the metals, each under the special governance of one of the seven planetary spheres. These metals were gifts from the planets and rather than citizens of our earth should be regarded as guests.[1] The metals were designated: gold, the gift of the sun, silver of moon, copper related to Venus, iron to Mars, tin to Jupiter, mercury (quicksilver) to Mercury, and lead to Saturn.

There existed then an understanding (proved today) that each metal has its own peculiar distribution on the earth. 'If we mark on the globe the various localities containing deposits of gold, copper, uranium etc., a different pattern arises for each metal. Something of an organic structure becomes visible and [as a correlation it is revealed that as well as other minerals] throughout the human organism we find gold, silver, mercury, tin etc. in minimal traces, each metal in a different distribution . . . in one organ more, in another less.'[2]

This living and dynamic connection with the stars and planets, their relationship to the earth and their correspondences within the human being faded as materialism appropriated the new scientific consciousness, preoccupied with only the visible and measurable. By the end of the nineteenth century the crucial role played by micro-nutrients was little heeded. Indeed, an 1897 textbook on human physiology deals with inorganic nutrients in less than two pages.[3] It was only in the twentieth century that the importance of these inorganic nutrients began to be researched. G. von Bunge started this new study when he identified seven mineral substances in mother's milk: potassium, sodium, calcium, magnesium, iron, phosphorus and chlorine. Less than a hundred years later a startling amount of information about minerals abounds in serious biochemical research, in popular books and magazines – not only the 'macro-minerals' listed above but hundreds of micronutrients as well.

Not only do we now have to be knowledgeable about our intake of fats, proteins, carbohydrates, and calories, but it appears that we need to know if we are zinc- or selenium-deficient, or deficient in any number of hitherto unheard-of substances. The manufacture of vitamins and food supplements has become a very lucrative industry and with it comes a new generation of nutritionists trained mainly in the prescribing of dietary supplements – pills, capsules and colloidal solutions of specific mineral combinations. Many people swear by them; it is for sure that they are paying more than they would for a kilo of biodynamically grown rice and some vegetables.

This is a mystery I have tried to penetrate for some years. I make no claim to have understood the biochemical information, which is often either confusing or contradictory, but one has to be aware that it is becoming a more and more controversial issue. Some years ago I came across a prediction of Rudolf Steiner's that human beings would in time be creating mineral blueprints of plant foods (Berlin, 4 November 1905). Later at Koberwitz in 1924, when he delivered the lectures to farmers on agriculture, he was speaking about mineral fertilizers and could clearly see the potential outcomes of their misuse:

> The materialistic farmer who thinks about these things can calculate about how many decades it will be in this century before agricultural products have degenerated so far that they can no longer nourish the human being adequately. With the materialistic world conception, agriculture has come the furthest from rational principles.[4]

I do feel that in mineral supplements we are witnessing a phenomenon that represents the tip of an iceberg pointing to something very important beneath. One aspect appears to be the deficiency of these nutrients in conventionally grown produce. In a sense, however, it seems that by promoting such supplements we are attempting to bypass the importance of good husbandry, of creating vital soils providing the full range of nutrition required for plant, animal and human. Shouldn't we ask ourselves: how are good soils formed?

A good soil consists of sand, clay, silt and humus in good balance. Aside from nitrates, all soils originate from weathered rock fragments. The sizes of the mineral particles determine the type of soil. For example, sandy soils, which mainly consist of particles of quartz, are said to be 'light', because the particles are relatively large, loosely packed and easily workable; they drain readily but are not able to hold nutrients very well. In a clay soil, fine particles predominate. They consist mainly of aluminium silicates arranged to form a layered crystal structure. Clay particles tend to aggregate together to form sticky clods, resulting in waterlogging and poor aeration; such a soil is said to be heavy. But clay soils are richer in nutrients, and their texture and drainage can be improved by adding both lime and humus — a dark, soft, moist material derived from leaf litter along with other decaying plant and animal remains and animal excrement.

Without humus soil cannot hold water or plant nutrients. Both humus and clay particles form colloids (i.e. states intermediate between suspensions and solutions), that adsorb dissolved nutrients. Humus improves sandy soils too, because its colloidal properties enable it to retain water.

A good soil will have an appropriate acid/alkali balance (pH6–6.5), the ideal being slightly acid for most plants (too much calcium can lock up other nutrients). Some plants, however, thrive in acid conditions, while some are lime-tolerant. Acidity in a soil is more likely to occur if the parent rock material from which it was derived has a low calcium content.

Plants require six major elements from the soil: nitrogen, phosphorus and potassium, and, in lower amounts, magnesium, calcium and sulphur. These and a range of essential trace elements are taken up in solution by the plant roots. Most of the nitrogen in the soil is in the form of decomposing organic matter, which must first be broken down to ammonium ions and then finally to nitrates by soil bacteria before it can become available to the plant. The work of earthworms is important here too. The worm digests matter in the soil, coating the material that passes through its body with a kind of gel. Worm castings not only improve the crumb structure of the soil, but also liberate chemicals that plants can use for nourishment. Some nitrogen compounds enter the soil with rain, after being formed in the air by lightning flashes; additional nitrogen compounds are synthesized by certain bacteria living in the soil. Good husbandry will conserve and replenish plant nutrients through proper composting and crop rotation.

An estimated 90 per cent of flowering plants, including grasses and trees, and also the conifers and ferns, increase the amount of nutrients they are able to access by means of an intimate relationship (symbiosis) with what are known as mycorrhizal fungi (myco = fungus, rhiza = root). The fungus is found inside the plant root system, but also spreads out its filaments (hyphae) from the root surface into the surrounding soil. Because these hyphae form a large network below ground, much wider than the plant roots can spread, they are able to increase the amount of soil nutrients available to the plant. In return, the fungus receives sugar synthesized by the plant. Mycorrhizal hyphae and bacteria also produce a gluelike substance that helps improve soil structure and soil nutrient retention by binding the soil particles and aggregates together.

The dissolved minerals taken up by roots of plants are carried upwards into stem, leaf and flower or fruit in the flow of the sap. In this way the mineral is released from its normal gravitational field and becomes vitalized. Rudolf Steiner spoke about crystal formation:

> The ability to crystallize manifests a higher formative force than is found in amorphous substances ... We shall also consider the actual formative forces within which the mineral appears as an expression of the world of substance which has developed over a vast period of time. What appears today as mineral substance is in fact an end product of the organic world ... just as coal originates from living plants, so too the mineral.[5]

In the same way the human organism must constantly transform or dissolve these crystalline substances and bring them into the stream of its life; only out of this ordered, dynamic, mineralized cellular fluid can it form its own crystals, as found in the skeleton, the teeth and the pineal gland. For this a specific degree of warmth is needed. Failure to do it in a healthy way can lead to the formation of stones or uric acid crystals. Though calcium has been known about for many years as the most abundant mineral in the human skeleton (see pp. 232–6 on silica and lime), knowledge of the activity of a trace mineral such as zinc is fairly recent. It reveals such subtle and almost magical properties that we are reminded of the alchemists' teachings. The other trace elements (micronutrients), required by plants as well as by the human body, include iron, boron, manganese, cobalt, copper, molybdenum.

Here is one example of the vital catalytic action of a micronutrient:

> During the one second that the blood is racing through the tiny capillaries of the lung, the single atom of zinc that is set in the centre of the enzyme carbonic anhydrase is brought into contact with 600,000 of its target molecules (carbonic acid). The result is that each is broken into one water and one carbon dioxide molecule. Only because of the rapidity of the enzyme's action can the carbon dioxide be freed fast enough from its compounds to leave the blood during that moment in the alveolus, when it is separated from the air by the thinnest of membranes. So our ability to rid ourselves of CO_2 is thus dependent on these critically located atoms of zinc![6]

Though the mineral in its resting form may be considered dead (as, for example, when it remains behind in plant or animal after fats, carbohydrates and proteins have been burnt off), as soon as it is incorporated into a life-system of a plant or animal it can initiate movement at vast speeds. Dr Schmidt explains: 'The mineral which has expelled warmth and life out of itself is not resting, it is in constant motion, directing processes between the earth and the cosmos [. . .] This is the power of the Phoenix, as it appears in mythology [. . .] Minerals thus provide the most extensive stimulation of the highest human activity, that of the ego-organization.'[7]

When we realize that the utilization of all substances and their effect on the organism is dependent upon the relationship of substances one to another – on the one hand of the minerals to each other and on the other hand on their relationship to the type and amount of primary nutrients – we will begin to realize that this living complexity is impossible to replicate under laboratory conditions. For example, nutritional calcium can only be utilized when in the right composition and in the right combination with other minerals, particularly sodium, potassium and magnesium.

In a healthy food plant these vital substances are embedded in a matrix of related substances and so they are perfectly organized to be accessible to the human digestion, in balance with nutrients that come in specific seasonal packaging. Consequently, 'To recommend the use of one isolated element of a complex family of protective compounds is a result of very materialistic and reductionist thinking.'[8]

All this leads us to ask the question again, why all these dietary supplements? Their use is often ridiculed by the medical profession, as shown by a typical *Daily Telegraph* headline (5 July 2002): 'Vitamin pills a waste of time and money, says study'. This study looked at the claims of cholesterol-lowering statins and a cocktail of vitamins C and E and beta carotene to reduce risk of heart disease, cancers and mental decline. Dr Jane Armitage of Oxford University said in *The Lancet*, 'This study found that they [the supplements] are a waste of money. People would be far better off spending the money on fresh fruit and vegetables!' And Paul Pitchford says: 'How well nutrients work when they are synthetically derived is questionable. Even "natural" vitamin supplements are usually more than 90% synthetic.'[9] These revelations lead us back to the related question: 'What about our farming practices?'

Independent research has shown that there has indeed been a declining mineral content in fruits, grains and vegetables over the past 50 years. Comparison of the mineral content of 20 fruits and 20 vegetables grown in the 1930s and 1980s shows several marked reductions in mineral content –

statistically significant reductions in the levels of calcium, magnesium, copper and potassium in vegetables, and magnesium, iron, copper, potassium in fruit. The only mineral that showed no significant difference over 50 years was phosphorus. Water content increased and dry matter decreased.[10]

To endorse these losses of nutrients, data from DEFRA (the Department of the Environment, Food and Rural Affairs) show that between 1940 and 1991 there was a 76 per cent fall in the trace mineral content of foods, this figure being supported by similar research carried out by USDA. The report also showed that organic produce has higher levels of certain plant chemicals – phenolics, terpenes, alkaloids and sulphur compounds, some of which are related to natural plant defence mechanisms. The possible nutritional value of these substances and the fact that they can be as much as 50 per cent higher in organic produce raises important questions for future investigation.[11]

Although DEFRA has recently brought out an 'Action Plan to Develop Organic Food and Farming in England' which on most issues rates organic farming as being better (a welcome development), it remains to be seen how quickly and practically it can be implemented, considering prevailing conditions and the fact that it takes 30 years for mycorrhizae to become completely reinstated in soils that have been badly overgrazed, tilled too much, or treated with fungicides.

The effects of chemical farming on food, its flavour and its nutritional value are added to by the effects of refining processes in the food industry. One example of this is that in the digestion of white bread chromium is required to assimilate the starches. Chromium is removed in the milling process, therefore the body has to supply it and will eventually become depleted. This is true for all refined foods. It is only recently that we have been exposed to these refining practices; previously our species had only used wholefoods. So we see from the example of chromium that when refined or synthetic substances are ingested the body is obliged to rob itself of nutrients to complete the incomplete products. It is quite simple, nature is extremely economic and efficient.

It is a logical deduction that the multitude of supermarket aisles devoted to spicy sauces, chutneys, pickles and relishes are a response to the fact that most foods today, vegetables or fruits, and especially pre-prepared foods, are dismally lacking in flavour, aroma and vitality.

Minerals also contribute to the colour of the plant, as well as its structure.

Most of us have had the experience of growing crystals from, say, a saturated solution of copper sulphate. You start with a crystal and suspend it in the solution and watch it grow; it will continue to grow only so far as the matrix of the particular crystalline substance allows. When we slice a carrot or a courgette the crystalline forms revealed correspond to the minute mineral trace elements that help the shaping forces of the plant (see below). When a vegetable lacks form and harmonious structure this points to certain deficiencies in mineral and fibrous content. The public are, unfortunately, now used to pale, sad fruits and vegetables that lack flavour and vibrancy.

Silica and lime

Rudolf Steiner spoke a great deal about the polarities of silica (silicon dioxide) and lime (calcium hydroxide), particularly in his agriculture lectures. They work together sculpting matter and have tremendous catalytic powers. According to Karl König[12] wherever silica is found, there is light and colour, working from without inwards from the periphery to the centre, gently forming layer after layer. Where we find lime/calcium there is movement, and the gesture is from within working outwards, hungrily radiating out and filling the silica layers with calcium, to form shell after shell. The dynamic relationship of the two forces is essentially that of circle and radius.

Silica (silicon dioxide) occurs in nature in crystalline forms, such as quartz. Waterglass — a viscous solution of sodium or potassium silicate in water — is a colloid. This is a labile state that can change for instance into the gelatinous condition of a hydrogel. Where we had solid silica particles in water we now have a liquid containing hollows in a solid mass of silica. Opals, for instance, are simply hardened silica jelly. Silica-gel is thus a structure made of 'skins' and internal energy.

All colloids are in this sense energy carriers. They have a maximum of reactive surfaces, always an essential factor in biological processes. As carrier of life, all the fluids in human, animal and plant are colloidal. (Aloe vera is a good example, also birds — the creatures closest to the silica process — whose feathers are composed of around 77% silica.)

Lime is a base — it gives a different picture, of dryness and aridity. Have you ever watched quicklime (calcium oxide) being changed to slaked lime (calcium hydroxide) by pouring water onto it, how it sucks up the water

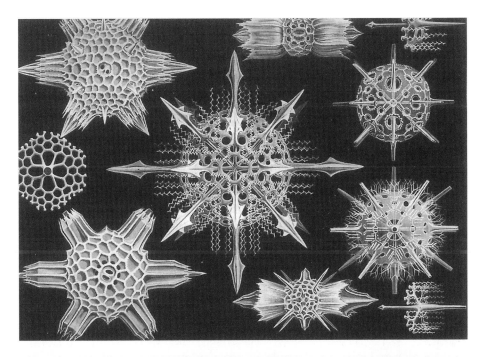

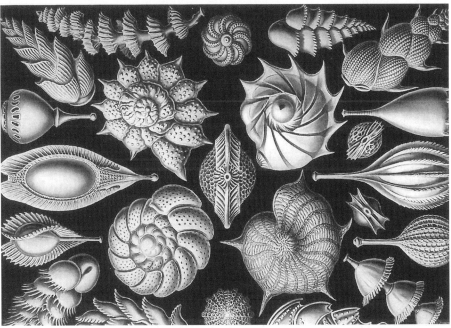

Radiolaria (above) and Foraminifera (below), drawings of microscopic marine protozoa from Ernst Haeckel's book Kunstformen. *They can be seen to demonstrate the 'gestures' of silica and lime*

with such ferocity, causing clouds of steam, heat and hissings? The mixture then takes more carbonic acid from the air and becomes hardened stone (calcium carbonate). Slaked lime plus sand is used as a mortar in building. Our skeleton is thus given stability and relationship to gravity, through this calcium/silica process, and our skin and organ sheaths are built out of a 'cosmic silica process' with its sphere-forming and light-reflecting properties. Although our skeleton is built out of calcium, the form into which it has been precipitated is created originally from this silica process. As the calcium hardens, the silica that has provided the strong structural lattice framework recedes.

In the plant families the cereals are particularly rich in silica, as are vegetables, in particular the carrot, and leafy greens and fruits. These elements, however, need to be in balance, otherwise there would be a tendency for plants either to be all fleshy like cacti (a preponderance of lime) or spindly climbing tendrils (a preponderance of silica).

Calcium/Lime: An example of the workings of a biodynamic preparation by Richard Smith, biodynamic farmer in South Devon

The greater diversity of the BD farm serves to hold a wide range of minerals in the life sphere of the farm as they are released from the breakdown of a variety of decaying plants and animal manures.

The abandoning of diversity and the use of artificial fertilizers in conventional systems has a detrimental effect on the life of the soil and particularly on the mycorrhizal fungi; this creates mineral deficiencies as well as increasing soil acidity. Earthworms disappear. To return the soil to a more balanced pH it becomes necessary to apply lime. Lime also has the effect of hastening the breakdown of humus in the soil, releasing accumulated fertility and causing a huge boost in yields.

There is a saying, however, that 'lime makes rich fathers but poor sons'. After 3–4 years acidity will have risen again and it will be necessary to apply lime once more; this time greater amounts are needed to maximize the contribution to the plants of the breakdown of residual humus. Over the years the amount of humus becomes less and since it also binds fine particles of soil as well as acting like a sponge for rainfall, the soil is now unstable and drought-susceptible. This is the case for well over half of the soils in this country which are in the initial stages of desertification. The plants now depend very much for growth and mineral content on what they are fed from a bag.

So it is that life becomes exhausted, mineral levels are reduced and deficiency diseases become common. Businesses have sprung up selling powdered mineral compounds for spreading on the land. But at this stage they need raising up into the 'life-process', being more akin to sub-soil that has not been worked through by worms and humus content.

On the biodynamic farm the emphasis is on feeding the life of the soil, building up humus levels, rather than exhausting their reserves. The soils thus become the environment for an abundance of earthworms which, possessing calcareous glands, bring calcium to the soil in an ideal condition to nourish the plant. Calcium in this form is far more effective than a normal pH assessment would indicate. We can now see a 'calcium process' at work. Levels rise and fall, becoming higher in the spring and autumn when soil temperatures are optimum.

The biodynamic preparations are particularly effective as catalysts that can trigger processes, raising substance into a more potent and permeable condition. So in one way this process is not dissimilar to the process of potentizing in homoeopathy – only a tiny amount of the preparation is needed to initiate a powerful response.[13] The basis for the calcium preparation comes from the bark of the oak tree. The oak 'surrounds' itself with calcium in its bark, comprising 70 per cent of its bark. This is grated off and rotted down in special conditions and tiny amounts (along with other preparations) are inserted into the compost heap so that wherever the compost is used the calcium process in the soil is strengthened. As I collect a bucket of powdered oak bark each autumn (which is enough to maintain the correct calcium condition of the soil on my 120-acre farm) I am truly grateful for the wisdom of this method. In the spring conventional farmers will have lime spread on their fields so that the land turns white. They pay in many ways for this service – the quarry and the contractors with specialist equipment, and by the further depletion of their land which may make their sons the poorer. In BD farming for the most part the farmer does not need to look far beyond the farm for the ingredients used in these preparations, all of which can be made and applied with the help of a few friends.

The acid/alkaline basis of human physiology

One of the most important mineral-based processes in human physiology is the acid/alkaline balance in human blood plasma. We have touched on this to a certain extent earlier in the chapter on salt. Equilibrium must be maintained and a fine balance kept, where the blood needs to be slightly alkaline to be a fit arena for the individuality – the ego – to work. (The astral quality has an acidic tendency.)

The margin of tolerance in a healthy acid/alkaline balance is indeed very slim, shown clearly in the following table of blood pH:

		NORMAL		
6	7	7.35 7.45	7.8 8	9
DEATH	ACIDOSIS		ALKALOSIS	DEATH

In the action of the alkali we are more passive and inward, remaining within ourselves; with acids we externalize ourselves, becoming active, even aggressive (active muscles form lactic acid).

The danger of acidosis is greater in our society than that of alkalosis. A diet rich in meat, dairy products, eggs, coffee, alcohol, sugar, nightshades and spices will tend towards the acidic. It is true that fruits are often acidic but they are neutralized by our digestion. Grains have a certain acidity but this is offset by the buffering effects of phytin (a compound common in many seeds, thought to store phosphorus). Acid foods can be counteracted by eating alkaline foods at the same meal, i.e. raw fruits and vegetables. And we should remember that we do need a certain amount of acidic foods, for example, lactic acid found in sauerkraut is beneficial to gut flora.

16

HERBS AND SPICES

Herbs and spices have been used for thousands of years – in ritual, in embalming the dead, in healing and in cooking. Since most spices could not be grown in the cooler climates, they were brought to the Mediterranean regions and then to the rest of Europe, for at least five thousand years, along the caravan routes passing through the Middle East. Their origins might be anywhere from China to southern Asia, Indonesia or Persia; Phoenicians, Arabs and Italians all grew rich in turn. Spices were particularly experimented with in the Middle Ages. The plant seeds, roots or bark all encapsulate dynamic digestible 'messages'.

The herbs, too, which are more gentle in their effects, point to their role as being somewhere between medicine and food. They were understood to be much more potent if found growing wild. Some of the most remarkable scholars in the Middle Ages were the herbalists whose tradition can be traced back through works of medieval Arab writers to the Greeks themselves. These healers, as well as being versed in botany and medicine, would also be experts in Latin, Greek, art, philosophy, literature and music. Dr Hauschka notes: 'Seasonings have come into increasing use the more that human development has enabled man to enter into full possession of his body and experience it in all its inner differentiation.'[1]

Spices and herbs, like salt have a special role, that of awakening sensibilities and heightening awareness both inwardly and outwardly. If used in enough quantity (as they surely were on many occasions) they can mask the evidence of putrefaction.

Everyone will have memories of tasting certain flavours for the first time. I can remember the first time I tasted fresh coriander (it had taken me over 40 years to find my way to this one). Every detail around the occasion is so vivid: the Vietnamese restaurant in Chartres, the waiter who had a wall eye, the wallpaper ... but the coriander! The merest sprinkling in a soup was so pungent, slightly soapy, really hard to describe in words. But now it is a favourite in my kitchen. This is what such seasonings can do, all the world enters into an alchemical fusion in our organs of smell and taste.

Flavouring our food is a very artistic activity, using herbs and spices as one would use notes in a symphony, letting them blend and converse. Often the secret of a chef lies in the subtle combination of very tiny amounts of herbs and spices individually almost unrecognizable if it has been done well. It is possible to choose from a range of around 85 common spices, 15 green and 10 dried herbs. In the ingenious combinations of certain of these flavourings we discover the character of any culture's cuisine. Eating a dish it is possible to travel to its country, in a manner of speaking, to that culture, to that very place. (In my Japanese cooking classes I was taught that orientals use combinations of herbs or spices in odd numbers, i.e., 3, 5 ,7, which is more dynamic than using even numbers, say 2, 4 or 6. I do believe there is a truth in this.)

The families of plants that produce these herbs and spices typify the capacities of 'salt-forming', 'oil-forming', 'mineralizing' and 'sublimating', all of which carry warmth characteristics. The oils of the plants arise as a result of a sun-ripening process, where etheric oils are released in aroma. This process has the most sublime and spiritual aspect, as the character of the plant is then released in a gaseous state.

There are seven areas of taste registered on the tongue.

Sweet – as in honey, sugars, ripe fruits, malt, beetroot and carrot
Oily – nuts, olives
Sour – capers, lemons, vinegar, lemon-grass, sorrel, unripe fruit
Sharp – pepper, chilli, horseradish, mustard, curry, pepper, garlic
Astringent (purifying) – parsley, marjoram, sage, thyme, basil, rosemary
Salty – salt, caraway, fennel, celery, lovage, summer savoury
Bitter – yarrow, chicory, wormwood, cinnamon, rue

To these we could also add as a taste 'metallic', which we can surely identify separately.

I will now describe a selection of herbs and then spices, the ones that I tend to use most. In some cases I have supplied the planetary and zodiacal influences from *Culpeper's Herbal*. The zodiac was held to govern the external anatomy of human beings, while the planets dominated the viscera, and the moon, as it affected tides, caused humoural fluids to increase and decrease.

Herbs

Basil (*Labiatae*)

'A herb of Mars — under Scorpio, giving it that little sharp undertone.'

Basil comes from Greek *basilikos* = royal. It originated in India where it is seldom used in cooking, but a version of it, *tulsi,* was considered so holy that Hindus would be prepared to swear an oath upon it. Many poems and stories speak of basil and its properties (famously, Keats's 'The Pot of Basil'). Old ladies in Majorca take a bunch with them when they stroll in the evening *paseo* to keep mosquitoes away.

Basil is warm and spicy with just that little surprising twist of sharpness; its fragrance is unique, penetrating and quickening the blood; it has a particular affinity with tomatoes. Tear the leaves off rather than cut them. Storage is best in olive oil in the form of pesto.

Bay (*Lauracae*)

'The Tree of the sun, under the celestial sign of Leo (a potent resistance to witchcraft).'

The bay is a small tree with tough laurel-like leaves, usually glossy. It is thought to come originally from Asia Minor but was soon well established around the Mediterranean. The crown of laurel leaves was the 'sun-symbol' of victory and glory in ancient Greece and Rome, worn by emperors and warriors. One of its properties was especially to keep away lightning. It has a strong, pungent and slightly bitter taste; it is used in a bouquet garni with thyme, sage and parsley. No kitchen should be without bay; its healing properties are more directed to the nervous system.

Chives (*Liliacae*)

'They are under the dominion of Mars, hot and dry. Prepared by the art of the alchemist they may be made into an excellent remedy for the stopping of excess urine.'

Chives are of the onion family. Again used extensively in the Middle Ages, they are more delicate than onion or spring onion. They have thin, hollow, grasslike stems and virtually no bulb. The flowers are a decorative pinkish-purple pom-pom, which can also be used discreetly in a salad. It is best to scissor the chives; they make a wonderful garnish for soups and salads.

Coriander (*Umbelliferae*)

Not in Culpeper. This annual herb grows wild throughout the Mediterranean area. It was introduced to China about AD 600, and is now cultivated all over the world, including Britain, but does best in warmer climates. In Exodus xvi.31 we read that when the Lord sent food to the Children of Israel, 'the house of Israel called the name thereof manna and it was like coriander seed, white, and the taste of it was like wafers made with honey'. Obviously coriander was highly appreciated.

The flavour of the fresh leaf is quite different to that of the dried seed. Green coriander was used in English kitchens during Elizabethan times but fell out of fashion. Now it is becoming popular again with the spread of Thai and Middle Eastern cooking and in curries. It adds a great deal to curry, both the seed and the green leaf. If you are using the green leaf it is best to add it towards the end of the cooking so that it retains its fresh flavour. The seed is better cooked into the food longer. Chilli, garlic, coriander and ginger ground together make a wonderful chutney. Coriander is also good in marinades for *à la greque* dishes.

Dill (*Umbelliferae*)

'Mercury has dominion over this plant and therefore to be sure, it strengthens the brain.'

Dill was important to the Greeks and Romans. Like fennel, dill has feathery leaves, seeds that are pungent because of their oils, and a rather aniseed-like flavour. Dill is used more in Scandinavia and Russia in pickled cucumber (both seed and the leafy herb). It goes well with sour cream in a cucumber salad, and is used in sauces with salmon. Dill water syrup is an old remedy for soothing digestive problems in babies.

Lovage (*Umbelliferae*)

'A herb of the Sun ... under the sign of Taurus.'

Lovage is one of the many herbs coming from the mountains of Persia and was used prodigiously by the Romans who called it 'the great *culinarius*'. The luxuriant foliage opens towards the sun in triangular serrated leaflets and grows up to seven foot tall. It has a lemony flavour, similar to celery, and is rich in mineral salts (as most herbs are). The seeds are also good in an infusion for the throat. Although somewhat neglected, it is definitely worth experimenting with. I use it in soups and have invented a nice butter bean and lovage pâté.

Marjoram, Origanum (*Labiatae*)

'It is the herb of Mercury and under Aries … excellent for the brain!'

Native to the Mediterranean, it has been cultivated as a flowering herb since ancient times. Growing about one to two foot high in 'knots' with small, bright green heart-shaped leaves, it is strongly aromatic. The flavour is in the same spectrum as thyme but sweeter. It is delicate, so better added towards the end of the cooking process. Use in all dishes as you would thyme. Can be grown in pots.

Mint (*Labiatae*)

'Herb of Venus. Drying, healing, soothing to the stomach.'

A refreshing summer herb, mint enjoys great popularity and has many varieties, is propagated by division of roots and likes a damp place. In English cooking it is often used in the cooking water for new potatoes (bringing needed warmth) and peas. Mint sauce with lamb dishes originated in Persia and the Middle East where a common drink is very sweet, strong mint tea. Varieties include: applemint, peppermint, spearmint, watermint, Eau de Cologne mint. Lovely in hummus and falafels.

Parsley (*Umbelliferae*)

'Under the dominion of Mercury.'

Parsley is a much loved and ubiquitous herb. It was used as a ceremonial herb in Greek and Roman temple rituals. Many dishes would not be the same without parsley, chopped finely and tenderly sprinkled on salads, vegetables and grain dishes. It stimulates kidney function, and helps excretion and circulation. Distilled parsley water is a familiar Culpeper remedy for wind. Parsley has always continued to be cultivated when other herbs have lost their popularity. There are several varieties. Flat-leafed parsley is more often found in the Mediterranean and Middle East; the curly variety is more familiar here in Britain. As it is a biennial it is best always to make new sowings for the following season.

Rosemary (*Labiatae*)

'The Sun claims privilege in it and it is under the celestial Sun.'

A native of the Mediterranean region and Asia Minor, rosemary is an ever-green shrub with grey-green, needle-shaped leaves and pale blue, typical labiate flowers. A beautiful astringent aroma permeates the whole plant. The stalks are cuboid in this family, signifying their earthy capacity to transform mineral salts. The flowers have the appearance of giving themselves out into the atmosphere. Rosemary can be seen as a portal to the morning; a bath or shower with rosemary essence will refresh and awaken, whereas its sister lavender is more soothing and calming and can ensure a restful sleep. Rosemary is wonderful for flavouring soups and stews and good with roasted vegetables. Carrots cooked with rosemary and honey make a dish fit for a king. Rosemary enhances both lamb and fish. It will lighten heaviness and aid digestion.

Sage (*Labiatae*)

'Jupiter, planet of wisdom, claims this herb.'

Garden sage is also a native of the north Mediterranean coasts – it grows wild in Greece, Yugoslavia and Provence. It prefers well-drained soils. The flavour is a little reminiscent of camphor. Bees love the purplish-blue flowers and produce a renowned rich honey. Italians particularly love sage which they use with meat and pasta. We use it in stuffings such as sage and onion and in nut roasts; it is good with both pulses and lentils. Sage is good for the health of the liver and the blood. In a drink with lemon and honey it heals sore throats. In the medical school of Salerno sage was regarded as the 'reconciler' of man and nature, and the Arabs had a saying, 'How can a man die when he has sage in his garden?' (Maria Geuter) The flowers can be scattered in salads for beauty and for medicine, but only a few, as they are pungent!

Sorrel (*Polygonacae*)

'Under the dominion of Venus.'

Garden sorrel and herb patience are both derived from common wild sorrels. The Egyptians and Romans used sorrel to offset the richness of their food. It has a refreshing lemony, sour taste. Chop it only with a stainless steel knife as it is high in oxalic acid and would be stained by a carbon steel knife. Sorrel needs little cooking. It is excellent in a purée for sorrel soup, thickened with spring onion and potatoes, and goes well with a dish of Le Puy lentils. It is also excellent with watercress in a green mayonnaise to accompany salmon, or on an egg salad with asparagus.

Tarragon (*Compositae*)

'Dedicated to Artemisia, goddess of nature.'

Really one of the great culinary herbs and related to wormwood and mugwort. It will become shrubby in the right situation. Tarragon has a unique, slightly bitter flavour that goes well with eggs, fish and salads of tomato, cucumber, chicory or beetroot. Tarragon vinegar is essential for sauce Béarnaise and can be made by filling a bottle with fresh leaves (before flowering) and filling it with white wine vinegar. Decant after two months.

> Plants create most of our reality and many of our dreams. They are a source of our nourishment and health, pleasures and ecstasies; they sustain religions, cultures, civilizations. In the end they can kill us (as the hemlock did with Socrates) and return us to the soil upon which they themselves feed.[2]

Spices

Cardamon (*Zingiberaceae*)

A perennial of the ginger family originating in India, and is said to have been grown in the royal gardens of Babylon. It has a strong, cool flavour, perhaps faintly reminiscent of eucalyptus. The seed pods, unusually, grow from the base of the plant at ground level. The small pale green pods are triangular in section, and can vary in quality; the seeds should be somewhat sticky when the outer covering is peeled back. The Arabs often put a cardamon pod into the spouts of their coffee pots to perfume the coffee.

Cardamon is used in curries, pilaus, sweet desserts like custard or rice puddings, and mulled wine. The Swedes use a quarter of the Indian harvest, and amongst other things use it in their pickled herrings. The fibrous pods need to be cracked to release the tiny black seeds, which contain all the flavour. A few whole cardamon pods slipped into a pot of brown rice for the cooking time will add a delicious fragrance.

Cayenne, chilli powder (*Solanaceae*)

'Red' or 'Cayenne' pepper is made from the powdered dried fruits of several varieties of capsicum that have been developed to be especially hot and pungent. They are a digestive stimulant and antiseptic when eaten in moderation but can cause blistering to mouth, throat and tongue if used in excess. People who eat chilli regularly can become desensitized to the heat factor which is sometimes used to disguise putrefaction, but they can also become desensitized to other subtleties in their food. This can arise when young children eat overly spiced food when it is not part of their culture.

The best chilli powder is home-ground. The dried chillies are first lightly roasted, then ground in a pestle and mortar or electric grinder. The seeds are usually the hottest part, so remove them if you want less heat. Chilli is much used in Indian, Indonesian and African cuisine, and in Mexican dishes like chilli con carne.

Cinnamon and Cassia (*Lauraceae*)

Cinnamon and cassia trees are closely related. Their dried inner bark has been amongst the oldest and most valued spices. The use of cassia is recorded in China from 2500 BC and in Egypt in 1600 BC. Cinnamon has a more delicate flavour and is more expensive than cassia. The quills of dried bark can be used to flavour puddings, sauces and mulled punches. Ground cinnamon (again, best if freshly ground) is used in cakes, buns, and puddings, and in Indian curries. It is one of the ingredients in the Chinese 'five spice' seasoning. Cinnamon has a warming, expansive effect which particularly enhances sweet dishes, as do cardamon, nutmeg, coriander and ginger.

Cloves (*Myrtaceae*)

Cloves are the dried pink flower buds of a tropical evergreen tree originally from the Moluccas but now widely grown in Zanzibar, Madagascar and the West Indies. The trees flourish best near the coast. The essential oil is a powerful antiseptic as we may recognize from our visits to the dentist where it is used as the basis for a powerful mouthwash. The oil is also numbing and used on the gums for toothache as a home cure. So we have to be delicate when we are using cloves in cooking because the smallest amount can be overpowering. An onion stuck with six or so cloves is essential in making a good bread sauce; an apple stuck with cloves likewise spices a dish of red cabbage. Used like this they can be taken out when the flavour is strong enough. Whole cloves, which should be plump and well formed, conserve their flavour better than the ground powder. But cloves are difficult to grind at home, so try to find a good organic source of ground cloves if you need powder for baking.

Coriander (*Umbelliferae*)
A slender annual plant native to southern Europe and the Middle East. The seeds are small, pale and slightly oval and the flavour is quite distinct from the leaf, being more sweet, mild and aromatic, especially when roasted. In England it has been used for centuries as a pickling spice, but it is used in large quantities in Indian, Malaysian and Indonesian cooking in both curries and sweet dishes. It is also used in a marinade for meat, fish and vegetable *à la grecque* dishes.

Cumin (*Umbelliferae*)
An annual and native of the Mediterranean region, but cultivated also in Asia. Cumin seeds were used by the Romans as a substitute for pepper. Medicinally cumin was said to encourage a pale skin. Its unique and pungent flavour makes it very popular in the cooking of North Africa and the Middle East, and it is also an ingredient in Indian curries, Mexican dishes and certain marinades.

Ginger (*Zingiberaceae*)
A native of tropical South East Asia, but widely grown in other tropical areas, such as Jamaica. The plant has beautiful golden yellow flowers with a purple lip and fat rhizomes – the part that has been sought after for millennia. Used originally in China and India, it was one of the first spices to reach Europe, where it became used not only as a flavouring but as a medicine in many

circumstances. It was used as an antidote for the Black Death, for it induces sweating to cleanse the body. Ginger applied as a poultice has a tremendous healing capacity where heat is needed in the body.

Fresh ginger is milder than dried ginger. Fine slices pickled in brine or rice vinegar are used in Japanese sushi. Stem ginger crystallized in syrup was a sweetmeat for the Chinese. In Europe, it appears in many dishes, mostly sweet, such as gingerbread or biscuits, in parkin, ginger creams and puddings. It also appears in drinks such as ginger beer and ginger wine. Ginger is often served powdered as a table condiment, to enliven slices of melon or peaches.

Mustard (*Cruciferae*)

Mustard was used by the ancient Greeks and Romans, and is mentioned on several occasions in the Bible. There are two basic types of mustard seed, brown (from *Brassica nigra*) and white (*B. alba*). Mustard came to be particularly developed in Dijon, southern France, where the mustard makers were given the exclusive right to make mustard with an *appellation controlée*. Today Dijon is still a great mustard-making area supplying half the world's mustard.

English mustard was made famous in the early nineteenth century by Jeremiah Colman, a young miller from Norwich. A mixture of white and brown mustard seed was ground finely, then sifted through fine cloth and mixed with a little wheat flour as an improver. It was sold as a dry powder and made freshly as required. The real pungency of the crushed mustard seed only emerges when its essential oils are mixed with water – the flavour takes a few minutes to develop.

Mustard was traditionally served with meats to help digestion and cut the fat, and in mayonnaise it helps as a stabilizer. Used carefully in bland dishes like cauliflower cheese, Welsh rarebit, sauces and salad dressings, it brings a sharpness and piquancy. Mustard seeds are used whole in pickling spices and in Indian curries (mustard seed oil is also used).

Mustard poultices and foot-baths are ancient remedies for colds, fevers and sciatica. It is clearly very warming, pungent, stimulating and has diuretic properties. Traditionally mustard is also used to strengthen digestion and loosen stools.

Mace and nutmeg (*Myristicaceae*)

Mace and nutmeg are products from the same large tropical evergreen tree, a native of the Molucca Islands but grown in other tropical countries from the eighteenth century onwards. The nutmeg is the seed and mace the bright red outer casing. These spices when dried and therefore transportable became popular in Europe after the Portuguese discovered the Spice Islands.

Nutmeg is both a stimulant and a carminative (for colic and flatulence). Some claim it has aphrodisiac properties. It goes particularly well with cheese and milk dishes, both sweet and savoury, and makes a very good addition to onion sauce. It also complements spinach (the Italians are particularly fond of this combination). We are familiar with it in cakes and hot mulled punches.

Pepper (*Piperaceae*)

Peppercorns grow on a climbing vine which grows in South East Asia. Pepper used to be so precious it was used for barter, for ransom and for gifts. Although previously rare and expensive, it is worth noting how pepper is now used as an ingredient in most cultures and will appear with any airline meal alongside the salt.

The alkaloid piperine found in pepper is a stimulant to saliva and gastric enzymes. The typical pungent quality is due to a resinous compound that is somewhat volatile, so it makes more sense to add freshly ground pepper at the end of the cooking to maintain its bouquet.

For black peppercorns, the berries are picked when they are green and unripe and then dried in the sun, when the outer skin becomes black and wrinkled. For white pepper, the berries are picked when they have ripened, when they are red in colour. They are then soaked to get rid of the husk and the inner seed is then dried and ground to powder. Many peppercorns are roasted these days, which tends to make their action more of an irritant, so do try to seek out a good quality product. Pepper used judiciously has a warming effect and counteracts food poisoning.

Saffron (*Iridaceae*)

One of the most rare and expensive spices, saffron comes from a crocus flower native to Europe and Asia, and was used by the ancient Persians, the Phoenicians, the Greeks and Romans. It is derived from the stamens which have to be hand-picked, hence the costliness. Saffron became very popular in medieval times, and made the Essex town of Saffron Walden famous. The growers were known as 'crokers'. Culpeper called it 'a herb of the sun –

refreshing the spirits and good against fainting fits and palpitations of the heart'.

The essential oils in saffron give it a warming effect with a slight undercurrent of bitterness. As well as a unique flavour, saffron imparts to certain dishes a beautiful golden hue, e.g. the traditional Cornish saffron cakes. Saffron is an important ingredient in bouillabaisse, a classic French fish soup, in Spanish paella and *arroz brut*, and in an Indian saffron coloured rice pudding with cardamon and pistachios, sweetened with honey.

It is best to buy saffron in threads and to infuse them in hot liquid to disperse the colour and flavour before using.

Vanilla (*Orchidaceae*)

The vanilla pod is the fruit of a climbing orchid, a native of the humid forests of Central America. The golden flowers are followed by flat pods which only develop the characteristic vanilla flavour through a curing process, changing the flavour through a chemical-enzymatic process, a kind of sweating carried out in airtight boxes. The perfume of genuine vanilla is sweet and penetrating; note that there is no substitute for the real vanilla pod. The pods are expensive and so they should be. But it is possible to slice a pod down the middle, use it to perfume custards or puddings, then after rinsing dry it and reuse it several times. At the end of its life it can be tucked into the sugar jar and used on that special occasion to make vanilla ice cream. (Montezuma chocolate is flavoured with real vanilla.)

Garlic (*Alliaceae*)

Though perhaps neither herb nor spice, garlic is in its own class as a flavouring agent, so we must include it.

Garlic is believed to have originated from a plant that grows wild in central Asia. It was used abundantly by the ancient Egyptians in many differing ways. Garlands of garlic were hung around the necks of their children to drive out worms. The workmen engaged in the building of the pyramids were given generous daily rations of garlic by the Pharoah Cheops for strength and protection from any plagues. Though the ancient Greeks and Romans used garlic liberally, it was forbidden to the acolytes of the temples of Cybele as it stimulates, excites and taints the breath. Until quite recently, farmers in Sweden used to fasten a garlic clove around the necks of cattle and horses to protect them against trolls.

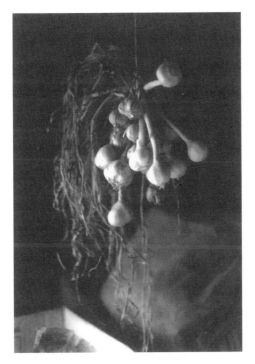

Garlic

Garlic contains antiseptic substances and also sulphur compounds that make it warming and tone up the digestive process. It is known to reduce blood pressure and reduces the risk of heart disease by clearing cholesterol deposits. Garlic also helps clear bronchitis, and is good for colds. (Garlic, cayenne and ginger in a soup is wonderful for colds.)

Raw and cooked garlic have quite different flavours and properties. It is possible to roast any amount of garlic cloves (in their skins, or whole cloves sliced through the 'equator') in olive oil, with root vegetables or squash. Their flavour is sweet and mild and you can eat a lot. But half a teaspoonful of finely chopped *raw* garlic can be enough to flavour the salad dressing for eight servings. So again, caution with raw garlic, but be generous in certain cooked dishes.

Horseradish (*Cruciferae*)

Since this root has been used for over 2000 years I thought it worth including. It can be a very helpful appetite stimulant, finely grated with cream and apple. It has the same essential oils as mustard, is extremely hot and pungent, but being a root has some mineral content too. A little in a beetroot salad can give a special twist.

Flowers in cooking

The following flowers are edible and can be used in salads, desserts, and as garnishes. They are colourful and add the 'blossom element': borage, marigold, rosemary, lavender, cowslip, nasturtium, camomile, mallow, chives, origano, viola, day lily, sage, rose petals, sweet woodruff, sweet cicely, primrose, elderflower.

Medieval herbalists saw food as medicine; daily dishes would then contain many of the herbs, spices and flowers that I have listed. Today we know that these plants have complex combinations of ingredients, including important phyto-chemicals that cannot be synthesized.

Herbs are choosy about the conditions in which they like to grow and, as herbalists know, the wild varieties tend to have more potency. However, I encourage you to experiment and see what these wonderful gifts of nature can bring to your cooking and to your health.

17

STIMULANTS: COFFEE, TEA AND CHOCOLATE

Too much tea drinking turns noses red, but that is not the reason why Mormons and others ban the leaf. It is rather because tea, like coffee, stimulates the mind, trespassing, however softly, on that inner part of man which is seen as his private, inalienable core. What some people prohibit, however, most others enjoy as a mild fillip in the day's routine, drinking ... without obvious decline some hundred thousand cups of one or the other beverage in a lifetime. Certainly these and other plant-based drinks have a hold on us, a hold which has had its effect on history.

Brendan Lehane in The Power of Plants[1]

Coffee, tea and chocolate were the last of the new discoveries brought in to stimulate and excite the European (and later the North American) palate in the 300 years after the voyages of Christopher Columbus and Vasco Da Gama. Let us look more closely at their history and their effects.

Coffee

Coffee appears to have originated in Kenya or Ethiopia. But how its growth and use spread to become the favourite drink of the Near East is still something of a mystery. An ancient legend tells of an Abyssinian goatherd called Kaldi who noticed that his goats became very frisky after eating from the coffee plant. He decided to experiment and discovered one of the properties many of us are now familiar with – a seemingly enhanced mental acuity. The use of the plant spread and by the fifteenth century the people of Constantinople would honour their guests with a drink called *coffa*, brewed from a blackish seed and served hot and sweet. The drink prevented those who partook of it from feeling drowsy, according to Pietro della Valle.[2]

Avicenna, the fifteenth-century Arab philosopher, termed it 'the wine of Islam'. Bedouins poured only enough for four sips at a time. To fill up a cup would mean to the guest 'Drink now and depart!' Such was its growing popularity that religious and political authorities attempted various purges. In 1553 coffee houses were closed down in Cairo, whereas by the mid-sixteenth century they had become popular in England. However, in 1675 Charles II closed 3000 of them in England as 'seminaries of sedition', but was forced to rescind his edict within only a few days as a result of public pressure. In 1690 the Dutch introduced coffee into Java, thus founding the basis of the East India coffee trade.

The introduction of coffee, tea and cocoa shops in Europe furnished an alternative to the bawdy alehouses, and they were considered more genteel. The only problem was that these drinks were often bitter and crude and needed sugar to make them more palatable – another factor that increased the sugar trade.

Whilst there are around one hundred species of coffee tree the two most widely cultivated are *Coffea arabica* and *Coffea canephora*. They have shiny evergreen leaves and are pruned to stay within the reach of pickers. White, perfumed flowers are followed by berries ripening from green to yellow to red. At present Brazil and Columbia are the greatest coffee producers. America and Germany are the largest consumers, the USA importing over one million metric tons per annum (one-third of the coffee grown in the world).[3]

Coffea canephora, known as 'robusta', is largely produced in Africa, India, Latin America and Indonesia. This species is cultivated because of its hardiness, disease resistance and rapid growth. It has a higher yield and twice as much caffeine as the *arabicas,* but the flavour and aroma are inferior to the arabicas. It is therefore usually blended with arabicas in an attempt to improve the flavour but impart the maximum caffeine 'thrust'.

Raw coffee beans are quite tasteless; the roasting imparts the flavour and aroma. Coffee is very complex in its effective total composition.[4] Through the science of gas chromatography over 300 aromatic substances have been identified and many more remain unidentified.

Caffeine

Caffeine is the principal active substance that has made coffee so desirable. It is an odourless, slightly bitter tasting alkaloid (i.e. mildly poisonous) found naturally in several plants, with the highest content in coffee. It dissolves readily in water or alcohol and has crystals 'that look like needles'.

The main site of activity of caffeine is the brain and the central nervous system: 'Caffeine stimulates the functions of the cerebral cortex, which is responsible for the smooth-running occurrences of certain mental processes ... Experiments demonstrate that it facilitates the transmission of impulses across synapses, which in turn explains the facilitation of thought connections; it also facilitates the impression of numbers.'[5]

The alkaloid caffeine overrides brain receptors designed for adenosine, a natural sedative that informs the body when to slow down. This allows the person to experience artificially an enhanced degree of mental alertness, even when they are in fact experiencing fatigue. This capacity to override normal body signals makes coffee potentially addictive and thus a danger to health when its use is abused. As well as causing an increase in heart and pulse activity, caffeine can inhibit the absorption of both calcium and iron. When taken in excess it can cause many adverse symptoms, manifesting as irritability and nervousness, hyperactivity and digestive problems, to name but a few.

Taken in moderation and when its quality is good (organically grown and preferably fairly traded), it is unlikely to cause major health problems for most adults. Rudolf Steiner spoke of coffee as being 'the drink of the journalist or the person of letters'. He described the action of coffee on the subtle bodies of the human being thus:

> The effect of coffee on the human organism is to lift the etheric body slightly out of the physical body, but in such a way that the physical body is experienced as a solid foundation for the etheric body ... because logical, consistent thinking arises from the structure and form of the physical body, the characteristic effect of coffee emphasizes the physical structure and physically promotes a logical consistency of thought ... thus it seems quite natural that the professional writer who cannot quite find the logical sequence in his writing would turn to coffee for stimulation.[6]

He did however point out that anything that we use as a crutch to enhance our consciousness was likely to be ultimately weakening to our capacities to develop our own focused and concentrated powers of thinking.

But the problem with coffee drinking, as with any addictive substances, is the tendency to need more and more in order to continue getting the same effect that was initially experienced. Thus the habit may gradually grow without a person being aware that they may have a problem. (See under Addiction, p. 257).

A cup of espresso coffee may contain as much as 300 mg of caffeine, whereas a cup of instant coffee contains 75 mg. When sugar is added to this and a cigarette smoked as an accompaniment on a regular basis, the body chemistry starts to change, challenging its capacity to maintain a healthy acid/alkaline balance.

Decaffeinated coffee can be an alternative but we should be aware that the decaffeination process is usually done using such solvents as methylene chloride, which may leave residues. The decaffeinated coffees that have been produced through a water method are less abrasive. (A sad little story but a telling one: house spiders given caffeine were shown to be incapable of spinning an orderly web.[7])

Tea

The most famous legend surrounding tea tells how a Chinese Buddhist had become quite tired during a nine-year meditation and had fallen asleep. When he awoke with shame and was filled with guilt for his lack of concentration he proceeded to cut off his eyelids to assure an end to such sinful behaviour. These severed eyelids fell upon the ground and sprouted as the tea plant *Camellia sinensis*, an evergreen shrub native to south and east Asia, producing a drink that is refreshing and stimulating and also contains caffeine. Tea had been popular in China since the T'ang period (tenth century); it was considered medicinal and to enhance longevity. However, tea may have come to Europe from Japan.

The first public tea sale in England was in 1657 and three years later Samuel Pepys wrote about his 'first cup of tee'. By the nineteenth century, with the opening up of the trans-Siberian railway, Russia became one of the greatest nations of tea drinkers with the famous *samovar* in its bain-marie continually steeping away. In the USA the famous Boston Tea Party happened in 1773, the incident that led to the American War of Independence. However, London still remains the tea capital of the world, and though habits are changing with younger people, still an average of five cups per person are drunk in Britain daily.

Tea was originally used in Burma as a vegetable relish, served as a pickle. Certain Mongolian tribes add a pinch of salt to their tea, and Tibetans stir in some yak butter. Elaborate tea ceremonies are traditionally practised in China and Japan, requiring lengthy training. Taoists include it in their elixir of immortality. Although tea by weight contains almost twice as much caffeine as coffee, this is more diluted in the drinking. One pound of coffee yields 40 cups, whereas one pound of tea can yield 250–300 cups.

Tea does not contain the same sorts of harmful oils and acids which all coffee contains, decaffeinated or not, and tea has not been subjugated to the same kind of caffeine manipulation that the robusta coffee has. However the alkaloid theophylline, a diuretic found in tea, takes longer to metabolize than the caffeine in coffee, which tends to be excreted more readily. Tea also contains tannins (used in leather tanning) and oils that are important for their aroma. In 1684, M. Dufour commented: 'One of the most important advantages of tea is that it has a sobering effect on drunks. It also purifies the brain. The Chinese who drink so much tea never spit or blow their noses, their brains are free of all excesses!'[8]

Despite the caffeine content, the action of tea on the human being is different to that of coffee. Rudolf Steiner posited: 'Though they both share the relative effects of loosening from the physical body, tea presses the liberated thinking into the fantastic, the unsolid, the fluctuating.'[9] He characterized tea as 'the drink of diplomats, who need to be witty, scintillating and sometimes superficial'.

Finally, we must not forget what the Chinese knew and passed on to the Japanese, that the finesse of tea was to be decided not only by the tea itself but, equally importantly, the quality of the water with which it is made, preferably from a pure spring or fast flowing stream.

Cocoa

The cocoa tree was cultivated by the Mayans and the Aztecs. The Mexicans and Peruvians, as well as using cocoa as a beverage and in their cooking, used it as currency. The Spaniards reported that the Aztec emperor Montezuma would drink no other drink than chocolate and then only served in ceremonial golden goblets. The offering of chocolate signified 'Welcome!'

Today in our culture chocolate is to be found everywhere – in newsagents, supermarkets, cinemas and petrol stations. British consumers spend around £3 billion on chocolate, mostly bought by women and children, and usually as a very different product from the one favoured by the Emperor Montezuma. It is increasingly used as a tempting coating on confectionery and ice-cream.

Chocolate bars may by law contain as little as 20 per cent cocoa solids, and may be packed out with cheap palm oil, sugar, colourants, antioxidants and emulsifiers. In a few years' time they may well contain cocoa butter that was not harvested from trees but was genetically engineered in a laboratory.

What is it that makes people chocoholics? Unlike tea and coffee, real chocolate does have some nutritional value in that the roasted bean contains 50% fat, 25% carbohydrates, 15% proteins and 1.5% theobromine, a stimulant related to caffeine. Another substance, anandamide, is thought to intensify the sensory properties of chocolate, encouraging a sense of well-being that fleetingly mimics the feeling of being in love. Pure chocolate literally melts in the mouth at body temperature, providing a pleasant sensation, so its texture as well proves seductive.

Chocolate taken as a drink was mentioned briefly by Rudolf Steiner as the celebratory beverage of comfortable German bourgeoisie for weddings and christenings, and possibly encouraging 'philistinism'. In Steiner's times chocolate abuse and the degradation of the product was hardly possible – it was still a treat. Now through advertising, promotion and availability it is largely bought on impulse. In our society £92 million in a year is spent on advertising chocolate, frequently employing sensual and sexual motifs, and often personified by slender models. The shiny foil packaging (usually made of aluminium) adds to this provocative image, but the sad fact is that chocolate is the number one binge item, particularly for people with eating disorders.

Behind the glamorous advertisements lies a much less publicized aspect of all of these products – vast plantations of monoculture for luxury goods, using the labour of women whose daily wages often amount to no more than £3, certainly not enough to buy the chocolate they harvest for export to the North. Usually these crops are heavily sprayed with 32 pesticides, some of which are on the Dirty Dozen list.[10] Added to this, we need to consider the land being used. More tropical forests in Brazil, Indonesia and Malaysia are being cleared to grow crops such as cocoa. Can we really justify the exploitation of land and people to supply non-essential luxury items for our society?

Addiction

Caffeine addiction is increased by the production of cola drinks, consumed in vast quantities by the most vulnerable sector of our society – our children and young people, and containing caffeine often extracted from robusta coffee. We are an addictive society and perhaps need to ask ourselves whether some of the addictions start with such seemingly innocuous substances. It is not my brief to go further into the question of addictions – a growing problem – but I will leave us with some more words from Brendan Lehane:

> There is more. Some plant stimulants burnish the emotions, giving joy, merriment, wonder and nostalgia a greater intensity. Some appear to quicken the wits, or sharpen desire, or enhance sensual pleasure. Some bring drowsy forgetfulness, sleep, visions. In a field of opium poppies lie a million dreams, and as many perceptions of another world.
>
> These amiable charms hide a harsher core. When plants insinuate their enchantments into the human mind, they secure their advance with steel batons. Pleasure is replaced by chains, obsessions, an enslavement which the years strengthen. At times it is no longer bearable, and then it kills. Many plants bring mundane blessings. A few go further. They seem to offer a glimpse of paradise. But we have enough tormented testimony to know that a mirage of heaven may curtain the gateway to hell.[11]

18

WATER

I am convinced that one of the gateways to consciousness is the micro-structure of water. Water is a very abundant and mysterious liquid ... the most researched and the least understood substance on the planet.

Alan Hall, founder of the Live Water Trust

Water is essentially the element of life, wherever possible it wrests life from death. It is the great healer of all that is sick and has lost its living poise ... bringing together elements that are hostile to one another, constantly creating something new out of them. In itself water remains chemically neutral but it does unite with other substances where the solid element is too much in opposition to life.

Theodor Schwenk

(Both cited in *Living Lightly*, Issue 17)

We all surely know how important water is in our lives and our nutrition; it is also the medium through which the etheric works. The sale of bottled water increases, and no wonder when we are told that in London the tap water has been through at least 13 people's organisms before it gets to yours! Then there is the extremely doubtful practice of adding fluorine – a by-product of aluminium production – to domestic supplies against mounting evidence of harm.

Great rivers are dammed to provide electricity, their banks are straightened, industrial and human wastes have been dumped into our rivers and our seas. All these practices show a lack of understanding of water's intrinsic nature and the extent to which everything in nature depends upon it. It is known that the human body is mainly composed of fluids.

Dr Gerhard Schmidt points out: 'All bodily fluids are mineral water, related to the mineral springs of the earth, or can be seen as the human being's "inner sea". These fluids are instrumental in allowing us to live in opposition to gravity, helping us to achieve a kind of buoyancy (particularly our brain in its surrounding fluid).'[1]

Biologists are now shifting their view of cells away from being no more than a membranous bag containing water with enzymes, other macro-molecules and ions in a free solution. Cells are now regarded as containing a 'structured water' matrix that holds enzyme systems and other macro-molecules in complexes with sodium and potassium ions. An important conclusion from this research is that the more 'structured' water there is in the system the better the enzyme systems function and the more readily the beneficial nutrients with their life forces are assimilated.[2] In general we will find more 'structured' or 'dynamized' water in biological systems than, say, tap water. For instance fruits and vegetables, particularly those grown bio-dynamically or organically, will contain a high proportion of this type of water, bearing valuable solutions of plant sugars and micronutrients.

PART FOUR

19

COOKING AND MENU-PLANNING

Just as there's no human society that doesn't have a spoken language, there's no human society which doesn't cook in some way. Like language, cooking is a prerequisite of culture; and the key feature of cooking is *its transformation of raw materials by fire*. Fire is the agent by which nature (raw food) is transformed into culture (cooked food) [my italics].[1]

That great systematizer Aristotle saw cooking as the continuation of a natural sun-ripening process — heat influencing matter, perfecting and maturing it. He called the process *pepsis,* which involves a softening, a kind of 'predigestion' through cooking. His view, which has survived for over 2000 years, had an important influence on alchemists who thought precious metals were incubated in the earth's belly by the sun's heat. So by using fire and crucible, the alchemists were always attempting to reproduce those conditions.

Significantly the alchemists also describe their art as 'cooking'. But the kind of cooking I wish to speak about is a little more social than the alchemist's lonely enterprise. Nevertheless every time we create in our kitchens we are engaging in that original alchemy which later became the basis of the study of chemistry and physics. We are also entering into a kind of Genesis situation where substances are prepared, then they interact and transform each other through the agency of heat in a creative process. What actually happens in the intricate energetic relationships of cells when cut up and combined with other substances in this cooking is still a mystery. Our reductionist thinking cannot grasp the matter by a description of actions of proteins, starches and fats. It is beyond analysis, because though cooking is certainly a science and a craft, it is also an art where the inspiration, imagination and knowledge of the cook give an immeasurable input. Then, when we have created, we have to give away the results of our efforts and this is the very social nature of cooking.

I have always loved cooking, graduating from the early age of mud pies garnished with cowslips to ambitious banquets. I have been endlessly fascinated by every aspect of cooking, from the growing of food to the eating of it – even the washing up doesn't put me off! But it seems that not everyone shares this love. In the West we seem to be more concerned with results than process, so it is little wonder that many women, and possibly men, see only a pile of washing up as the result of a two or more hours' cooking session (the food having taken a matter of minutes to eat) rather than the enjoyment of the process. This is surely why convenience foods have such an appeal?

That the business of eating has been relegated to simply 'refuelling the machine' and meal-times are a 'pit-stop' pause, something to be got through as quickly as possible, has led to the kind of rushed eating called 'grabbing a bite', 'eating on the hoof' or 'grazing'. I am convinced that these practices (and I am aware that there are many people who do not live like this) are responsible for certain deteriorating social problems.

Until recently the family meal has been the cornerstone of community building, and I am glad to see that it still is in many cultures, particularly Third World countries where there has been little opportunity for them to become blasé about food. The act of eating together can bring such a wonderful feeling of being nurtured, of gratitude for the gifts of the earth skilfully combined to bring 'companionship' (from the Latin *cum panis*, with bread). So in breaking bread together we become companions. The meal table is also where many social skills can be learned – the skills of conversation, how to look after each other's needs and to welcome guest and stranger. In Eastern traditions it was a time to honour the gods; the central portion of the rice pot would be placed on the shrine for the family deities. The kitchen would be next to the meditation room, and the wisest person was entrusted with the cooking and therefore the health of the household.

In Victorian and Edwardian households the kitchen seems to have been banished to below stairs, an unseen realm of chopping, boiling, roasting, and polishing – somewhat like our metabolic processes, warm, dark and unconscious. Occasionally the children of the house would secretly find their way into this enchanted and magical world and have it change their lives, but more often than not they were confined to the nursery floor – all the important activities in the house of the bourgeoisie were firmly segregated.

Perhaps the aftermath of a seemingly joyless attitude to cooking and even eating, in terms of restrictive social interactions, has contributed to the situation that we see today. However, one might be encouraged to think that Britain had become entranced with the art of cooking in recent times, judging by the number of cooking programmes that have sprung up on the television. Upon enquiry, I am led to believe that many people watch them whilst eating their microwaved pre-prepared meal, having a vicarious experience. Let us hope there are others who are experimenting, but, in view of the statistic that in Britain we buy over 80 per cent of our food from supermarkets, this doesn't leave much margin for the kind of freshly harvested local produce that I'm advocating. As I see it, these TV programmes generally tend to treat food as a kind of plaything; vegetables are often just a garnish, the main course being a large portion of fish or meat, and grains and salads are much less in evidence.

I lament that children and young people are, generally speaking, no longer being taught cookery either at home or at school. They might be doing Food Technology, but this seldom seems to involve hands on preparing a meal. Many young people leave university still unable to boil an egg! Now if education does not give young people practical life skills, what hope do we have of a strong, useful and creative society? What happens if all this technology and imported food for some reason cannot be sustained? Could Britain feed and sustain herself? We saw the results of short-sightedness at the beginning of the last World War when Britain only had enough grain and sugar to last for three weeks. If we have generations who can neither cook a meal nor grow a lettuce we have again put ourselves in a rather vulnerable situation.

Do we have to lose something in order to know, too late, that we have lost it? The fish only realizes the importance of his watery environment when he is flapping about on the kitchen table. Do we have to lose the human skills and our delicately balanced environment in order to know to what extent we are dependent upon them? The sad reality is that many people feel that they have little power to change the juggernaut impact of factory farming and supermarket monopolies. But we *can* bring about change, and the process starts in our own homes, our own kitchens, our own gardens. *We need to inform ourselves, experiment, retrieve our own authority back from the hands of the 'experts'. We have so much of our own wisdom, our own common sense – common to all of us, until recently. We need to look with new eyes, for the more we look the more we will see, and the more we see the better we will know where to look.*

When I was working in an energetic Waldorf school in Sussex it was clear to see the effect of good food on the young people and the staff. We had wonderful biodynamically grown vegetables, biodynamic milk, yoghourt and freshly made bread. Often the young people would come after having left the school and say, 'I've just popped in for one of your BD meals and brown rice!' The food too had become an important part of their education. The ones who went home to mothers with a freshly cooked meal or home baked bread also were discernible; it seemed to give them an extra 'shine'.

So having come thus far with me on my philosophical journey I shall assume that you, too, share something of my passion for the subject of nourishing ourselves, and that you too want something other than a meal-time that is a motley of tin-foil containers.

Let us consider some of the aspects of choosing a balanced diet.

Root, leaf, stem and fruit

In Chapter 7 I spoke of the threefold nature of the plant, corresponding to the threefold nature of the human being, and showed these relationships:

Human being	Plant
Nervous system (head)	Root
Rhythmic, breathing system (heart and lungs)	Leaf and stem
Metabolic and limb system (intestines and limbs)	Fruit, seeds, nuts, blossoms

If we plan a meal to include these various elements, a useful guide to proportions is given in human teeth (see Chapter 6, p. 135). You will also be aware that I have made several references to acid/alkaline ratio, which I will mention again at the end because this is another important consideration.

Usually wholegrains will play a central part in the meal; their balanced nutrient content helps to reduce the desire for meat. So a good general ratio of foods would look like this:

35–60% wholegrains;
25% vegetables;
5–10% legumes, lentils, nuts and seeds;
15% fruits and salads;
10–15% animal products (dairy, fish, meat).

This is not to be taken as a formula; the ratios will change according to the climate one lives in and according to where one might be in one's own nutritional journey. We have choices that many of our antecedents did not, and which are not available to most of the human family. That means that our choice of food has an enormous moral/ethical impact, not only on our own health but on other people's livelihoods and consequently on the health of our planet. To align ourselves both inwardly and outwardly towards a fair and just way of eating will affect our whole outlook on life and ultimately our lifestyle, as we become more sensitive to life-enhancing qualities rather than those that are life-diminishing.

The place of raw food

I always aim to have a salad as part of the meal. Fresh salads are full of etheric forces; they can be colourful, and provide texture and stimulus for the digestion. I would obviously use more salads and fresh fruits in the summer when they are more plentiful (I often serve salad as a beginning to the meal). Rudolf Steiner saw raw food more in the light of a therapeutic function; we have to 'cook' the raw food with our own body temperature, which requires more forces but the effort involved is usually valuable. I can imagine that salads and raw foods were not so popular in Steiner's time, but one should use one's discretion, depending on the people we are cooking for. The elderly may have more difficulty in masticating and digesting raw foods, but for young children some raw carrots or raw apple and celery grated together are very nutritious.

Instead of fasting it can be a real rest for the body to have one day in the week when one only eats one food, raw, like apples or carrots. It is better to attempt something like this than be constantly experimenting with different diets, which can confuse the body's own intelligence. *More than anything, the body, soul and spirit thrive on rhythm.*

Colour in food preparation

Each coloured food energizes, cleanses, builds, heals and re-balances the glands, organs and nerve centres associated with its coloured-related chakra ... and each food has a specific energetic frequency and field of resonance. The colour of a food indicates a great deal about its properties.[2]

We all know how colour affects us and various experiments have been done with colouring food in an abnormal way, such as blue mashed potato, bright red rice pudding, pink cabbage. The result was a deleterious effect on people's digestion, nausea often arising at the very sight of such unnatural tones. Naturally occurring colours have healing and nourishing properties, so artificial colours are, I feel, very harmful not only visually but nutritionally too. It is important to think of the colour aspect of a food in such a way that not only will the eye be delighted but the inner organs are also able to discern colour quality in a subtle way.

1. *Base chakra*   Colour: red
   Red foods: red currants, raspberries, strawberries, red apples, beets, cherries.
2. *Hypogastric chakra*   Colour: orange
   Orange foods: oranges, carrots, tomatoes, mango, papaya, pumpkins, persimmons, satsumas, clementines.
3. *Solar plexus*   Colour: yellow
   Yellow foods: bananas, lemons, maize, yellow squash (and their flowers), yellow zucchini, pears.
4. *Heart and thymus*   Colour: green/gold
   Green foods: spinach, lettuce, kale, cabbage, celery, herbs, gooseberries, cucumber, kiwi fruit, golden wheat, nuts and seeds.
5. *Throat and thyroid*   Colour: blue
   Blue foods: blueberries, grapes, blue corn, blue sage.
6. *Ajna* (brow centre and pituitary)   Colour: indigo
   Indigo foods: olives, figs.
7. *Head chakra*   Colour: purple
   Purple foods: blackberries, damsons, black currants, purple plums.

Once again, I would like to stress that these ideas should not be used in a formulistic way – you will possibly run into contradictions if you interpret them literally. Use the concepts if they are of artistic interest; the more we understand our ingredients and our bodies the more we will know intuitively what to do.

Planning the menu

How do we plan a meal? Or do we ever plan? If we want to be thoughtful about the subject then there are many considerations. In the beginning it may seem arduous to take on board the various points I am about to suggest. The exercise, however, does soon become second nature, an intuitive process, and once one starts to get it right the results can be so gratifying that one will just want to keep building on positive experiences.

Some of these considerations are:

- What is in season and therefore available locally?
- What is the age and ethnicity of the diners and what are their professions? Are they farmers, office workers, children, elderly people?
- What is the budget?
- What are the time constraints?
- What are your own capacities? (Best not to be overly ambitious in the beginning)
- What is the temperature outside?
- What time of the day is the meal?

Last, but not least,

- What do they like?

It's important that the meal is enjoyed so, no matter how potentially nourishing it might be, if the meal is all brown and unappetizing it may not be a success. It is a delicate balance in preparing something that you know is healthful but is also delicious and attractive – not necessarily mutually antagonistic.

The sooner you start food education, particularly with children, the better it is. It is amazing how quickly they can lose a sense of what is good for them once they start snacking on crisps and junk food. In order to get away from merely looking at the constituents of foods, one of my intentions has been to look at foods 'energetically', to look at where they grow, which part of the plant has been exclusively developed, what is the 'gesture' of the plant and what it tells us about itself. What colour is it? What energetic values does it represent? For instance, when we look at a hen's egg rather than seeing a conglomeration of fats, proteins, water and minerals, can we not also see that it also contains the necessities for creating a whole new chicken? Similarly, a cereal grain is the potential for a whole new plant, and it has been estimated that one pound of natural honey requires a bee-journey equivalent in distance to encircling the earth. This imaginative process will help us to picture the forces we are working with in a more holistic way.

In substances like whole cereals and whole milk (when produced in a natural way) we have foods that nourish the whole human being. The rest tend to nourish or stimulate particular aspects of the organism. When I speak about 'one-sidedness' in a food or a plant it is not necessarily a criticism; I wish simply to indicate that we need to use our understanding when we combine that food with others and use a cooking method and appropriate flavourings and seasoning to bring a balance.

I have worked for over 25 years using a concept of menu-planning based on the inclusion of something of the root, leaf, stem and fruit of various plants. If these categories are observed properly one should have a properly balanced meal without having to agonize about proteins, starches and fats. I find this so much more artistic and 'painterly' and now this way of planning seems like second nature to me. To the central plant-based menu we can add, in smaller proportion, dairy products, eggs, fish or meat if still enjoyed.

If, as I did at Emerson College, you find yourself catering for an international group of 200 people, the task is helped by having a wide repertoire of multi-cultural dishes to choose from. My cookery education has been varied, starting at home, then at school and later doing several short courses, including one in Paris and with the Japanese Zen teacher Aveline Kushi, who did everything as a meditation. I also have had the good fortune to eat in some excellent restaurants and often ask to visit the kitchens — always a revelation. One can never stop learning — there is always some new practical lesson to be tried. So I do urge you to experiment and find joy in this important activity. Joy is contagious and will permeate your food, but so will anxiety and rush. Please try to slow down.

Ingredients

If you have the great good fortune to have your own organic kitchen garden then you couldn't be in a better position for having optimum nutritional and tasty bases for your meals. Being able to harvest vegetables, salads and herbs early in the morning when the dew is still fresh upon them is such a delight, but sadly not everybody's lot these days The next best thing is to make a relationship with your local farm shop. They may not be organic but then one has to weigh up the differences between buying supermarkets' organic fruit and vegetables, possibly from Brazil or South Africa with all the air pollution that involves, and supporting local agriculture.

Many farmers are preparing themselves to change to meet the growing demands for organically grown food. I myself do extend what is available seasonally with a little imported food for variety, but I love living with the seasons and know that we are given exactly the appropriate foods by nature to support our needs as we go through the year. These fresh, local foods are full of phyto-chemicals and riboflavonoids[3] very much under scrutiny by present nutritional science. Right now (May) I am really enjoying the wonderful mineral-rich flavour of globe artichokes and asparagus with home-made mayonnaise; sautéd fennel has the same nourishing and cleansing sweet aniseed flavour too. Let's be honest, asparagus would not taste so good in December and would not be what my body needs either.

I do think it important to seek out a good supply of organic or, better, biodynamic produce. Despite what scientists tell us, it is more delicious and more nutritious for us (see research mentioned in Chapter 6), and better for the land. It may be a little more expensive, but this is the best investment one can make because it is going inside us, forming our health and our ideas. I am amazed that so many people are prepared to spend large amounts of money on clothes, cars, holidays and homes, but for something as important and intimate as food – they want it cheap! Once one knows what goes into growing a lettuce it does not appear cheap. The French spend 18% of their income on their food budget (it used to be 33%). In the EU as a whole, in 1993 just over 20% of income was being spent on food, according to an OECD report of 1996. The Americans too are allocating a declining percentage of their income on food, from 14.2% to 11.7% between 1980 and 1992, but individual income did rise faster than food prices.[4]

I spend about 25% of my modest income on food and tend to entertain on a small scale. In my store cupboard you will find: a good selection of all the grains (though I do tend to use more rice than the others); a variety of flours; pastas; a selection of beans and lentils, nuts, seeds and sun-dried fruits and tomatoes; seaweeds (kelp, *wakame*, dulse) and *nori* for Japanese sushi; good virgin olive oil, hazelnut, sesame and walnut oil, organic refined sunflower oil for deep frying on rare occasions; tamari, soya sauce; good quality honey; maple syrup; malt; muscovado sugar; vanilla sugar; grey moist sel de mer (sea salt); a good selection of organic herbs and spices (many commercial varieties have been irradiated); good cider, rice and wine vinegar; salted Japanese plums (*omeboshi*); and rose-water and sweet wine for cooking. I get fruit and vegetables and dairy produce from my local farm shop twice weekly (they also run the most successful 'veggie box' scheme in the country).

The importance of soups

Soup with its liquid, salty nature is reminiscent of the briny oceans and our blood. Soups are nourishing and warming or they can be cool and refreshing. Because the soluble constituents of the vegetables are dissolved into the liquid, soups are very easy to assimilate and are good for invalids and small children too. They can be chunky and filling, constituting a whole meal with some good bread, or they can be delicate and stimulating to the appetite at the beginning of a meal. A soup like the Spanish gazpacho is really a liquified salad and would traditionally be kept cool in a shady part of the courtyard in a big earthenware crock, ready to refresh those returning from work on the land.

Keeping a stockpot

When you are cooking regularly for a family it is a good idea to keep a vegetable stockpot, into which can go vegetable trimmings and herbs, a piece of *kombu* or kelp (the vegetarian equivalent of the stock bones), plus any water from cooking vegetables for soups or sauces. Nothing need be wasted; any vegetable remains can be recycled into the compost heap.

Pots and pans

Saucepans and cooking vessels are important 'sheaths' for cooking, mediating between the fire and the food, and most cooks have their favourites. I favour heavy cast iron, enamelled Le Creuset cooking pots for cooking grains, stews and bean dishes, which need slow sustained cooking on a low flame, and a small copper saucepan for sauces. Copper has a special capacity for conducting heat, but it must be lined. For vegetables I use stainless steel with heavy bottoms and glass lids so that I can see what's going on inside. And for lasagnes or casseroles I have lovely earthenware dishes (*greixoneras*) from Majorca, made of an open bodied grogged clay that can be also used directly on the flame. They are also very reasonably priced.

For stirring, wooden spoons and spatulas are best. We want to put as much gentleness into the food as possible and metal spoons are squeaky and can scratch the bottom of enamelled pots.

Cutting and chopping

I use Japanese vegetable-cutting knives for much of the vegetable and fruit cutting. It takes seven years of apprenticeship in Japan before you can make one of these knives, so they are seriously efficient and have a lovely weight; I always take mine whenever I travel. You will need other sharp vegetable knives, including a serrated one for slicing tomatoes, and a zester for zesting citrus fruits. I have a food processor, which I use for finely chopping nuts and liquidizing soups, but I don't use it for pastry making, cake making or for slicing vegetables. Machines bring heat into slicing vegetables; they also cannot honour their shape and tend to really destroy vital forces. (However, I would recommend a small grain mill to provide freshly ground or flaked grains.) One has to prioritize, and for me hand-cutting food is a definite priority even if there are a lot of people to feed.

There is a real science in the activity of cutting vegetables in a conscious way. My Japanese teacher said, 'You can always tell the state of mind of the cook by looking at the way the vegetables and fruits have been cut!' (It should be orderly and not chaotic.) The Japanese and Chinese cooks developed this to a high art.

If we look at each well-grown vegetable we will see that they have their own intrinsic shape and there should be a good rhythmical structure of fibrous material. When we cut them we are rearranging energy pathways and this should be done in a way that enhances the potency of the food. The way we cut influences not only the visual, but also the nutritional aspect of the food. It also affects the cooking time. If we want the flavours to go into a soup or sauce then we cut small and regular, whereas for long cooking we need larger chunks like the 'roll-cut' (see drawing). When cutting a vegetable, say an onion, we can cut half-moons in a way that each slice has something of the quality of the root end as well as the shoot. Cutting should also have a 'musical' aspect (in a way, all matter is frozen music), and we should try to unlock that musical energy. Our knives should be sharp and 'sing' on the wooden chopping board. Wipe this board after each vegetable, as they each have different smells and colours which we will mix later in the pot. All these considerations may seem strange but they turn cooking into a meditative art.

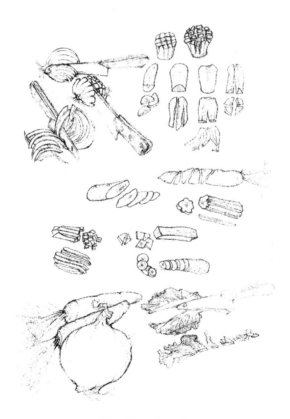

Vegetable chopping

Let's choose our menu and cook

So now we are all set to have a nice undisturbed session in the kitchen. It is good to start off with a clean and tidy kitchen and to wash up as one goes along – order is important and will be imprinted on the food. If one starts off feeling a little chaotic, it is amazing how soothing working with good fresh ingredients and the dance in the saucepan can be; one will soon be feeling grounded.

So start with washing hands, putting on a clean apron, tying hair back, then we plan our work schedule, thinking of all the things that will take the longest time. Does everything need to be in the oven? Leave salads and fruits as late as possible so as not to lose those delicate vital forces, the vitamins. I find that I enter a kind of time warp when I am cooking, because one is in a world of process where every substance has its own laws and timing. Of course it is possible to hurry processes up and slow them down (our Western world is obsessed with this kind of manipulation), but when I cook I try to honour those special inbuilt time laws, which include pauses. If we can put time and spaciousness into our food, that will be passed on in subtle ways to the diners. Cyclical time has spaciousness and when entered into can help to free us from the normal strictures of clock time.

When I had a houseful and a job, I used to spend Saturday morning making various dishes that I could build on during the week, such as a rich home-made tomato and vegetable sauce, a pot of rice (which keeps well), a béchamel sauce, which could become a spinach soufflé or Welsh rarebit. Rice pilaff and pizzas were also favourites with the young people, so I had the basis of several potential meals at the ready. Having said this, my best intention is to start each meal from scratch. Reheated food just does not have the same vitality, but sometimes one has to make compromises.

Now I have planned a series of menus that use the grain of the day, the root, leaf, stem and fruit concept, with an attention to colour, texture and flavours. I have designed these menus for different seasons and some of them include desserts. They are perhaps not exactly the kind of meal that you would make every day, but they could be modified. They are all vegetarian, but a little meat or fish could be added in all cases. One of my missions is to show how wonderful vegetarian food can be and to stimulate people to explore a more plant-based nutrition. (I lived by vegetarian principles during the macrobiotic phase but when we went to Majorca and had our own animals, eating meat and fish occasionally seemed in keeping with our way of life and this is how I have continued to live, as long as I can get free-range products.)

Monday: Moon day   Rice
Parsnip and spinach curry – Orange dhal – Whole Basmati rice – Chapati (optional) – Cucumber and yoghourt raita – Coriander and mango chutney (autumn/winter) – Apple and rose petal jelly.
Colours: green, white, orange, gold.

Tuesday: Mars day   Oats
Pumpkin, chestnut and porcini croustade with oat and cheese herb topping – Spiced red cabbage and watercress and chicory salad – Sautéd leeks (autumn/winter) – Seasonal fruit (any season depending on produce).
Colours: magenta, orange, gold, green.

Wednesday: Mercury day   Millet
Millet, leek and walnut croquettes with ginger tamari sauce – Beetroot salad with lemon glaze and sesame seeds garnished with rocket and lamb's lettuce (autumn) – Stewed fruit *compote* (dried figs, apricots, apples).
Colours: yellow, green, magenta.

Thursday: Jupiter day   Rye
A summer *Salade niçoise* with potatoes (rye bread is wonderful but whole rye is difficult to digest and everyone likes potatoes at some point!) – Strawberries with hazelnut biscuits. (*Salade niçoise*: new potatoes, green beans, capers, hard-boiled eggs, roasted red peppers, olives, roasted pine nuts and crispy lettuce with home-made mayonnaise).
Colours: green, white, red, black, yellow.

Friday: Venus day   Barley
Middle Eastern barley and yoghourt salad – Beetroot soup (*borscht*) with sour cream and chives – Baked apples stuffed with dates and cinnamon.
Colours: orange, gold, beige, green, red, brown (winter)

Saturday: Saturn day   Maize
Souffléd polenta pie – Rich tomato sauce – Refried beans – guacamole with shredded lettuce – Poached pears or seasonal fruit (spring or autumn).
Colours: yellow, red, green, maroon.

Sunday: Sun day   Wheat
Tri-colour pasta with saffron cream sauce (pasta is a popular way to serve wheat) – Sautéd fennel and carrots – Three-leaf salad – Majorcan almond cake with raspberries (summer).
Colours: green, red, gold/orange, white.

The connecting of each of the seven grains to a planet is a help in bringing rhythm into menu planning – particularly so if you are working in a community where you would like to introduce the seven whole grains. It is also important to reconnect ourselves to the starry worlds. However, anything that becomes formulistic or passed on as esoteric knowledge without an appropriate background is questionable to my mind. I admit, though, to being surprised at my own attachment to what I considered 'my system' when I did a course on cereal cooking that included a class on the planetary connections. The barley grain which I had associated with Venus was ascribed to Mars, with apparently good reason. Nevertheless, after 20 years of using the version presented here I found it quite difficult to abandon the connection between barley and Venus, and oats and Mars. So it just goes to show it is often difficult to be completely objective! Perhaps others will help to solve this problem, or maybe it's not a problem.

Recipes

Below is a selection of dishes from the menus. Unfortunately, space prohibits more than a few. For these recipes, I would recommend (to save repetition) that wherever possible all vegetables and fruits, flours, grains and pulses should be fresh and organically grown (or, even better, biodynamic). The eggs should be free-range, the olive oil virgin cold-pressed, and always use sea salt.

All the recipes serve six approximately.

Monday (The moon – rice)

Whole Basmati rice and vegetable curry with dhal, yoghourt and cucumber raita, chutney and poppadoms. Apple and rose petal jelly.

For vegetable curry see Madhur Jaffrey's or any good Indian cookbook. I do recommend roasting and grinding your own spices – it makes a world of difference. I also don't like overcooked vegetables, so I cook spinach or courgettes separately, frying them with ground coriander and cumin and adding them to the main vegetable curry right at the end.

Here is a nice chutney:

Apricot, sultana and coriander chutney
8 oz (200 g) dried apricots
2 oz seedless sultanas
1 pint (10 fl oz) apple juice, heated
1 red onion, finely chopped
2 oz muscovado sugar
1 teaspoon coriander seeds
2 tablespoons wine vinegar
salt and pepper to taste

Method:
1. Soak the dried apricots and sultanas in the hot apple juice for $\frac{1}{2}$ an hour.
2. Add the other ingredients and bring to the boil, turn down the heat and simmer for another $\frac{1}{2}$ hour or until the apricots are really tender and all the flavours combined beautifully. It should be thick by the end of the cooking.

Apple and rose petal jelly
$1\frac{1}{2}$ lb (700 g) eating apples, peeled and sliced (the peel can be used for apple tea)
$\frac{1}{2}$ pint (275 ml) elderflower cordial, with $1\frac{1}{3}$ pint (725 ml) water (could also be blackcurrant or rosehip syrup)
zest of a lemon
honey or maple syrup if needed
2 tablespoons rose water
1 sachet (6 g) Vege-gel (vegetarian gelatine substitute, seaweed based)

Method:

1. Cook apple slices in the syrup water (1 pint altogether) until tender
2. Strain off the fruit and taste the remaining juice for sweetness. Add maple syrup or honey if needed. Allow to cool.
3. Add the Vege-gel to the juice (1 pint) and bring to the boil, stirring vigorously. It should start to set if you test a little on a cold plate.
4. Pour the jelly onto the apple slices arranged nicely in a glass bowl and decorate with crystallized rose petals.

(This jelly can be prepared with any kind of fruit. Children usually love jelly.)

For crystallized rose petals (they do look pretty and children will enjoy preparing them) —
Rose petals, egg white and caster sugar.
Paint the petals (pink ones look good) with egg white and dredge them with unrefined caster sugar. Leave in a dry place to harden. They will keep for two days in an airtight box.

Tuesday (Mars — oats, or could be barley depending on which system you favour)
Pumpkin, chestnut and porcini croustade (oat and cheese herb topping) with braised spiced red cabbage and sautéd leeks

Pumpkin, chestnut and porcini croustade
Topping:
4 oz (110 g) oat flakes
3 oz (75 g) fresh breadcrumbs
1 tablespoon finely chopped herbs (sage, rosemary, thyme, or Provencal dried herbs)
3 oz (75 g) grated Emmenthal cheese (optional)
salt and pepper
1 teaspoon paprika.
3 oz (75 g) melted butter

Filling:
1½ lb (700 g) of peeled and sliced Hubbard or Hokkaido pumpkin (has the dense sweet flesh, not the watery, tasteless variety that the English usually think of as pumpkin)

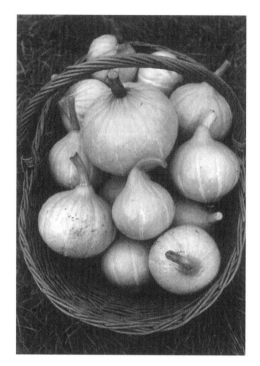

Basket of Hubbard squash

2 large onions
6 cloves of roasted garlic (it's good to roast several heads of garlic with oil, salt and rosemary when you have the oven going and then you have it to hand)
celeriac, small cubes (or 2 celery stalks)
2 oz (50 g) dried porcini (wild mushrooms) washed carefully and soaked in boiling water for $\frac{1}{2}$ hour
$\frac{1}{2}$ teaspoon cinnamon
$\frac{1}{2}$ teaspoon grated nutmeg
4 oz (110 g) dried chestnuts (soaked in boiling water for 1 hour or so, then cooked separately with a little salt for $\frac{1}{2}$ hour)
Olive oil and butter for sautéing

Method for topping:
Mix all the dry ingredients in a bowl, melt the butter and pour over them. Work it through with fingertips.

Method for filling:

1. Slice the onions finely and sauté in a mixture of butter and oil with a pinch of salt. Add garlic and sliced pumpkin, chestnuts, soaked porcini and celeriac.
2. Add 1 pint stock (20 fl oz) and the strained porcini liquor (being very careful not to include grit!). You may need a little more stock later on. Bring to the boil in a heavy bottomed pot.
3. Turn down heat to a minimum and allow to gently simmer for $\frac{3}{4}$ hour, until vegetables are tender. The stock should be absorbed and the vegetables dense. Adjust seasoning. It should have just a hint of spice, for the accompanying red cabbage dish is quite spicy.
4. Fill an oven-proof dish with the pumpkin mixture, top with the oat topping mixture, dot with butter. Bake in the oven at 180°C or gas mark 4 until golden for about $\frac{1}{2}$ hour.

Spiced red cabbage

1 head of red cabbage ($1\frac{1}{2}$ lb, 700 g, approx.)
1 red onion, sliced
1 small eating apple studded with about 10 cloves
1 heaped teaspoon ground cinnamon
1 teaspoon ground nutmeg
$\frac{1}{2}$ teaspoon cayenne (or to taste)
2 tablespoons muscovado sugar
1 teaspoon sea salt
$\frac{1}{4}$ (150 ml) pint wine vinegar
a little vegetable stock

Method:

1. Boil a kettle of water. Finely shred the red cabbage, removing tough stalks and inner core. Pour the boiling water onto the shredded cabbage and let it steep for 10 minutes or so. This removes excess sulphur qualities or 'yin' as in the macrobiotic scheme. Drain.
2. Sauté the red onion in a mixture of butter and olive oil (just enough to coat the bottom of the pan). Add spices and sugar, steeped cabbage, salt, vinegar and clove-studded apple and some stock if necessary. The liquid should not cover the cabbage mixture but the mixture must not boil dry.

3. Bring to boil and reduce heat to simmering. Depending on the quality of the cabbage, the cooking should take about $\frac{3}{4}$ hour and should be a gorgeous colour of magenta, tender and subtly 'pickled'.

Lightly sautéd leeks would be a fine accompaniment to this meal. Their delicate flavour and colour will balance the deeply earthy, rich and spicy main dishes.

Wednesday (Mercury – millet)

Millet, leek and walnut patties with ginger and tamari sauce, beetroot salad with lemon glaze and sesame seeds, garnished with rocket leaves. Stewed compote of dried fruits (Hunza apricots, pears, apples, etc.)

Millet, leek and walnut patties

10 oz (250 g) millet
3 oz (75 g) walnuts
2 tablespoons millet flakes
8 oz (225 g) cleaned and finely sliced young leeks
2 tablespoons quark or cream cheese
1 large egg for binding
1 oz (25 g) butter and 2 tablespoons olive oil for sautéing
1–1$\frac{1}{2}$ pints (800 ml) good vegetable stock

Method:

1. Measure the millet in a measuring jug. Wash and pick over the millet carefully. Allow to dry. Melt the butter and oil in a heavy bottomed pot and sauté the millet for 2–3 minutes until the grains are coated (this keeps them from clogging together too much). Pour on the double amount of hot vegetable stock, which should be appropriately seasoned. Allow to come to the boil, then turn down flame to minimum (perhaps use a flame-spreader to prevent scorching of the bottom of the pot). I use a Le Creuset pot for grains, and it is important to choose the right size pot. The grain will double in size, so make allowances for this, but at the same time the pot should not be too large because this will not bring good results. Do not stir during cooking. After 30 minutes the stock should be absorbed and the grains plump and fluffy. Add raw millet flakes (for binding). Allow to rest until cool enough to handle.

2. While the millet is cooking you can lightly roast the walnuts in a dry

frying pan (again, a cast iron one is best). Then grind them in a food processor, but not too finely — leave some texture.

3. Sauté shredded leeks in a little butter with oil until softened, but keep the emerald-green colour.
4. Add leeks, walnuts, Quark, egg. Adjust seasoning. The mixture now should be easy to form into firm patties. Makes 8–10. Dust with millet flakes and rest for 10 minutes. They should be cold now.
5. Fry in olive oil for approximately 5 minutes on each side. They should be golden brown.

Tamari, ginger and green onion sauce
1½ pints (800 ml) good vegetable stock (not too salty, as the tamari is salty)
2 teaspoons finely grated fresh ginger root
1 tablespoon tamari (soy sauce), more if necessary
bunch finely sliced green onions (scallions)
1½ tablespoons arrowroot mixed to a paste with a little cold water, no lumps

Method:
1. Heat stock until nearly boiling. Add ginger and tamari
2. Carefully add the arrowroot mixture, stirring briskly. The sauce should thicken to a pouring consistency. Add the shredded green onions and serve.

Thursday (Jupiter — Rye)
Hazelnut sables (biscuits)
7 oz (200 g) butter, softened
5 oz (150 g) unrefined caster sugar
3 oz (75 g) roasted and finely chopped hazelnuts
8 oz (225 g) unbleached self-raising flour
1 egg

Method:
1. Combine all the ingredients. Make into a sausage shape by wrapping in cling film.
2. Chill in the refrigerator until hard enough to slice.
3. Oil a baking tray and place slices on. Bake for 15 minutes at 200°C (gas mark 5).

Friday (Venus – barley)

Middle Eastern barley salad, beetroot soup (borscht) with sour cream and chives.

Rudolf Steiner extolled beetroot for their qualities of stimulating mind-brain function and excretion, and for acting as an excellent blood purifier. So we have here a hearty beetroot soup which includes other vegetables, served with a dramatic swirl of sour cream and chopped chives.

Barley salad

8 oz (200 g) whole barley
double the volume of good vegetable stock

Dressing:
$\frac{1}{2}$ pint Greek yoghourt
2 tablespoons olive oil
finely grated zest and juice of 1 lemon
1 tablespoon chopped mint
1 tablespoon chopped flat leaf parsley
$\frac{1}{2}$ teaspoon cumin
$\frac{1}{2}$ teaspoon cayenne
small red onion, finely chopped
diced cucumber for garnish

Method:
Soak the barley overnight or for a few hours, pour away soaking water. Cook in double quantity of stock. Do not stir during cooking. The grain should be plump, having absorbed all the stock, and tender. Leave to cool to room temperature. (Note many Middle Eastern dishes are served at room temperature.)

Dressing:
Whisk the olive oil into the yoghourt, add all the rest of the ingredients. Adjust seasoning. Garnish a bowl with crisp lettuce leaves and spoon in the barley salad. Sprinkle with parsley, chopped onion and a little paprika.

Beetroot soup (borscht)

$1\frac{1}{2}$ lb (700 g) raw beetroot (peeled)
8 oz (225 g) carrots

8 oz (225 g) potatoes
3 blades of celery or some celeriac
$\frac{1}{4}$ medium red cabbage
2 leeks (white part only)
4 cloves garlic
$\frac{1}{2}$ teaspoon cumin
$\frac{1}{2}$ teaspoon caraway seeds
salt and pepper to taste
1 tablespoon tomato concentrate
1 bay leaf
3 pints ($1\frac{1}{2}$ litres) good vegetable stock
oil and butter for sautéing
sour cream and chives for garnish

Method:
1. Slice all the vegetables finely but keep them separate.
2. Heat butter and oil in a heavy pot. Sauté onions and garlic first (this drives off excess sulphur). Add all the other vegetables, coating them with the oil by stirring over a low heat.
3. Add all other ingredients one by one, adding spices and some salt. Then add the stock and bring it to the boil.
4. Turn down the heat and let it simmer for approximately $\frac{3}{4}$ hour until the vegetables are all soft (the beetroot will take longest). Allow to rest for $\frac{1}{2}$ hour to let the flavours stabilize. Then blend in a food processor.
5. Adjust seasoning, bring to the boil again and serve with a dollop of sour cream and chopped chives.

A word on stirring. If you know about the stirring of the biodynamic preparations, you may begin to realize how potent is the way we move liquids and other mixtures about. In the same way, when we stir our food during the course of preparation it should be because it needs to be stirred, and in a consequent way, not just getting rid of our nervous energy. This applies to all our gestures towards the food.

Saturday (Saturn – maize)
Polenta from Italy, a rich and nutritious dish, with side dishes that give it a Mexican orientation.

Souffléed polenta pie
10 oz (275 g) yellow polenta
1 ¾ pints (1 litre) approx. hot water
4 large eggs, separated
1 red pepper, finely diced
1 green pepper, finely diced
1 large onion, finely diced
3 cloves of garlic (minced)
1 dessertspoon chopped sage
6 oz (175 g) freshly grated Parmesan cheese
salt and pepper to taste
pine kernels to sprinkle on the top
1 oz (25 g) butter and 3 tablespoons olive oil for sautéing

Method:
1. Prepare the polenta (a kind of porridge) by gently sautéing the grains in a little of the butter and oil in a heavy bottomed pot until coated. Then pour on hot water with the sea salt and bring to the boil, stirring briskly with a wooden spoon so that no lumps occur. Cook for 10–15 minutes, stirring from time to time so that it does not stick and burn. It should not be gritty by now and the grains should be cooked. Set aside to cool.
2. Sauté onions, garlic and peppers (in that order) with the chopped sage and a pinch of salt. Reserve a small quantity for garnish and add the rest to the polenta.
3. Add egg yolks and grated cheese, reserving a little for the top. Mix well.
4. Whip egg whites until soft peaks arise. Then fold in gently to the rest of the mixture. Sprinkle cheese, the reserved peppers and onions and pine nuts, also some oregano on top and put into an oven, 200°C, gas mark 5, till golden on top (about 20 minutes). Then turn down heat to 180°C, gas mark 4, for a further 20 minutes until set.
5. Serve with a rich tomato sauce

Rich tomato sauce
1 large onion finely chopped
4 garlic cloves, minced
1 large red pepper finely chopped
1 large green pepper finely chopped

3 sticks of celery finely chopped
3 carrots, grated
2 teaspoons *herbes de Provence*
1 400 g can of chopped tomatoes (or $1\frac{1}{2}$ lb, 770 g skinned fresh tomatoes)
2 teaspoons muscovado sugar
1 bay leaf
2 tablespoons tomato purée
Fresh basil to finish off
Salt and pepper to taste
Olive oil for sautéing

Method:
1. Sauté onions, garlic, herbs and all the rest of the vegetables in a heavy cast-iron pot, adding them one by one and gently softening them.
2. Add the rest of the ingredients and stir. Bring to the boil, then turn down the heat and allow to simmer for approx $\frac{3}{4}$ hour until all the vegetables are completely cooked and the flavours blended. Add basil right at the end.
(The carrot and celery help to alkalize the acidity of the peppers and tomatoes.) This keeps well in the refrigerator and will be enough for two meals.

Refried beans
1 lb ($\frac{1}{2}$ kilo) pinto or red kidney beans
a piece of kelp
herbs, celery and a piece of carrot for flavouring
$\frac{1}{2}$ teaspoon salt
1 large onion
1 dessertspoon olive oil
4 cloves of garlic
1 teaspoon ground cumin
1 dessertspoon soy sauce
chilli (optional)

Method:
1. Soak pinto or red kidney beans overnight with the piece of kelp. Throw away soaking water and cook in 3 pints of water with some herbs, celery and piece of carrot. Add $\frac{1}{2}$ teaspoon salt towards the end of the cooking time. Cook until soft (1 hr or more).

2. Slice the onion into fine rings and sauté in olive oil with the garlic cloves until soft. Add cumin and some soy sauce (about 1 dessertspoon). You could add some chilli too.
3. Add the onion mixture to the beans and continue to cook, mashing the beans but leaving some whole for texture.

Guacamole
3 ripe avocados
3 cloves garlic, crushed
salt and pepper
small red onion, finely minced
juice of $\frac{1}{2}$ lemon
2 tablespoons olive oil
1–2 tablespoons fresh coriander, chopped

Method:
1. Peel and stone the avocados and mash with the lemon juice to prevent discoloration.
2. Add the garlic, onion and coriander, olive oil, salt and pepper. Chill and decorate with coriander leaves.

Sunday (The Sun – Wheat)
Tri-colour conchiglie (pasta shells) with saffron cream sauce, sautéd carrots and fennel, accompanied by three-leaf salad with lemon olive oil dressing. Majorcan almond cake with raspberries for dessert.

Saffron cream sauce
$1\frac{1}{2}$ pints (30 fl oz, 900 ml) whole milk
Infusion: 2 bay leaves, 2 teaspoons whole black peppercorns, a few slices of onion, carrot, celery
parsley stalks
3 oz (75 g) butter
3 oz (75 g) unbleached white flour (for roux)
$\frac{1}{4}$ pint (150 ml) single cream
wineglass of Amontillado sherry (or white wine)
1 teaspoon saffron threads, soaked in small quantity boiling water for 10 minutes or so

Salt and pepper to taste
Bunch of spring onions, finely sliced and sautéd in butter

Method:
1. Put milk and infusion ingredients in a heavy bottomed saucepan. Bring slowly to the boil. Turn off heat and allow to infuse for 10 minutes or so.
2. Melt butter in a saucepan, add flour and cook gently, stirring with a wooden spoon until it thickens. Start straining the hot milk into the roux (flour and butter mixture). Now you need a strong whisk to keep stirring this mixture briskly so that it does not lump. Keep adding the milk until it has all been absorbed. You should now have a thick, velvety sauce free of lumps.
3. Add cream, sherry and saffron. Continue to cook until bubbling gently. Add the sautéd spring onions.
4. Pour over cooked pasta and sautéd carrot and fennel slices.
5. Serve with three-leaf salad of 'Lollo Rosso' and cos lettuces and rocket, scattered with a few pecans for crunch, and a lemon, garlic and oil dressing.

Majorcan almond cake
At the end of January the island of Majorca begins to be covered with a frothy bridal veil of almond blossom. This cake makes me think of the exotic Moorish culture – with its taste for almonds and citrus – that created the exquisite palace of Alhambra in Granada. I imagine beautiful veiled women eating snips of this cake in a setting of tinkling fountains and jasmine-scented patios. It is very rich so you only need a little. It goes well with a fruit compote, fresh raspberries and/or crème fraîche. It has no butter or flour in it so can be offered to those with gluten problems. Will keep well.

11 oz (350 g) ground almonds
10 oz (325 g) unrefined castor sugar
grated zest of 2 unwaxed lemons
1 heaped teaspoon cinnamon
7 eggs (separated)
a few drops of real almond essence

Method:

1. Line a 9-inch (24 cm) loose-bottomed cake tin with baking parchment. Set oven at 180°C (gas mark 4)
2. Beat egg yolks and sugar (an electric hand-beater is useful here) until thick and pale yellow.
3. Add lemon rind, cinnamon and a few drops of almond essence. Combine well.
4. Whip egg whites with a pinch of salt in a large metal bowl, until soft peaks form.
5. Gently combine the two mixtures together. (I find hands best for this. You don't want to knock the air out of the egg whites but you do need the mixture to be homogenous.) Gradually sprinkle in the ground almonds.
6. Spoon into the cake tin and cook for $\frac{3}{4}$ hour. Allow to cool gently. It will still be moist in the centre.

The qualities of fire and its uses in cooking

'Culture grows out of the mastery of fire,' writes John Davy.[5]

How did human beings first discover its enormous benefits as well as its dangers? The Greek legend of Prometheus tells us how he (the son of Iapetus and the ocean nymph Clymene) was the benefactor of man. It was said that Zeus, having been tricked by Prometheus over his share of sacrificial ox, denied mankind the use of fire. Prometheus then *stole* the fire from Vulcan to save the human race. For this he was chained to Mount Caucasus, where an eagle preyed on his liver all day, but was renewed every night. (The liver is one of the most indestructible of organs, whose forces are regenerated at night. See the section on rhythms in the family meal, p. 305–8). He was eventually released by Hercules who slew the eagle. It was to revenge the theft of fire by Prometheus that Zeus sent Pandora to earth with all her box of ills; the only quality that stayed in the box when it was opened was Hope. ('Promethean Fire' was the vital principle, fire, with which Prometheus quickened his clay figures, from which came the first human beings.)[6]

Some of the earliest evidence of human control over fire was found in the ancient hearths of Peking Man. Whatever these beginnings may have been, we can see it as a great determining step in the development of human capacities. However, we do need to remember that in the Greek legend it was *stolen,* and the price to pay was the liberation of the contents of Pandora's box, which amongst other ills probably contained those sub-earthly 'shadow forces' of fire – nuclear and atomic energy. ('We passed through the gates of hell,' said scientists at Los Alamos after the first test of a nuclear bomb.)

But the fire we wish to consider here, whether released from wood, coal or gas, is directly or indirectly a gift of the sun – it is a solar event. All these substances come from a kind of ripening process that has taken place in growing organisms, producing usable energy. When we cook with sensitivity and insight we should be continuing that *ripening* process, rendering foods more digestible and flavourful.

It has been said, 'Cooking is one of the oldest arts in the world, and was one of the highest crafts of men and women. Temples and mystery centres were its cradle, as mythology and legends of all races show us, when often gods have been said to have given it as a divine gift and revelation to humanity.'[7] The early stages of cookery must have been full of surprises, even the laying of the piece of grain paste next to the fire and finding that it develops an appetizing crisp brown exterior led people on to greater experiment.

As we saw, the home was centred on the hearth in those earliest of settlements, such as Çatal Hüyük. Later we see the Greeks honouring the goddess of the communal hearth, Hestia; the principle that all hearths were shared with the gods was known as Hestiatoria. Citizens were instructed that when setting out to found new colonies (eighth and seventh centuries BC) they must take some of this central fire with them. And so it was in the home, down the years, that the woman was entrusted with the hearth but the men dealt with the roasting of animals on spits, which naturally required more physical strength and certain practical skills.

I can certainly say that I was brought up with the hearth as the centre of the home. We had one of those cast iron ranges that had an open coal fire with ovens at either side. It needed blackleading (polishing with special black polish) every week, and mornings began with the sounds of the hearth being cleared and a new fire being started or stoked up again. I remember gazing into the fire night after night, seeing the whole of creation taking place in the red embers, and then came the 'salamanders' who continued to flare up and sparkle even when the fire seemed to have gone out. This was our television set.

Bread was baked in the ovens from time to time; I began to realize that it was no mean thing to know how to gauge the temperature, because sometimes the bread was scorched on one side. We had a gas oven, too, and that would take preference as it was easier to handle. This experience, however, laid the basis for my interest in differing kinds of heat for cooking. When I lived in Majorca I was delighted to see that most village houses and farmhouses invariably had outdoor stone bread ovens, many of which were still used. The people had a real appreciation for food cooked in them – the result was much more flavourful.

Such baking is an art and I don't pretend to have become mistress of it, but I certainly tried it and in the attempt developed real respect for those village bakers and farmers who continued to fire their ovens with wood. (I am delighted to see that many Waldorf schools with the help of the Hiram Trust are building clay ovens and using them to make pizzas, and thus the children learn how to handle true fire.)

In times gone by country folk developed real sensitivities to the different qualities of woods burnt in their hearths and stoves. Here is a charming traditional verse, full of insight about these differing burning qualities:

Oak logs will warm you well
If they're old and dry.
Larch logs of pinewood smell
But the sparks will fly.
Beech logs for Christmas time,
Yew logs heat well.
Scotch logs it is a crime
For anyone to sell.
Birch logs burn too fast,
Chestnut scarce at all.
Hawthorn logs are good to last
If you cut them in the fall.
Holly logs will burn like wax,
You should burn them green.
Elm logs like smouldering flax,
No flame to be seen.
Pear logs and apple logs,
They will scent your room.
Cherry logs across the dogs

Smell like flowers in bloom.
But ash logs, all smooth and grey,
Burn them green or old;
Buy up all that come your way,
They're worth their weight in gold!

This kind of traditional wisdom in verse form would be taught to children, so they came to recognize the differences between sources of wood and the fire they produced.

Another unforgettable experience for me was being present at the creation of a *luau* in Hawaii. A *luau* must be one of the oldest kinds of cooking known to humanity. It involves the digging of a pit (by the men) which is then lined with volcanic fire-proof pebbles. A fire is started in the bottom, then the food – which could be a pig, *taro*, yams and other root vegetables wrapped by the women in banana leaves – is laid on top of banana stalks which also cover the food. Then a tarpaulin is laid on top and covered with earth and left for five hours (you certainly have to know about fires to build this one properly). The whole procedure is part of the festival, with songs and dances being sung to celebrate the life of the pig. Garlands of fresh flowers are made and appetites build up while stories are told. The food eventually is uncovered, needing great art to know when it is truly cooked, the process being a mixture of roasting, steaming and smoking. Then more singing and dancing. Ritual accompanies the whole event and everyone is involved, children and grandparents together, bringing cultural richness and showing clearly the community-building activity of a shared festival meal. In Hawaii healing rituals often are practised in the traditional way with a shared *luau*. The food is chosen for its special colours and each family member goes before the sick person and asks, 'What may I have done to cause your sickness?' Tremendous insight, humility and compassion are shown here, and at the centre is the fire.

It is becoming quite rare now to go into a home, particularly in the city, and see a fire. There may be a simulated one, but a real one – seldom. Nasty, dirty, dangerous things! If we proceed into the kitchen we might be met by enough technology to perplex a seasoned astronaut. It is usually powered by electricity, with not a flame to be seen. Electricity is an inescapable force in our lives; we are almost buried in a matrix of it. There are overhead and underground cables, flickering television and computer screens, fluorescent light-bulbs, deep-freezers. And now there are microwaves, which add to the invisible pollution. Often we have little idea what it has taken to provide this convenient push-button energy.

Although heat is measured in calories, and no one would dispute that 100 calories provided by a wood fire could be different from 100 calories provided by an electric fire, we intuitively know there is a *qualitative* difference.

What is the nature of electricity? Perhaps we can perceive something of its quality when we suffer from an electric shock: '... like meeting a mysterious and foreign will, which shakes our bodies in strange contortions; it is not a force with which we feel comfortable, it is like a trapped energy, emerging from the hidden depths of nature, full of tension and buried violence.'[8]

Do we have choices? Some may and others may not. One of the ways to redeem a less than ideal situation is to show gratitude towards it. To despise something whilst we use it for something as important as cooking will not improve things. My ideal would be an Aga solid fuel cooker, which is a cast iron stove that usually heats the water and radiators. It gives a real presence in the home. I would like to have a wood fire and a gas range, too, for differing kinds of cooking, but this is a dream at the moment. I think gas is most practical since one can still really experience and have control over the flame, and it responds quickly.

Lastly we should not forget the old-fashioned but wonderfully gentle hay-box cooker for certain dishes like porridge. One soaks the oat flakes and then gently brings them to a rolling boil. Then one takes them off the heat, wraps the heavy pot in a blanket and places it overnight in a box, packed around with hay. This produces the most wonderful porridge. You can also 'rest' grain dishes in a hay-box cooker when they have cooked and only need to carry on expanding a little.

Microwaves used for food are dealt with in a separate section below, but I must share an experience I had not long ago of going into a restaurant with my daughter. The menu was long and quite complex. Whilst waiting to be served I went to the cloakroom, passing the kitchen on my way. I peered in, as I am wont to do, and was dismayed to see a virtually empty kitchen, displaying a kind of funereal absence of food preparation. All that was visible was a deep-freezer, a microwave oven and a timer. We decided not to stay. I believe that there are many such establishments.

So what has happened to Hestia and the principal of Hestiatoria, of sharing our hearths with the gods and the salamanders? When we do not acquaint ourselves with the *being* of fire, we may deny our own qualities of fire, of passion, the warmth of enthusiasm. And what happens when we banish something out of our lives — where does it go? Underground? Into the unconscious, where all our fears percolate, eventually emerging into the way we live our lives? Will not the banished Hestia conspire with the contents of Pandora's box to give us fire, but of a sub-earthly quality? I think it is time for the feminine principle at last to retrieve the fire and tame it. For when Promethean man gets hold of the fire he has a tendency to create guns and bombs and wreaks havoc on nature. Just think what could happen if all that huge potential of energy could be directed into creative activity and solar-sourced power. We must believe that it *can* be done.

Types of cooking

When we cook, whether using coal, charcoal, wood or gas, let us remember that it is a transformed gift of the sun, and cooking furthers the sun process of ripening. The warmth comes from the outside and penetrates inwards (in microwave 'cooking' this process is reversed), proceeding through conduction and convection. Starches expand, proteins harden or soften according to cooking, cellulose softens, sugars change, salts dissolve and certain nutrients become more available for digestion — all this at their own specific temperatures. Of course, we can damage certain foods through heat, by overcooking, and that is why we need to understand the nature of our ingredients.

Why cook at all? Would you wish to eat rice raw? (Perhaps only if you were suffering from worms.) Or potatoes, dried beans or flour? There are many things that need to be cooked and are greatly improved by it. They are also enhanced by coming into contact with other influences, such as water, oils, herbs and sometimes spices which can only do their dance in the pot stimulated by the flame enthusing their passions.

Different kinds of cooking are more appropriate for different seasons. In the autumn and winter in the northern climes we need longer, slower cooking methods which bring more heat, such as *casseroling, braising, stewing, roasting* and *baking*. Our ingredients tend to be more dense and fibrous than in the summer — grains, dried beans, pulses and roots, all of which require a longer cooking time, as they slowly expand, absorbing the flavours of the liquids they are being cooked in. Some people like to use pressure cookers, but I prefer not to try to speed up processes which naturally have their own time framework, rather like the germination process in plants.

Braising and casseroling can start off with the ingredients being gently sautéd in oil, adding stock and finishing the dish in a slow oven. Stewing involves cooking the ingredients in a flavoured liquid on top of the range on a medium to low heat. With roasting, the ingredients are lightly coated with oil and cooked in the oven at quite a high temperature (depending on the density) to produce a browning and crisping of the surface. *Baking*, which we tend to do throughout the year, requires dry oven heat; it produces bread, cakes, biscuits, pies and tarts. Moderately high temperatures are needed to bring about the browning and crisping result from caramelized sugars, creating the flavours and textures we find so appetizing. French scientist Louis-Camille Maillard did much research in 1912 into this browning process in cooking. At that time the malting process in beer-making was one of his studies. What he found was a combination of complex factors: plant cellulose, sugars, pyrazines, amino acids, sulphides. Later, food chemists seized on this research saying, 'The Maillard work may provide a means of chemically synthesizing some flavours which will nearly approximate the natural flavours.'[9] In the later section on microwaves you will see to what lengths food chemists and manufacturers will go to try and synthesize this natural, sought-after crispy browning, the nutty flavour and texture that proper baking produces.

Lighter methods of cooking, possibly more suitable for spring and summer are: *sautéing, steaming, steam-sautéing* and *stir-frying*. Steaming is quite a gentle and delicate way to cook vegetables. (Also Japanese rice cakes. Until recently the Japanese did not use ovens, so everything was cooked in either stacked up bamboo steamers or woks and skillets.) Start with about 1 inch of lightly salted water in the bottom of the pan. Steam for ten minutes or so in a bamboo steamer (French beans, carrot sticks, mangetout peas, broccoli florets are ideal); the vegetables should be *al dente* and have kept the intensity of colour.

To sauté-steam

Sauté vegetables in a tablespoonful of olive oil to which has been added a knob of butter. To this add seasoning. The sautéing seals in some of the flavour. Then add half a cup of water and gently simmer until tender. (In both cases keep the resulting cooking liquid, which is full of soluble nutrients for a sauce or soup.)

To stir-fry

Use hot oil (but not smoking), as this sears in the natural flavours of the finely sliced vegetables. Keep them in constant motion by wooden chopsticks.

The high temperatures of fats and oils reached in *frying* and particularly *deep-frying* cause oxidized fatty acids to accumulate and many of these can cause DNA damage, so the reuse of frying oils is not to be recommended. These last methods of cooking should be only used very occasionally, in my opinion.

Grilling

Uses a dry but fierce heat. Char-grilled vegetables are very delicious sometimes, if you have a charcoal grill.

Other kinds of food preparation do involve a kind of cooking but don't need more than room temperature, such as pickling in salt – the lactic acid process – for sauerkraut, or marinating, with oil, wine and spices.

Microwave ovens

The invention of microwave ovens dates from the Second World War and is thought to have originated as a means of food preparation in German submarines. It was then taken up in the USA by a company called Raytheon who marketed the first ovens for the public in 1952. Microwave ovens have been promoted world-wide with virtually no research until the 1970s, when histological studies showed that the molecular structures of nutrients were damaged to the point of destroying cell walls, which conventional cookery left intact.

In 1989 a Swiss food scientist, Dr Hans-Ulrich Hertel, did some research the results of which were suppressed following a complaint filed by the Swiss Association of Dealers for Electro-apparatus for Households and Industry. Dr Hertel's findings showed, 'Any food eaten that has been cooked or defrosted in a microwave oven can cause changes in the blood indicative of a developing pathological process that is also found in cancer.' Hertel goes on, 'When food is microwaved the oven exerts a power input of about 1000 watts or more. The resulting destruction and deformation of food molecules produces a new radiolytic compound, unknown in nature.'[10]

How a microwave oven works

A device called a magnetron tube causes an electron beam to oscillate at very high frequencies producing microwave (MV) radiation. Domestic ovens use a frequency of 2.45 gigahertz (GHz) because water absorbs electromagnetic energy quickest at this frequency, thus allowing food containing water to be heated quickly. The molecules within the food are forced to align themselves with the very rapidly alternating field and to oscillate around their axis. Heat is produced from the *intense intermolecular friction*. Microwaves are beamed from the magnetron in the oven compartment where they heat the food *from the inside out*. Heating from the inside first can give rise to cold spots, hence the need to constantly rotate the dish.

Research in Russia showed microwaves to have many serious effects that denature the nutritional factors in food: significant decreases in the bio-availability of B-complex vitamins, vitamin C and E, essential minerals and lipotrophics; lowering of the metabolic activity of alkaloids, glucosides, galactosides and nitrilosides (all basic plant substances); and marked acceleration of structural disintegration in all foods. As a result microwave ovens were banned in Russia in 1976; the ban was however lifted after *Perestroika*.

Research at Stanford University in California revealed that the levels of anti-infective factors in human milk even at low temperatures were severely decreased by microwaves. Indeed, any milk heated in microwave ovens can suffer significant molecular change, considerably reducing the nutritional value. Reheating left-over food is also potentially dangerous.

Since microwaved food has a tendency to be low in colour and flavour, new technology produced 'susceptors' to produce flavour. By gluing these devices to the packaging of microwavable foods local areas of high temperature could be achieved, so browning the foods. The glues from these 'susceptors' have been shown to release toxic chemicals into the food.[11] There is no space for me to elaborate further on the dangers of microwave cooking, and we have not touched upon the question of leakage of radiation in faulty installations, or what it takes to recycle such a piece of equipment. I hope you will be able to put this information into some perspective alongside my section on different qualities of heat.

Food irradiation

Food irradiation is the treatment of food with high doses of ionizing radiation. It is used to delay ripening of fruit, to inhibit the sprouting of vegetables, to kill bacteria that can cause food spoilage or food poisoning, and to kill insects that infest foods. There is growing international pressure from the irradiation industry and from some international organizations to increase the irradiation of food, but the process has many potential dangers for workers, for animal welfare and the environment. A major decision will soon be taken over which foods will be allowed to be irradiated. Up until now member states of the European Union have made their own rules over which food they permit and at what doses. The new Directives aim to harmonize the member states' national laws, which means that irradiated foods can be freely traded within the EU. At the moment the one category allowed is dried aromatic herbs, spices and seasonings. Many more foods are on the list for proposed inclusion.

There are many arguments against this technology, an outcome of Eisenhower's Atoms for Peace campaign in 1953 seeking to devise industries that could use up waste products from the nuclear industry, such as dying isotopes. Why do consumers oppose irradiation?

Food irradiation can cover up poor hygiene practices and so provides no incentive to clean up food processing, which should take the first priority. It destroys essential vitamins and nutrients in food, and this damage is further increased by the longer storage times of irradiated foods. This is not in the interests of consumers and could be particularly harmful for impoverished nations or sections of society already struggling to obtain adequate nutrition, such as the elderly, the young, the sick and the poor. Irradiation also creates radiolytic by-products in food, some of which have known or suspected carcinogenic and mutagenic properties.

Food irradiation does not deactivate dangerous toxins already produced by bacteria prior to irradiation, so it does not prevent recontamination afterwards. Altogether there seems to be little to recommend this technology and a great deal to suggest it is not designed with the benefit of the consumers in mind but only the producers' interests. Yet another invisible process added to all the others that have been described.

In the story of Snow White, she is offered a delicious looking, shiny red apple by the jealous queen, disguised as an old woman. One bite of the poisoned fruit is enough to send her into a coma for a hundred years until rescued by the prince (or could it be her common sense?). This really seems to be a story of our time, a cautionary tale. We can protect ourselves by training all our sense perceptions to become sensitive to these death-dealing forces within shiny apples that have no flavour, aroma, texture or taste. We must seek out real food. (If you buy herbs because you cannot grow your own and dry them, do enquire whether they have been irradiated. Try to seek out non-irradiated sources from organic suppliers.)

(Information taken from The Food Commission UK Ltd. leaflet *Attitudes to Food Irradiation in Europe*.)

Freezing

Freezing is a method of food preservation often used today that is still expanding. Freezing converts the water in food into ice crystals. Commercially blast freezers are usually employed. Food is placed on refrigerated shelves and cold air at below $-30°C$ is blown through. Sometimes foods are immersed in or sprayed with liquid nitrogen, when the freezing is extremely rapid and outer appearance and shape are kept.

Frozen food is stored at temperatures of $-18°C$ in the freezing compartment of a refrigerator. Blanching foods before freezing destroys certain enzymes and though we are told that frozen food has all the food values intact, according to Dr Gerhard Schmidt,[12] we have in frozen food a 'dead image of life, a mere semblance ... life has withdrawn, enzymatic processes stopped, most bacteria killed (though some can become reactivated when the thawing process takes place), cells are ruptured and the total structure decays rapidly.'

Eaten occasionally, frozen foods are not harmful. The best way to have frozen food is for it to have been home-grown and frozen quickly whilst still fresh. But on a daily basis it would have some deleterious effect. The same applies to ice cream (apart from what might be in it); it is a question of temperature. The human being is a creature whose organism, though robust and able to withstand many hardships, has a very finely calibrated temperature control, not assisted by too many dietary extremes. Even raw food has to be 'cooked' within the organism, so a lot of very cold food is a shock to the system. In view of all this it seems sensible to recommend that little children not be given ice cream or frozen lollipops frequently.

The family meal, the shared meal

I wonder what memories my readers may have of family mealtimes. Were they colourful, unhurried, delicious? Or the opposite? Or non-existent? I must say that I've listened to some sad personal accounts during food biography workshops — of childhood mealtimes spent eating alone in the

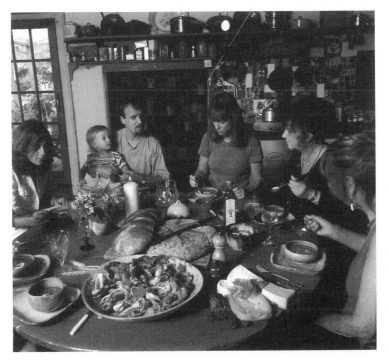

A family meal in Janet's kitchen, including grown-up Daisy and Lucy

kitchen, being left to forage in the fridge for food, or surviving on a diet of peanut butter sandwiches. Then there is the other extreme where a mother is so anxious about her child's nourishment that she engenders real food phobias and antipathies by her exaggerated attitude. At all events mealtimes can provide an enduring experience of a real sense of well-being and community, of vitality and connectedness to nature, or the opposite, of alienation, restriction, lack of care.

In this small section I also want to look at how and where meals take place because it's an area seldom touched upon in books on nutrition. The whole art and etiquette of eating together has accompanied the human food journey, becoming more refined or ritualized depending on the culture. (Earlier I touched on such customs as placing a guest above or below the salt or of the Victorians measuring two feet between place settings.) But in our culture, this central human activity anchored traditionally in the family is being seriously eroded. A big factor is the return of mothers to the workplace and being too tired to want to cook. I do sympathize, although I personally find cooking extremely therapeutic, even when a bit 'frazzled'; working with plants and with the hands can be very renewing. I realize that is not the exclusive domain of the woman these days, and it's good to see men taking more of a participative role in cooking.

Perhaps it's possible, however, to make a ritual even if the food is pre-prepared, and to make meals from something really simple but of good quality, like good bread, salad, cheeses, fresh or dried fruits. But first let us look at some situations we might consider to be nearer the ideal.

The setting

I personally prefer kitchens that are big enough and nice enough to both cook and eat in. A kitchen where an Aga or a wood-burning stove radiates its warm and benign presence is lovely in colder climates (although I've only managed that in one of our homes). But no matter, kitchen or dining room, we do need a table – preferably a round one. A round table allows parity for all and does away with the often threatening Victorian image of the Head of the Table, emphasized by an oblong table. I hope new social ideals are more blessed by the circle, allowing more equality. Again I didn't manage this myself, although I did have a lovely large, oblong pine table which for years was scrubbed and bleached ceremoniously on Saturday mornings. This table had been witness to so many wonderful meals and conversations which I swear had impregnated its very fibre, I could not bear to see it go when I was down-sizing my homes, so daughter Daisy took it on, and being an excellent cook carries on the tradition.

Serving dishes

I have a passion for hand-made ceramic bowls to serve the food in and to eat from. What we eat from has a definite bearing on the nutritional uptake. You can have the most delicious food, but served on plastic plates its quality will be significantly depleted.

Tablecloths seem to be a thing of the past, but I confess to loving white linen and lace, and I have a couple made by my grandmother which come out for special occasions. I always try to have an arrangement of fresh seasonal flowers on the table, candles and a beautiful crystal for decoration.

A lovely practice, traditional in Japan, is to echo the seasons and festivals with a centrepiece on the table, but not so tall that you can't see people over it. It is particularly helpful for children learning to appreciate and respect the specialness of certain times and the constant changes taking place in nature if these are reflected in the table decoration and on their plates. Children can be encouraged to bring their own discovered treasures to add.

All this may sound very élite and expensive, but it need not be so. For instance, the pottery from my local potter in Majorca, a glossy deep caramel-brown, strong and enduring, is cheaper than Woolworth's. Wooden plates and bowls for the small children are softer and gentler than pottery and help to cut down on the 'clatter'. Wooden chopsticks are also good to experiment with on appropriate occasions (they certainly help to slow one down substantially, which is a good thing). If you can, it is a good idea to paint the walls of the dining space with a colour that enhances the digestive process. One of the colours most suited to this is a warm peach or apricot.

The absence of television and loud music will certainly be helpful if we want to develop an attentiveness to food and to conversation. Soft music which doesn't get the pulse and breathing overactive and which really *is* in the background is best, if you have it at all. Constant sensory overload is contributing to the rise in stress and ADD (attention deficit disorder) in both children and adults, so anything we can do as parents to reduce sound and unnecessary image levels, especially when eating, is vital.

The enjoyment of food requires that one comes to the table with a proper appetite, stimulated by adequate physical exercise and not spoilt by constant snacking (usually a sign of unbalanced nutrition as well as other imbalances). Encourage children to help prepare the meal as this can stimulate their interest; get them to harvest a lettuce (if you're lucky enough to have a kitchen garden), lay the table or pick some flowers for a centrepiece. If you grow up knowing what is involved in growing a lettuce, harvesting and washing it, the chances are that you will have more respect for the process. It needs to be made fun and interesting to combat the resistance in our society to any tasks of a manual nature, but if these values and practices can be embodied in the parents' attitude it will percolate into the children, for small children love to imitate.

Saying a blessing
Human beings, unlike animals, can actually hold back on gratifying their desires, but this kind of delayed gratification has to be learned. Becoming quiet around the table to say a blessing on the meal can be difficult for little children (not to mention many adults), but children do often display a real sense of reverence and will respond to a mood if generated by those around them. We don't realize how important this pause of preparation is — to wait, slow down, let go of some of the anxieties and frustrations of the day in order to be present in gratitude. Eating is an act we are privileged to engage in, remembering that there are many who are hungry.

The food has taken a whole season to grow and maybe a couple of hours to prepare, so reflecting on this time-investment by nature and the cook on our behalf prepares us to enjoy the experience of chewing, tasting and relishing it. The saying of a blessing acknowledges all the unseen work that has gone into providing us with that meal.

Here I offer a selection of possible pieces to use:

The silver rain,
The shining sun,
And fields where scarlet poppies run,
And all the ripples of the wheat,
Are in the bread that I do eat.
So when I sit for every meal
And say a grace, I always feel
That I am eating rain and sun,
And fields where scarlet poppies run.

Before the flour the mill,
Before the mill the grain,
Before the grain, the sun, the earth, the rain,
The beauty of creation.

Blessings on the blossom,
Blessings on the fruit,
Blessings on the leaf and stem,
And blessings on the root,
Blessings on the meal.

We may think deeply of the ways and means
By which our food has come,
And consider our merit in accepting it.
By excluding greed from our minds
We help to protect ourselves from error.
We accept this food so that we may become enlightened:
Homage to Christ,
Homage to the Divine Law,
Homage to Humanity,
Homage to the Buddha,
Homage to the Dharma,
Homage to the Sangha.

Mealtimes and the question of rhythm

How does rhythm differ from routine? I think that good rhythms taken from biological or natural rhythms are life enhancing, whereas routine can be very mechanical. However, at present I think we are witnessing the breakdown of the latter in our culture. English society in general seems to suffer from a lack of ability for true enjoyment, relaxation and the appropriate sensuality, particularly around mealtimes. A 'workaholic' attitude, plus the long hours worked, tend to put eating into a category of 'refuelling', no longer an enjoyable and relaxed part of the day.

This was one of the reasons I went to live in the Mediterranean, frustrated at witnessing daily in the Waldorf school the fruits of our labour downed in

20 minutes, while business was intently discussed. I could picture the digestive enzymes battling against these poor life habits! It wasn't the teacher's or pupil's fault, it was the system, the routine of anti-enjoyment impressed upon the English folk-soul, not knowing what might be truly good for us.

In the Mediterranean (and thank goodness this still prevails) most shops and activities shut down in the middle of the day for two to three hours, depending on the time of the year, while people eat. This pause is not only about eating; it's also about meeting, and the enjoyment usually perceptible at most of these occasions is a real lesson in living. Then they have a siesta or a stroll. On all the saints' days they stop work, dress up, go to church and have special meals together. The Majorcans, whose life-rhythms I have been lucky enough to participate in, know how to work hard and relax with equal application. It is to these rhythms that we should look when we want to evaluate a culture's health (it's not just a matter of eating olive oil and plenty of vegetables). In these countries the intensity of the sun mainly dictates such sensible practices. The people's vitality is also surely enhanced by living largely outdoors. Talking about rhythms dictated by the sun, on a recent visit to South Africa I was astonished to see that in many situations British routines had been grafted entirely inappropriately on a culture living with fierce sunshine much of the time.

So what are appropriate rhythms in a society whose routines are pretty much fixed by school times and work times, school holidays and summer breaks? (These are often spent in trying to undo the effects of such imprisoning schedules, even by other excesses.) Since we've spent so much of our creativity designing a world of technological innovations that allows us on the whole to bypass the vagaries of climate or lack of daylight, it would be really hard to get back (or go forward) into natural bio-rhythms, to listen to our bodies and to work with what nature might be saying to us. However, in many traditional spiritual practices these human and seasonal rhythms were observed and daily life, work and meditation times arranged around them. If you have ever experienced for a while what it is like, to live within the rhythms of a monastery or an ashram, I think you might agree how different and life-enhancing it is. Although some aspects might be possible, for most people the whole routine is just out of the question. Rhythm is certainly emphasized in Waldorf schools, despite the truncated mealtimes, and these rhythms, starting in pre-school and kindergarten, make children feel secure. Some of them are based on human bio-rhythms.

The activity of the liver and production of bile are influenced by the cir-cadian rhythm (a cyclical variation of intensity which occurs about every 24 hours), which in turn is influenced by the alternating levels of light and darkness with day and night. Peak activity in the liver is usually around 3 a.m. (a time when some people find themselves waking up and some monasteries start their meditative practices). The blood-sugar handling activity of the liver changes again and 'troughs' at around 3 p.m., when many feel a low in energy and may reach for some stimulating, sugar-sweetened drink rather than rest or doing something a little more gentle. So, the further away from peak liver activity the meal is taken, the more completely can the liver perform its manifold functions.

The stomach's peak activity is from 7–9 a.m. When we realize that foods such as grains and legumes tend to stay in the stomach for up to three hours, it is clear that the practice of eating later than 6 p.m. (which many of us do) can prove burdensome to the digestion. (Again, the kind of metabolism one has influences the rate of digestion, so it is a complex matter.) So the maxim, 'Eat like a king in the morning, like a prince in the middle of the day, and like a pauper for supper' might be seen as based on wisdom. Many spiritual practices recommend eating the last meal of the day before sundown, around 6 p.m. This is still an hour observed by many families in England; in my upbringing it was known as high tea. But for many this is impractical and the main meal may be eaten somewhere between 7 p.m. and 8.30 p.m. So much depends on the schedules of the parents and the ages of any children. I think we have to do the best we can in our own individual circumstances. But every effort to have a daily or a weekly rhythm that works and holds the etheric body of the family together will bring rewards.

I have just been discussing this with my daughter and she very much valued our eating together in the evenings at a more or less set time. We used to discuss the day's events and often had time to share a 'magic moment' – something that had made that day special. On holiday we would gather for breakfast under the vine and share dreams.

The psycho-physiological state in which one eats is crucial for proper digestion; so many later illnesses can be laid down for later life around the family table, from peptic ulcers to gallstones. Perhaps that is why we're witnessing the disintegration of the mealtime – people's distressing memories around shared food. It was a wise rule that suggested 'No heated discussion about religion, politics or money at table amongst polite society'. I think Rudolf Steiner commented in a similar vein, though his recommendation was for people at table not to get involved in controversy, wherever possible. We can all sense that the adrenalin often generated by argument just does not foster ideal conditions for the nutritive process. If we are eating wholefoods we need to remember that they require extra forces, proper mastication and an awareness of what we are doing.

Cooking for children

I admit to feeling somewhat reticent in giving advice for the feeding of children, first of all because my children had their fair share of fish fingers and spaghetti hoops in their earlier years (as well as fresh vegetables and fruits). I didn't know then what I know now. It was only when Daisy at the age of seven decided to be a vegetarian that I started to explore the field of nutrition and vegetarian cookery. Also, despite this strong protest from my young daughter (which was, after all, in the direction of health and ethics), I think children were not so exposed to seduction by advertising companies in the late sixties. Now I honestly don't know how I would cope with the tantrums that some parents face from their children over food issues.

I have been aware of the 'wars' being fought between parents, teachers and children over the question of sweets and crisps in their lunch-boxes, showing the degree to which sugar and salt addiction has taken hold. Many parents just tend to give in for the sake of peace. It is a complex subject and part of the problem is that many people have lost any kind of healthy instinct and simply do not know any more what is right either for themselves or their children. They may be reluctant to create boundaries that then need consistency to keep in place. As little children learn by imitation they will naturally want to copy what they see in their environment. If they are exposed to a lot of television and trips to the supermarket, they will probably want brand names and breakfast cereals with plastic toys in them. If much of the family shopping is done in the local farm shop or health food store they will be surrounded by a very different ambience – different colours, shapes and smells – all of which become part of their food sensory experience, helping them learn to distinguish what is authentic and what is counterfeit.

Recently I spent one day a week observing in a local Waldorf kindergarten where the teacher was particularly keen on having healthy food habits as

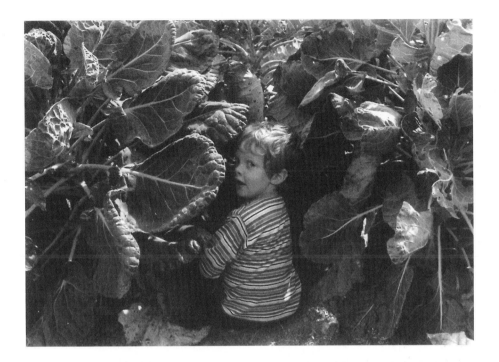

part of the learning process in his classroom. Every day a different cereal dish was created for the mid-morning break: apple crumble, oat porridge with molasses, millet patties, barley and wheat bread. The children were allowed to participate in the preparation, as and when they wanted to. They always played vigorously before the break and smelling the food cooking usually stimulated their appetites.

There were about 16 children; when the time came the tables were nested together, laid with napkins, a candle and flowers. Then the children went through a hand-washing ritual while a song was sung with their own name mentioned in it. When seated they said a simple grace and two of the children took the food around to each child. Spoons were the last item to be handed out so that they could start together (and practise a little delayed gratification). They drank herb tea made from herbs that they had collected from their kindergarten garden. It was so touching to witness the beginnings of conversation and caring for each other's needs. The bowls were emptied and the ones with really healthy appetites usually wanted second helpings. If there was a grumble it was met by some creative response by their teacher who used humour often to make them laugh and see another way of looking at matters.

I was very impressed by the whole experience. Children are like blotting paper, absorbing much of the influences around them. By the end of their first seven-year period, when the second teeth have come in, much of their physical basis for life and their orientation towards the world has been set in place. The Jesuits used to say, 'Give me a child for seven years, and I'll give you the man,' and we can see that there is much in this. Traditionally royal children were fed only vegetarian food for the first seven years of life.

The first three years of a child's life are also very important. We have spoken about the importance of breast milk as a beginning in life, then starting with solids around six months or when the baby indicates a readiness. We should remember that each new food represents a complete

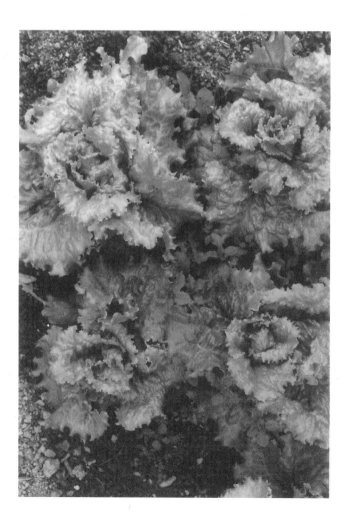

new world to the little child. You give them a spoon of fruit purée for the first time and a look of puzzlement or delight comes over their face. You spoon it back in – 'What is this you are giving me of the world? How does it taste?' So it continues, adding new substances gradually one by one. Puréed fruits from the *Rosaceae* family that are ripe, and gently cooked if necessary, are a fitting introduction to solids, followed by a cereal gruel. 'Holle' is a brand of biodynamic prepared cereal especially for young babies. To it can be added the 'fruiting' type vegetables such as courgettes, pumpkin (puréed), then leafy vegetables, bearing in mind the importance of seasonality. The roots, carrots and parsnips may come next, and later some cooked beetroot, though this may be rejected at first. A little honey or butter can be gradually included, but substances such as salt, refined sugar, the nightshade family and beans are best kept back for later.

Eggs have the potential ingredients – fats and proteins – to grow a whole new chicken. They are therefore a very concentrated food consisting of strong reproductive protein, so use only a little at a time. As for mushrooms, observe how they grow, quickly and at night, bypassing the chlorophyll processes. So they are not a 'sun' food. Save them too until later.

The process I am advocating aims to keep the child as 'plastic and permeable' as possible, open to the forces of imagination, so that he can stay in touch with all his senses and come in a timely way to be a full earth citizen. Certain foods such as salt, sugar, meat, potatoes and spices can tend towards a 'hardening' effect on the child's etheric body and may interfere with a harmonious and balanced physical/spiritual development.

I can only present a small outline here. There are many books on the subject of child nutrition, but in the end we have to use our own discretion as parents. Eating the right foods does not always guarantee adequate nutrition – no two people eating the same diet will necessarily receive the same nutrients. The digestive system and its unique functioning are a product of one's constitution and one's temperament, and as we have pointed out in the section on the family meal, it is powerfully influenced by our emotional life. Most of all, food should wherever possible be freshly prepared and from biodynamic or organic sources – and served with joy.

CONCLUSIONS

When Rudolf Steiner was asked by Ehrenfried Pfeiffer why it was that despite the enormous amount of stimulus he gave to the people that came to hear his lectures there seemed to be little fruitful action at that time, he replied, 'This is a problem of nutrition. Nutrition as it is today [the 1920s] does not supply the strength necessary for manifesting the spirit in physical life. A bridge can no longer be built from thinking to will and action. Food plants no longer contain the forces that people need for this.'

This was 70 years ago, not long in the context of world evolution, but a highly accelerated time in terms of technological development. I have attempted to put us in a position to reconnect with our food history in order to understand better how this nutritional journey may have resulted in a weakening of the soil's capacity to nourish us as it once did. What part does vital (living) food play, not only in our physical health, but our more subtle and spiritual aspects which include imagination and intuition and love? The statement that vital food is necessary to allow us to be able to 'walk our talk', to be able to integrate ideation and action, is very important. It seems a very real possibility that certain so-called 'foods' or stimulants have exacerbated a tendency towards a one-sided intellectual development and altered human and soil chemistry in an unbalanced way.

This focusing on the power of the mind in the Western scientific paradigm has gradually de-emphasized the more feeling, sensitive, artistic and com-passionate human qualities in favour of the rational. A kind of desensitizing and hardening seems to be the result. Art, science and religion have gone their separate ways until quite recently and have not known what the other is doing. It is encouraging now to see scientists and mystics talking to each other. This is not to deny that development of reason and rationality has been very important, but with what losses? We note that most cultures have manifested arrogant and myopic tendencies at their apparent climax. Not knowing when to stop and evaluate where they might be going, the seeds of decline are sown within the very successes of that culture.

We too seem to be in danger of losing the whole picture. But by our culture and our excesses the whole planet is affected. Often it appears that the human being's magnificent achievements in the outer world have not led to an expansion of the spaces within. We may be intellectually brighter, but we are also brittle and narrow. We have imposed a dangerous and fragile format onto what was a matrix full of wisdom, beauty and strength. Materialism – dualistic thinking – chains the mind as a bird to a post, from which it seeks in vain to fly to its freedom, its liberty, but exhausted keeps returning to the post. We need to learn to live with paradox.

Dr Twentyman says:

Today the human 'ego' feels enormously insecure, inferior and bereft of that support from the spiritual dimension which a younger mankind felt. Psychologically this shows itself in all the arrogant self-assertion, male chauvinism or feminism of our time. The individual retreats into his castle and puts up an important show of force. The organic expression of this seems to be an even greater dependence on the whole immune system, until it begins to break down.[1]

The monetarization of most human transactions must encourage a further sense of insecurity. As people become more and more separate from manual skills and a true sense of vocation, their reliance on money to buy everything they need often requires them to do work that is not deeply satisfying. And the dissatisfaction can rarely be assuaged by material objects. King Midas in the end asked for his capacity to turn everything to gold to be taken away by the gods. He discovered that in the end you cannot eat gold.

Are we intelligent enough to stop and reflect, to stop tinkering around the edges, only dealing with symptoms instead of causes? Can we retrieve a vision, not of the human as 'the ghost in the machine', but a worthy one that includes soul and spirit, this time with new insights into the exquisite and awe-inspiring creativity of the universe? Can we restore the hope that Pandora had retained in her box?

There are now more human beings on the earth than there ever have been before. Are we to feel this as a terrible threat, or as the most wonderful resource and potential for creative sharing with our fellow creatures — an opportunity for inter-fecundity? Can we recognize that we can all live in a symbiosis that is finely tuned? There is plenty for all if we choose to live within our needs rather than by our greed.

What as individuals can we do? There are so many wonderful projects that seek to reinstate ethical and spiritual values into the way we farm, eat, share our food and creative skills. They often do not get much publicity, but they are multiplying, that is certain. We can start to cook and garden again and restore the community-building activity of the shared meal. Let us be generous and hospitable, as nature is. She never holds back on giving of her best! We can *do* less and enjoy it more. Slow down and breathe deeply. Support our local farmers, take an interest in what they are doing, their particular problems — they have had a very challenging time, 'between a rock and a hard place'. Actively seek biodynamic or organic food — it is better for all levels of life. Try to develop a relationship with a piece of land — share an allotment. Make compost wherever you can and deal with your garbage in a conscious way; it is an aspect of our soul-life and we should only allow it to proliferate as little as possible. So take baskets with you when you go shopping; refuse packaging wherever you can. Explore the possibilities of community supported agriculture (CSA). Use money in a creative way like seeds; though it is totally artificial and man-made it can be used to the good when kept in healthy circulation. Let's try to be conscious of what we are supporting when we spend it. Try to be active in local decision-making. Develop friendships (they are better than bank accounts). Try to treat others in a way that you would like to be treated. This means loving yourself, having a sensitivity to the workings of one's body, soul and spirit as they affect one another, treating yourself with compassion, patience and understanding; thus we can retrieve our own authority from the grip of materialistic science.

With the emphasis on materialism in the West, we should be interested enough in matter to want to enquire into its role in the universe and how it wants to be used wisely. This is an important part of spiritual practice, I think. Many people are taking up a life of voluntary simplicity. Perhaps they have seen the ravages of excesses and know that that is not the way forward. We can join forces with an emerging system that is developing impetus and relies on human *participation*. Our higher ego is being formed by the way we make choices in life and by the motives behind them. When we are fortunate enough to have choices (and there are many who do not), can we make them from the perspective of 'What is ultimately good for me is also good for the rest of the world', so that out of egotism we can rise to a new kind of ego-hood that is self-governing and aligned to the good of the whole? As Mother Teresa said: 'Love until it hurts.' The purpose of the world is Love.

NOTES

Preface

1 Emerson College in Sussex is an adult training college for anthroposophical studies.

Chapter 1

1 Rudolf Steiner, *Man in the Past, Present and Future*, Rudolf Steiner Press, 1982.

2 Reay Tannahill, *Food in History*, Stein & Day, NY, 1973.

3 Rudolf Steiner, *Man in the Past, Present and Future*.

4 *Kapha* is one of the three *doshas*, basics of Ayurvedic medicine. It includes everything about the organism that is substantial, solid and heavy. Foods which give the body solidity are said to be 'kaphic'.

   The three *doshas* are dynamic factors which, when interacting, produce the whole person. They are:

   kapha – heavy, dense material: earth;
   vata – least perceptible, most active, erratic and unpredictable, often translated as 'wind';
   pitta – hot, quick and aggressive: fire.

   (Rudolph Ballentine of the Himalayan Institute, 1982.)

5 Reay Tannahill, *Food in History*.

6 J. Van Bemelen, *Zarathustra* (unpublished manuscript).

7 J. Mellaart, *Çatal Hüyük, A Neolithic Town in Anatolia*, Thames & Hudson, 1967.

8 Brendan Lehane, *The Power of Plants*, John Murray, 1977.

9 Something happens when we drink wine to displace the human 'I' – after heavy drinking we cannot remember the next day what happened. It is relevant that the grape is unusual in that the germinal power of the seed is very weak. Also that no seed can germinate in wine because it is 'mineralized' – it will preserve substances, but not allow new life. The grapevine is a crop that needs quantities of fungicides and insecticides.

10 Rudolf Steiner, *Turning Points in Spiritual History*, Spiritual Science Library, NY, 1987.

11 Gerhard Schmidt, *The Dynamics of Nutrition*, Biodynamic Literature, USA, 1980.

12 Phyllis Pray Bober, *Art, Culture and Cuisine*, University of Chicago Press, 1999.

13 Reay Tannahill, *Food in History*.

14 Joan P. Alcock, *Roman Food in Britain*, Tempus, 2001.

15 Richard Tarnas, *The Passion of the Western Mind*, Ballantine Books, 2001.

16 Andrew Welburn, *The Beginnings of Christianity*, Floris Books, 1991, p. 144.

17 The *Seder*, or Passover meal, is celebrated in the home on the night before the first day of the Passover. The house is cleared of all leaven and no leavening agents must be used in the feast. The meal should include, according to Leah W. Leonard in *Jewish Cookery*:

Afikomen Three matzos are placed separately in the folds of a napkin or special matzo cover. These represent the Sabbath loaves over which the benediction is pronounced and bear the special significance of symbolizing the 'bread of affliction', or slavery ...

Roasted lamb bone A piece of lamb shank or chicken leg bone is browned on the open flame and placed on a plate to symbolize the Paschal sacrifice of ancient days when each family brought its special offering.

Roasted hard cooked egg An egg is roasted in the shell and placed on the plate with the roasted bone. The egg symbolizes life, the perpetuation of existence.

Bitter herbs A horseradish top with some of the green leaves or sprouts, symbolizes the bitterness of Israel's bondage in the land of Egypt.

Morar Some grated horseradish, unflavoured or seasoned, is placed on a small dish. During the service some *morar* is placed between two pieces of matzo and passed to each member of the family circle.

Charoset Finely chopped nuts and apple, moistened with wine, represent the morsel of sweetness to lighten the burden of unhappy memory.

Hard cooked egg and salt water Hard cooked eggs in one dish and salted water in another are passed to everyone at the table during the service.

Greens Parsley, watercress, chicory, lettuce or other available greens are the herbs that symbolize hope and redemption of life. There should be salt water in a small bowl for each one at the table and some of the greens are placed alongside it.

Wine This is served in goblets and refilled four times during the service, symbolizing the fourfold promise of redemption.

Cup of Elijah A special goblet of wine is placed on the table towards the end of the service. At this time the door is opened and left ajar for the 'coming of Elijah', the coming of a more *perfect world of justice and joy for all mankind.*

18 Reay Tannahill, *Food in History.*
19 Titus Burckhardt, *Moorish Cultures in Spain*, Allen and Unwin, 1972.
20 There had long been connections with the Americas via Norway, but after the ninth century all contact was lost for several hundred years. Steiner implies that this was to protect Europe from the influences present in the Americas. (See 'Geographic Medicine', *Geographic Medicine and the Secret of the Double*, Mercury Press, Spring Valley, NY, 1986.)
21 Eric Schlosser, *Fast Food Nation*, Penguin, 2001.

Chapter 2

1 John Humphrys, *The Great Food Gamble*, Hodder & Stoughton, 2001, p. 11.
2 John Orr, *The History of British Agriculture*, Oxford University Press, 1922.
3 From paper *The Origins of the Common Agricultural Policy*, website access 2002Europa.EU.irt.
4 John Humphrys, *The Great Food Gamble.*
5 Unpublished essay, 2000.
6 George Monbiot, TV programme.
7 James Lovelock, *Gaia: The Practical Science of Planetary Medicine*, Gaia Books, 1991.
8 Ibid., p. 14.
9 Biodynamic preparations. Two preparations are made for the soil, one from cow manure buried in a cow horn over the winter, diluted and stirred in particular ways, and sprinkled on the land; the other is made from finely ground silica quartz, this time buried in a cow horn over the summer. In this takes place a strengthening of the forces of sunlight — sweetness, keeping quality and vitality of seeds. Wide areas of exhausted soil in Australia have benefited from the first preparation. Composting is also helped by special herbal preparations, enhancing the living processes taking place (chemicals are considered dead, end-products of a densifying process).
10 Personal communication.
11 Trauger Groh and Steve McFadden, 'Farms of Tomorrow: Community Supported Farms', in *Biodynamic Farming*, 1990, p. 41.
12 The Camphill Movement of schools and villages was founded by Dr Karl König. They are land-based communities which include people with learning difficulties, living and working together out of the ideal of anthroposophy.
13 Elm Farm Research Centre was founded in 1980 as an educational charity, the

Progressive Farming Trust Ltd. Based on a 232-acre farm in Berkshire, it provides three services: running a fully converted organic farm; undertaking a research programme; developing advisory and extension services.

Chapter 3

1 A movement for religious renewal, founded in 1922, following Steiner. It has churches or communities in many countries.
2 From an article on embryology in *Perspectives*, journal of the Christian Community, 1997.
3 Reproduced by permission of William Elkin Music Services on behalf of Thames Publishing.
4 Rupert Sheldrake, *A New Science of Life*, Blond & Briggs, 1981.
5 Quoted in Barbara Brennan, *Hands of Light*, Bantam Books, 1988.
6 Manly P. Hall, *Paracelsus*, The Philosophical Research Society, Los Angeles, 1980.
7 Franz Hartmann, *The Life of Paracelsus*, Wizards Bookshelf, 1997.
8 C.G. Jung, *Collected Works*, Routledge & Kegan Paul, 1979.
9 Ralph Twentyman, *The Science and Art of Healing*, Floris Books, 1992.
10 George Adams and Olive Whicher, *The Plant between Sun and Earth*, 2nd ed., Rudolf Steiner Press, 1980.
11 Ibid., p. 37.

Chapter 4

1 Maarten Ekama, unpublished article.
2 Bruce D. Smith, *The Emergence of Agriculture*, Scientific American Library, 1998.
3 Gerhard Schmidt, *The Essentials of Nutrition*, Biodynamic Literature, USA, 1980.
4 Robert Runnels, cited in Vicki Peterson, *The Natural Food Catalogue*, Macdonalds & Janes, 1978.

Chapter 5

1 Gerhard Schmidt, *The Dynamics of Nutrition*, Biodynamic Literature, USA, 1980.
2 Friedrich Husemann, edited and revised by Otto Wolff, *The Anthroposophical Approach to Medicine*, Vol. 1, Anthroposophical Press, Spring Valley, NY, 1982.
3 *The law of conservation of matter:* nothing is lost, nothing is created; everything is transformed.

   The atom is considered the smallest particle of matter and constant in nature. From this law it was assumed that no element could be created and no atom could disappear in nature. It has been applied to nutrition, which was considered a matter of combustion in which foods were seen as carriers of calorific energy which in conjunction with oxygen released energy in the digestive process. One needed simply to count the calories needed and select nutrients that had the matching number of calories.

The second law of thermodynamics states that all things are breaking down to their most simple and basic and stable forms and the total energy in a system moves from a more organized to a less organized form or state — a process called entropy.

It is in the dynamics of the most diverse processes that the human being lives, and it is in these processes that the principle of life can be found. In metabolism we find all the following polar processes: deposition — dissolution; contraction — expansion; anabolism — catabolism; inflammation — sclerosis; absorption, secretion and excretion; oxidation — reduction. In a healthy person there is continuing variation around an equilibrium maintained by the individual (the ego) as he or she matures.

4   Gerhard Schmidt, *The Essentials of Nutrition*, Biodynamic Literature, USA, 1980.

5   Protease: any enzyme involved in proteolysis (hydrolysis of proteins into simpler compounds).

6   Quoted in an article by E.M. Kranich, 'Planetary Influences upon Plants', in *Paidia*, No. 18.

7   Walter Holtzapfel, *The Human Organs*, Lanthorne Press, 1993.

8   Ibid.

9   Rudolf Steiner, *The Study of Man*, Rudolf Steiner Press, 1966.

10 Ibid.

11 Steve Levine and Paris Kidd, *Antioxidant Adaption, Its Role in Free Radical Pathology*, Avery Publishing Group, New York, 1986.

12 The chakras have been named according to their special qualities and effects upon the human body and soul. Clairvoyantly they are seen as vortices of whirling energy. Rudolf Steiner refers to them as 'lotus flowers'. They are usually described beginning from the lowest chakra:

Muladhara (root support), located at the base of the spine and corresponds to the pelvic plexus, testes and ovaries. Imbalance results from the desire for personal safety as the highest goal.
Swadisthana (one's own place), located just below the navel and corresponds to the hypogastric plexus, adrenal glands and kidneys. Imbalance produces an enlarged desire for personal and sensual pleasure.

Manipura (gem city), links with drives for power. It is located just above the navel and corresponds to the solar plexus, liver and pancreas.

Anahata (unstruck sound), located in the heart region and corresponds to the cardiac plexus and thymus gland. Balance here develops creativity and unconditional love.

Vishuddha (purity centre), located in the throat area and corresponds to the pharangeal plexus and thyroid gland. Balance in this chakra facilitates the integration of events and the development of inner harmony.

Ajna (non-knowledge), located between the eyes and corresponds to the naso-ciliary plexus and pituitary gland. Balance in the Ajna can enable Siddi-abilities.

Sahasrara (the thousand-petalled centre), located at the top of the head and corresponds to the cerebrum and pineal gland. Balance here can bring about a union of all levels of consciousness with the highest, known as enlightenment. (Taken from *Breath and Spirit* by Gunnel Minett, Aquarian Books, 1994.)

According to many yoga masters, most people today are unbalanced in their lower chakras. This can be witnessed in selfish acts which only consider the satisfaction of their own physical needs. This lack of spiritual insight and realization of our oneness with the universe can lead to conflicts and wars.

13 Gabriel Cousins, *Spiritual Nutrition and the Rainbow Diet*, Cassandra Press, 1986, p. 60.

14 Friedrich Husemann, revised by Otto Wolff et al., *The Anthroposophical Approach to Medicine*, Vol. 1, Anthroposophical Press, 1982, p. 294.

15 Jenny Luke, *On Fluoride Deposition in the Aged Human Pineal Gland*, research paper, 1999.

16 Karl König, *Earth and Man*, Biodynamic Literature, USA, 1982, pp. 225–6, 260, 265.

17 Steiner's twelve senses: touch, sense of life or well-being, sense of self-movement, balance, smell, taste, vision, sense of temperature or warmth, hearing, language, conceptual sense (thought), sense of ego (I am). (See Albert Soesman, *Our Twelve Senses*, Hawthorn Press, 1990.)

18 Parahamsa Yogananda, *Autobiography of a Yogi*, Rider, 1996.

Chapter 6

1 Cited in Janet Barkas, *The Vegetable Passion*, Camelot Press, 1975, p. 50.

2 Ibid.

3 Macrobiotic – macro = large, bio = life, so 'large, or long life'. It comes from the traditional Zen monastic way of living and eating, a cereal and vegetable-based diet that works with the dynamics of yin and yang to bring balance and harmony.

4   Rudolf Steiner, *Nutrition and Health: Lectures to the Workmen*, Anthroposophic Press, NY, 1987.

5   Janet Barkas, *The Vegetable Passion*, Camelot, 1975.

6   Quoted in Gerhard Schmidt, *The Dynamics of Nutrition*, Biodynamic Literature, USA, 1980, p. 141.

7   Quoted in K. Castellitz and B. Saunders-Davies, *Nutrition and Stimulants, Lectures and Extracts from Rudolf Steiner*, Biodynamic Literature, USA, 1997, p. 136.

8   Cited by Gabriel Cousins, *Spiritual Nutrition and the Rainbow Diet*, Cassandra Press, 1986.

9   Rudolf Steiner, *Nutrition and Health*.

10 Quoted in K. Castellitz and B. Saunders-Davies, *Nutrition and Stimulants*, 1990, p. 136.

11 Quoted in Gerhard Schmidt, *The Dynamics of Nutrition*, p. 133.

12 Friedrich Husemann, edited and revised by Otto Wolf, *The Anthroposophical Approach to Medicine*, Anthroposophical Press, Vol 1, 1982, p. 296.

13 From a lecture by Rudolf Steiner dated 17 December 1908. Quoted in K. Castellitz and B. Saunders-Davies.

14 Ursula Balzer-Graf, 'Quality Research with Picture-Forming Methods,' a paper in the proceedings of an IFOAM (International Federation of Organic Agriculture Movements) conference entitled: Quality Control and Communication for the Organic Market, 1999. (Dr Balzer-Graf is founder of The Vital Quality Research Institute in Frick, Switzerland.)

15 Schrödinger (1945), Popp (1989), research papers cited by Angelika Meier-Ploeger in *Food Quality Concepts and Methodology*, in Proceedings of the Colloquium organized by Elm Farm Research Centre in Association with the University of Kassel, 1993.

16 Gabriel Cousins, *Spiritual Nutrition and the Rainbow Diet*, Cassandra Press, 1986.

17 Marthe Kiley-Worthington, *Eco-Agriculture, Food First Farming*, Souvenir Press, 1988.

18 Unpublished article by Michael Schmundt.

19 Paul Pitchford, *Healing with Wholefoods*, North Atlantic Books, 1993, p. 90.

20 Peter J.D. d'Adamo and Catherine Whitney, *Eat Right for Your Type*, Century Press, 2001.

21 Paul Pitchford, *Healing with Wholefoods*.

22 Quoted in Gerhard Schmidt, *Essentials of Nutrition*, p. 91.

Chapter 7

1   Wolf D. Storl, *Culture and Horticulture, a Philosophy of Gardening*, Biodynamic Literature, USA, 1979.

2 Brendan Lehane, *The Power of Plants*, John Murray, 1977.
3 Gerhard Schmidt, *The Dynamics of Nutrition*, Biodynamic Literature, USA, 1980.
4 *Selected Poetry*, Penguin, 1986.
5 Andrew Weil, *Eating Well for Optimum Health*, Warner Books, 2000.
6 Gabriel Cousins, *Spiritual Nutrition and the Rainbow Diet*, Cassandra Press, 1986.

Chapter 8

1 Brian Swimme and Thomas Berry, *The Story of the Universe*, Harper, San Franciso, 1994.
2 Gerhard Schmidt, *The Essentials of Nutrition*, Biodynamic Literature, USA, 1987.
3 Gerhard Schmidt, *The Essentials of Nutrition*.
4 Henry Hobhouse, *Seeds of Change*, Pan Books, 1999.
5 Paul Pitchford, *Healing with Wholefoods*, North Atlantic Books, 1993, p. 331.
6 Henry Hobhouse, *Seeds of Change*.
7 Paul Pitchford, *Healing with Wholefoods*, p. 92.

Chapter 9

1 Bruce D. Smith, *The Emergence of Agriculture*, Scientific American Library, 1998, p. 88.
2 Reay Tannahill, *Food in History*, Stein & Day, NY, 1973.
3 Phyllis Pray Bober, *Art, Culture and Cuisine*, University of Chicago Press, 1999.
4 Fr. Schyre, compiled from indications given by Rudolf Steiner on various occasions, 1928. (Cited in K. Castellitz and B. Saunders-Davies, *Nutrition and Stimulants, Lectures and Extracts from Rudolf Steiner*, Biodynamic Literature, USA, 1991.)
5 Ibid.
6 Rudolf Hauschka, *Nutrition*, Rudolf Steiner Press, 1983.
7 Emil Bock, *The Three Years*, Floris Books, 1995.

Chapter 10

1 Rudolf Steiner, lecture given on 23 July 1924 at Arnheim. Quoted in K. Castellitz and B. Saunders-Davies, *Nutrition and Stimulants, Lectures and Extracts from Rudolf Steiner*, Biodynamic Literature, USA, 1991.
2 Rudolf Hauschka, *Nutrition*, Rudolf Steiner Press, 1983, p. 106.
3 Rudolf Steiner, a lecture given on 16 June 1924 at Koberwitz. Quoted in K. Castellitz and B. Saunders-Davies, *Nutrition and Stimulants*.
4 Vicki Edgson and Ian Marber, *The Food Doctor*, Collins & Brown, 1999.

Chapter 11

1 *Phaseolus vulgaris* (French or kidney bean) and *P. lunatus* (butter-bean).
2 Rudolf Steiner, *Agriculture*, Biodynamic Agricultural Association, 1993, p. 58.
3 Eugen Kolisko, *The Twelve Groups of Animals*, Kolisko Archive Productions, 1978.
4 Rudolph Ballentine, *Diet and Nutrition, A Holistic Approach*, Himalayan Institute, 1982.
5 Carol Simontaachi, *Crazymakers*, Putnam, NY, 2000.
6 Gerhard Schmidt, *The Essentials of Nutrition*, Biodynamic Literature, USA, 1987, p. 131.
7 Rudolph Ballentine, *Diet and Nutrition*.
8 Paul Pitchford, *Healing with Wholefoods*, North Atlantic Books, 1993.

Chapter 12

1 Rudolf Hauschka, *Nutrition*, Rudolf Steiner Press, 1983.
2 Reay Tannahill, *Food in History*, Stein & Day, NY, 1973.
3 Richard Smith, article in *Star and Furrow*, Journal of the Biodynamic Association, Winter 2001/2.
4 Rudolf Steiner, *The Effects of Esoteric Development*, Anthroposophic Press, 1997.
5 Rudolf Steiner, *A Study of Man*, 1966, p. 153.
6 Rudolf Hauschka, *The Nature of Substance*, 2nd ed, Rudolf Steiner Press, 1983, p. 176.
7 Michel Odent, *Entering the World, The De-medicalization of Childbirth*, Marion Boyars, 1984, p. 96.
8 A. and P. Stanway, *Breast is Best*, Pan Books, 1996, pp. 30–9.
9 Richard Smith in *Star and Furrow*, journal of the Biodynamic Association, Spring 2002.
10 Rudolph Ballentine, *Diet and Nutrition, A Holistic Approach*, Himalayan Institute, 1982.
11 Paavo Airola, *Are You Confused?*, Health Plus Publications, 1977, p. 87.
12 Gerhard Schmidt, *The Essentials of Nutrition*, Biodynamic Literature, USA, 1980.

Chapter 13

1 Chloroplast is a plastid containing chlorophyll and other pigments. It occurs in plants that carry out photosynthesis.
2 Gerhard Schmidt, *The Dynamics of Nutrition*, Biodynamic Literature, USA, 1980, p. 49.

3 See Chapter 1, Note 4.
4 The health of the people of the Mediterranean cannot be separated from their life-style which is sun-orientated. They live far more outside than we northerners, enjoy good rhythm in their days (siestas) and more physical activity.
5 Tomas Graves, *Bread and Oil*, Prospect Books, 2000.
6 Ibid.
7 Rudolf Steiner, *Nutrition and Health, Two Lectures Given to Workmen*, Anthroposophic Press, 1987.

Chapter 14
1 Rudolf Steiner, *Agriculture*, Biodynamic Agricultural Association, 1994.
2 Michael Crawford and David Marsh, *Nutrition and Evolution*, Keats Publishing, Connecticut, 1995, p. 62.
3 Gerhard Schmidt, *The Dynamics of Nutrition*, Biodynamic Literature, USA, 1980.
4 Rudolf Hauschka, *Nutrition*, Rudolf Steiner Press, 1983, p. 67.
5 In Paul Pitchford, *Healing with Wholefoods*, North Atlantic Books, 1993.
6 Gerhard Schmidt, *The Dynamics of Nutrition*, p. 127.
7 Walter Cloos, *The Living Earth*, Lanthorne Press, 1977.
8 Ibid.

Chapter 15
1 The existence of metals within the mineral world is mysterious. Gold, silver or platinum having the strength to endure the earth's processes, mankind has given them the rank of precious metals. Semi-precious metals such as copper, mercury or tin are released relatively easily from their ores, whereas more effort is needed to extract magnesium, aluminium and calcium and that has only been possible in more recent times. More technology has been required to extract the alkaline metals, which are very unstable and produced by the 'salt' nature of the earth, such as sodium and potassium and their relatives. Because of their softness, low melting-point and instability they have to be protected by glass walls or kept under petroleum, because every drop of water or breath of air threatens them. Wilhelm Pelikan's opinion is that, 'With full justification we may therefore conclude that the metallic quality is, fundamentally, a stranger to the earth. It is a guest rather that a citizen!' Wilhelm Pelikan, *The Secrets of Metals*, Anthroposophic Press, NY, 1973.
2 Ibid.

3 Cited in Gerhard Schmidt, *The Essentials of Nutrition*, Biodynamic Literature, USA, 1987.

4 Rudolf Steiner, *Agriculture*, Biodynamic Agricultural Association, 1994.

5 Quoted by Gerhard Schmidt, *The Essentials of Nutrition*.

6 Rudolph Ballentine, *Diet and Nutrition*, Himalayan Institute, 1982.

7 Gerhard Schmidt, *The Essentials of Nutrition*.

8 Andrew Weil, *Eating Well for Optimum Health*, Warner Books, 2000.

9 Paul Pitchford, *Healing with Wholefoods*, North Atlantic Books, 1993.

10 Anne-Marie Mayer, 'Historical Changes in the Mineral Content of Fruits and Vegetables', in *British Food Journal*, 1997.

11 Data from DEFRA cited by Richard Thornton-Smith, in article, 'Food Quality and Human Health', in *Soil Association Review*, August 2001.

12 Karl König, *Earth and Man*, Biodynamic Literature, USA, 1982.

13 Homeopathy: In the process of homoeopathic potentization, a dilution of a healing plant, mineral or metal substance is carried out in successive rhythmical steps until no measurable substance is left, so 'releasing the spiritual (etheric) ideal form from its prison house in earthly matter', i.e., the memory of its structure is left imprinted in the water molecules. (From Ralph Twentyman, *The Art of Healing*, Floris books.)

Chapter 16

1 Rudolf Hauschka, *Nutrition*, Rudolf Steiner Press, 2002.

2 Brendan Lehane, *The Power of Plants*, John Murray, 1977.

Chapter 17

1 Brendan Lehane, *The Power of Plants*, 1977.

2 Reay Tannahill, *Food in History*, Stein & Day, NY, 1973.

3 Charles F. Wetherall, *Kicking the Coffee Habit*, Wetherall Publications, Minneapolis.

4 Gerhard Schmidt, *The Dynamics of Nutrition*, Biodynamic Literature, USA, 1980.

5 Ibid.

6 Rudolf Steiner, *The Effects of Esoteric Development*, Anthroposophic Press, 1997.

7 Articles in *Majorca Daily Bulletin*: 'Chocoholism', and 'Drugged Spiders Give Coffee a Bad Name'.

8 Gerhard Schmidt, *The Dynamics of Nutrition*.

9 Rudolf Steiner, *The Effects of Esoteric Development*, Anthroposophic Press, 1997.

10 The Dirty Dozen are chemicals including lindane (1 tsp is fatal), paraquat (a

major method of suicide), parathion (an organophosphate insecticide), chlordane and heptachlor, dieldrin and methyl bromide. Information taken from a paper published by the Women's Environmental Network, April 1993.

11   Brendan Lehane, *The Power of Plants*.

Chapter 18

1   Gerhard Schmidt, *The Essentials of Nutrition*, Biodynamic LIterature, USA, 1987.

2   Cited by Gabriel Cousins, *Spiritual Nutrition and the Rainbow Diet*, Cassandra Press, 1986.

Chapter 19

1   Patrick Harpur, *Mercurius*, Macmillan, 1990.

2   Gabriel Cousins, *Spiritual Nutrition and the Rainbow Diet*, Cassandra Press, 1986.

3   Phyto-chemicals and flavonoids, of which there are several thousands (e.g. carotenoids which give the orange colour and flavour to carrots), are a group of plant pigments that possess some remarkable healing properties, restoring flexibility of connective tissue, helping circulation, bolstering the immune system and containing many powerful antioxidants. (See Andrew Weil, *Eating Well for Optimum Health*.)

4   Data from the Consumer Expenditure Survey conducted by the Bureau of Labor Statistics.

5   John Davy, *Hope, Evolution and Change*, Hawthorn Press, 1985.

6   *Brewer's Dictionary of Phrase and Fable*, Millennium edition, 1999.

7   Gertrude Meier, unpublished manuscript.

8   John Davy, *Hope, Evolution and Change*.

9   Harold McGee, *The Curious Cook*, North Point Press, 1990.

10   Much of this information was taken from an article by Simon Best in *What Doctors Don't Tell You*, Vol. 10, No. 12, March 2000, and an article by Julie Johnson in *New Scientist*, 18 January 1992.

11   Cited in *The Perils of Progress*. Zed Books, London, 1999.

12   Gerhard Schmidt, *The Dynamics of Nutrition*, Biodynamic Literature, USA, 1980.

Chapter 20

1   Ralph Twentyman, *The Essentials of Healing*, Floris Books, 1989.

SELECT BIBLIOGRAPHY

Abehsera, Michel, *Cooking for Life*, Swan House, 1970.

Airola, Paavo, *Are You Confused?*, Health Plus Publications, 1977.

Alcock, Joan P., *Food in Roman Britain*, Tempus, 2001.

Ballentine, Rudolph, *Diet and Nutrition, a Holistic Approach*, Himalayan Institute, 1982.

Barkas, Janet, *The Vegetable Passion*, Camelot Press, 1975.

Black, Maggie, *A Taste of History, 10,000 years of Food in Britain*, English Heritage, 1997.

Bock, Emil, *The Three Years*, Christian Community Press, 1955.

Brennan, Barbara Ann, *Hands of Light*, Bantam Books, 1988.

Brown, Kathy, *The Edible Flower Garden*, Lorenz Books, 1999.

Burkhardt, Titus, *Moorish Culture in Spain*, Allen & Unwin, 1972.

Castellitz, K., and Saunders-Davies, B., *Nutrition and Stimulants, Lectures and Extracts from Rudolf Steiner*, Biodynamic Literature, USA, 1991.

Chardin, Pierre Teilhard de, *The Phenomenon of Man*, Fontana Books, 1965.

Cloos, Walther, *The Living Earth*, Lanthorne Press, 1977.

Cousins, Gabriel, *Spiritual Nutrition and the Rainbow Diet*, Cassandra Press, 1986.

Crawford, Michael, and March, David, *Nutrition and Evolution*, Keats Publishing, Connecticut, 1995.

Crowe, Ivan, *The Quest for Food*, Tempus, 2000.

Culpeper's Complete Herbal, Wordsworth Reference, 1995.

D'Adamo, Peter J.D., & Whitney, Catherine, *Eat Right for Your Type*, Century Press, 2001.

DEFRA, *Action Plan to Develop Organic Food and Farming in England*, July 2002.

Dudley, Nigel, *Soil Association Consumer Guide to Food, Health and the Environment*.

Edgson, Vicki, and Marber, Ian, *The Food Doctor*, Collins & Brown, 1999.

Edmunds, L. Francis, *Quest for Meaning*, Continuum, NY, 1997.

Edwards, Lawrence, *The Vortex of Life*, Floris Books, 1993.

Elm Farm Research Centre, *Food Quality Concepts and Methodology*.

Geuter, Maria, *Herbs in Nutrition*, Biodynamic Agricultural Association, 1978.

Goodwin, Brian, *How the Leopard Changed its Spots*, Weidenfeld & Nicholson, 1994.

Graf, Emma, *Cooking with Grains*, InterActions, Stroud, 1996.

Graves, Tomas, *Bread and Oil*, Prospect Books, 2000.

Groh, Trauger M., and McFadden, Steven H., *Farms of Tomorrow: Community Supported Farms*, Biodynamic Farming, 1990.

Hall, Alan, *Water, Electricity and Health*, Hawthorn Press, 1998.

Hall, Manly P., *Paracelsus*, The Philosophical Research Society Inc., Los Angeles, 1980.

Harpur, Patrick, *Mercurius*, Macmillan, 1990.

Hartmann, Franz, *The Life of Paracelsus*, Wizards Bookshelf, 1997.

Hauschka, Rudolf, *Nutrition*, Rudolf Steiner Press, 1983.

Hauschka, Rudolf, *The Nature of Substance*, Rudolf Steiner Press, 1983.

Hobhouse, Henry, *Seeds of Change*, Pan Books, 1999.

Holford, Patrick, *The Optimum Nutrition Bible*, Piatkus, 1997.

Holtzapfel, Walter, *The Human Organs*, Lanthorne Press, 1993.

Humphrys, John, *The Great Food Gamble*, Hodder & Stoughton, 2002.

Husemann, Friedrich, edited and revised by Otto Wolff, *The Anthroposophical Approach to Medicine*, Vol. 1, Anthroposophical Press, Spring Valley, NY, 1982; Vol. 2, 1987.

Janson, H.W., *A History of Art*, Thames & Hudson, 1981.

Jayakar, Pupol, *Temenos Review*, No. 6.

Jenny, Hans, *Cymatics*, Macromedia, 2001.

Kiley-Worthington, Marthe, *Eco-Agriculture, Food First Farming*, Souvenir Press, 1993.

Kolisko, Eugen, *The Twelve Groups of Animals*, Kolisko Archive Productions, 1978.

König, Karl, *Earth and Man*, Biodynamic Literature, USA, 1982.

König, Karl, *A Living Physiology*, Camphill Books, 1999.

Kranich, Ernst-Michael, *Planetary Influences Upon Plants*, Biodynamic Literature, USA, 1984.

Kurlansky, Mark, *Salt*, Jonathan Cape, 2002.

Lehane, Brendan, *The Power of Plants*, John Murray, 1977.

Lehmann, Johannes, *The Hittites*, Collins, 1977.

Lovelock, James, *Gaia: The Practical Science of Planetary Medicine*, Gaia Books, 1991.

McGee, Harold, *The Curious Cook*, North Point Press, San Francisco, 1990.

McTaggart, Lynne, *What Doctors Don't Tell You*, Thorsons, 1996.

Mees, L.F.C., *Secrets of the Skeleton, Form in Metamorphosis*, Anthroposophic Press, NY, 1984.

Mehta, P.D., *Zarathustra, the Transcendental Vision*, Element Books, 1985.

Minett, Gunnel, *Breath and Spirit*, Aquarian/Thorsons, 1994.

Oldfield, Harry, *The Dark Side of the Brain*, Element Books, 1995.

Palaiseul, Jean, *Grandmother's Secrets*, Penguin, 1973.

Peterson, Vicki, *Natural Food Catalogue*, Macdonald & Janes, 1978.

Phillips, Roger, and Rix, Martyn, *Vegetables*, Pan, 1993.

Pitchford, Paul, *Healing with Wholefoods*, North Atlantic Books, 1993.

Polkinghorne, John, *Science and Creation, The Search for Understanding*, SPCK, 1988.

Pray Bober, Phyllis, *Art, Culture and Cuisine*, University of Chicago, 1999.

Robertson, Laurel, *Laurel's Kitchen Bread Book*, Random House, NY, 1974.

Salter, Joan, *The Incarnating Child*, Hawthorn Press, 1987.

Saltzmann, Joanne, *Amazing Grains*, H.J. Kramer Inc., 1990.

Schauss, Alexander, *Diet, Crime and Delinquency*, Parker House, 1981.

Schlosser, Eric, *Fast Food Nation*, The Penguin Press, 2001.

Schmidt, Gerhard, *The Dynamics of Nutrition*, Biodynamic Literature, USA, 1980.

Schmidt, Gerhard, *The Essentials of Nutrition*, Biodynamic Literature, USA, 1987.

Schwenk, Theodor, *Sensitive Chaos*, Rudolf Steiner Press, 1996.

Smith, Bruce D., *The Emergence of Agriculture*, Scientific American Library, 1998.

Simontaachi, Carol, *Crazymakers*, Penguin Putnam, NY, 2001.

Soesman, Albert, *Our Twelve Senses*, Hawthorn Press, 1990.

Soil Association, *Organic Farming, Food Quality and Human Health: A Review of the Evidence*.

Steiner, Rudolf, *Agriculture*, Biodynamic Agricultural Association, 1994.

Steiner, Rudolf, *The Effects of Esoteric Development*, Anthroposophic Press, 1997.

Steiner, Rudolf, *The Four Temperaments*, Anthroposophic Press, 1980.

Steiner, Rudolf, *From Beetroot to Buddhism, Answers to Questions*, Rudolf Steiner Press, 1999.

Steiner, Rudolf, *Man in the Past, Present and the Future and The Sun-Initiation of the Druid Priest*, Rudolf Steiner Press, London, 1982.

Steiner, Rudolf, *Nine Lectures on Bees*, Steinerbooks, USA, 1988.

Steiner, Rudolf, *Nutrition and Health, Two Lectures Given to Workmen*, Anthroposophic Press, 1987.

Steiner, Rudolf, *Turning Points in Spiritual History*, Spiritual Science Library, NY, 1987.

Stobart, Tom, *Herbs and Spices*, International Food and Wine Pub., 1970.

Storl, Wolf D., *Culture and Horticulture, a Philosophy of Gardening*, Biodynamic Literature, 1979.

Style, Sue, *Honey*, Chronicle Books, 1993.

Swimme, Brian, and Berry, Thomas, *The Story of the Universe*, Harper, San Francisco, 1994.

Symons, Michael, *A History of Cooks and Cooking*, Prospect Books, 2001.

Tannahill, Reay, *Food in History*, Stein & Day, NY, 1973.

Tarnas, Richard, *The Passion of the Western Mind*, Ballantine Books, 1991.

Teodorowicz, J., *Theresa Neumann*, R. Herder Book Co.

Thun, Maria, *Gardening for Life, the Biodynamic Way*, Hawthorn Press, 1999.

Time Life International, *The Epic of Man*, 1963.

Twentyman, Ralph, *The Science and Art of Healing*, Floris Books, 1992.

Van Bemelen, *Zarathustra* (unpublished manuscript).

Wachsmuth, G., *The Evolution of Mankind*, Philosophic-Anthroposophic Press, Dornach, 1961.

Weil, Andrew, *Eating Well for Optimum Health*, Warner Books, 1994.

Westland, Pamela, *Encyclopedia of Spices*, Marshall Cavendish, 1983.

Wetherall, F., *Kicking the Coffee Habit*, Wetherall Publishing.

Zaehner, R.C., *The Dawn and Twilight of Zoroastrianism*, Weidenfeld & Nicholson, 1961.

Zuckerman, Larry, *The Potato*, Macmillan, 1988; Chronicle Books, 1998.

INDEX

HILLSBORO PUBLIC LIBRARIES
Hillsboro, OR
Member of Washington County
COOPERATIVE LIBRARY SERVICES